Palliative Nursing

For Elsevier:

Commissioning Editors: Ninette Premdas, Steven Black
Development Editors: Mairi McCubbin, Clive Hewat
Project Manager: Kerrie-Anne Jarvis
Senior Designer: George Ajayi
Illustrator: Graeme Chambers
Illustration Manager: Merlyn Harvey

Palliative Nursing

Improving end-of-life care

Edited by

Shaun Kinghorn MSc BA(Hons) RGN CertEd RNT RCNT
LETTOL, ITOL

Online Learning Developments Lead, Marie Curie Cancer Care, Newcastle upon Tyne, UK

Sandra Gaines MEd PGD Ed PGD(Pain) RN DPSN

Senior Lecturer, Cancer and Palliative Care, Marie Curie Centre, Newcastle upon Tyne, UK

SECOND EDITION

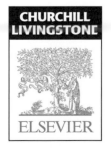

CHURCHILL
LIVINGSTONE

ELSEVIER

EDINBURGH   LONDON   NEW YORK   OXFORD   PHILADELPHIA   ST LOUIS   SYDNEY   TORONTO   2007

CHURCHILL LIVINGSTONE
ELSEVIER

An imprint of Elsevier Limited

First published 2001
Reprinted 2002, 2003, 2004

ISBN: 9780702028168

British Library Cataloguing in Publication Data
A catalogue record for this book is available from the British Library

Library of Congress Cataloging in Publication Data
A catalog record for this book is available from the Library of Congress

Note
Knowledge and best practice in this field are constantly changing. As new research and experience broaden our knowledge, changes in practice, treatment and drug therapy may become necessary or appropriate. Readers are advised to check the most current information provided (i) on procedures featured or (ii) by the manufacturer of each product to be administered, to verify the recommended dose or formula, the method and duration of administration, and contraindications. It is the responsibility of the practitioner, relying on their own experience and knowledge of the patient, to make diagnoses, to determine dosages and the best treatment for each individual patient, and to take all appropriate safety precautions. To the fullest extent of the law, neither the Publisher nor the editors assumes any liability for any injury and/or damage to persons or property arising out or related to any use of the material contained in this book.

The Publisher

Printed in China

Contents

Contributors

Robert Becker MSc Dip N(Lond) RMN RGN CertEd
(FE) FETC 730
Macmillan Senior Lecturer in Palliative Care,
Staffordshire University and Severn Hospice, Shropshire,
UK

Janet Brown MA Ad Dip Counselling BACPreg
Counsellor RGN RCNT
Freelance Counsellor, Trainer and Supervisor,
Scarborough, UK

Jacquelyn Chaplin PhD MN(Cancer Nursing) BA
RGN RCNT RNT
Lead Nurse (Scotland) Marie Curie Cancer Care,
Glasgow, UK

Simon Chippendale M Med Sc BSc(Hons) RGN RNT
Cert Ed Dip Pall Nurs
Senior Lecturer in Applied Health Studies (Palliative
Care), University of Gloucestershire, Gloucestershire;
Head of Education Leckhampton Court Hospice –
Sue Ryder Care, Cheltenham, UK

Alison Conner MSc, Pg Dip Cognitive Therapy RGN
Clinical Nurse Specialist in Palliative Care, Newcastle
upon Tyne Hospitals NHS Trust, Newcastle upon Tyne,
UK

Kevin Donaghy PhD BSc(Hons) PGCE PGCHET
Lecturer, Cancer and Palliative Care, Marie Curie Cancer
Centre, Belfast, UK

Graham Farley MSc BSc(Hons) PGDE RGN RNT
Practice Educator, Marie Curie Hospice, Bradford, UK

Keith Farrer RGN RNT BA(Hons) Nurse Education
Nurse Consultant in Cancer and Palliative Care,
NHS Orkney, Macmillan House, Balfour Hospital,
Orkney, UK

Valerie Forster RGN Dip Cancer Care BSc(Hons)
ENB998
Ward Sister, St Oswald's Hospice, Newcastle upon
Tyne, UK

Sandra Gaines MEd PGD Ed PGD(Pain) RN DPSN
C&G 730 LeTTOL Cert
Senior Lecturer, Marie Curie Cancer Care, Newcastle
upon Tyne, UK

Maureen Gambles BSc(Hons) Psychology
Senior Research Fellow, Marie Curie Palliative Care
Institute, Liverpool, UK

Tom Gordon MA BD
Chaplain, Marie Curie Hospice, Edinburgh, UK

Philippa E. Green MSc BA(Hons) DIP RGN
Community Macmillan Nurse Specialist, Northumberland
Care Trust, Cramlington, UK

Jacqueline Howard BA(Hons) MCLIP RGN
Librarian, Cherry Knowle Hospital, Northumberland,
Tyne and Wear NHS Trust, Sunderland, UK

April Joslin MB Ac C Dip Ac Northern College of
Acupuncture
Acupuncturist; Lecturer at the Northern College of
Acupuncture, York; formerly Acupuncturist and Head of
Services at Cancer Bridge, Hexham, Northumberland, UK

Shaun Kinghorn MSc BA(Hons) RGN CertEd RNT
RCNT, LETTOL, ITOL
Online Learning Developments Lead, Marie Curie Cancer
Care, Newcastle upon Tyne, UK

Pippa Lovell MBBS Dip Pall Med
Macmillan Medical Information Officer, Lifespan
Complementary, Ministeracres, Consett, County
Durham, UK

Rosemary McIntyre PhD, MN DipN (Lond), RGN, NDN, RNT
Research Fellow (funded by Macmillan Cancer Support), Napier University, Edinburgh, UK

Karen Merkin-Eyre BWY Teaching Diploma LFST Teaching Diploma IIHHT Diploma Bi-Aura Diploma
Yoga Therapist, formerly at Cancer Bridge, Hexam, Northumberland, UK

David Mitchell BD Dip P Theo MSc PG Cert HE
Parish Minister and Lecturer in Palliative Care, Church of Scotland, Tighnabruaich, UK

Michelle Muir BSc(Hons) PG DipMan PG Cert Man RGN
Clinical Nurse Specialist in Palliative Care, Newcastle upon Tyne Hospitals NHS Trust, Newcastle upon Tyne, UK

Helen Richardson MSC BSC (Hons) ITEC Diploma in Massage and Aromatherapy, 11R Diploma in Reflexology (Previously SRN RM)
Complementary Therapist at Northern Centre for Cancer Treatment, Newcastle General Hospital, Newcastle upon Tyne, UK

Anita Roberts MSc BSc(Hons) RGN RSCN
Education Lead, Liverpool Care Pathway, Marie Curie Palliative Care Institute, Liverpool, UK

Kathy Roberts Dip ISPA Reiki 4
Complementary Therapist, Lifespan Complementary, Consett, County Durham, UK

Audrey Rowe RGN BSc(Hons) PGCE LeTTol
Nursing Team Manager, Marie Curie Nursing Service (North East), Newcastle upon Tyne, UK

Gill Satterley RGN RMN RHV Dip Cancer Palliative Care Dip Cognitive Therapy
Nurse Manager, Day Services, Marie Curie Hospice, Newcastle upon Tyne, UK

Fiona Setch C&G730, CTP, CertEd, NLP Practitioner, LETTOL Cert
Company Director, Fiona Setch Motivational Training & Coaching, www.fionasetch.co.uk Newcastle upon Tyne, UK

Linden Tansley MA BA(Hons), Dip ISPA VAI Dip Reiki 3a
Complementary Therapist, Lifespan Complementary, Consett, County Durham, UK

Elizabeth Travers MSc BA RGN DN Cert Diploma is Cancer and Palliative Care RNT PGDipEd
Senior Education Manager, Marie Curie Hospice, Glasgow, UK

James Youll RGN ONC DipPallcare ENB100 931 FETC HEFC
Macmillan Clinical Nurse Specialist, South Tyneside District Hospital NHS Foundation Trust, South Shields, Tyne & Wear, UK

Preface

Palliative care has undergone significant development since the first edition of *Palliative Nursing: Bringing Comfort and Hope* was published in 2001, edited by Shaun Kinghorn and Richard Gamlin. We are delighted to report that this first edition has attracted global interest within the international community, with a Greek translation of *Palliative Nursing* being available and a distribution profile that spans the five continents. Some contributors from the first edition have moved on to pastures new and the responsibility to produce new versions of the chapters has been ably handled by our new contributors. We are grateful to Richard Gamlin and other chapter editors from the first edition whose support has ensured a successful roll-out of the first edition.

Changes in palliative care are reflected in this second edition of the text, which has embraced the need for new thinking and additional expertise. Firstly, Sandra Gaines has joined Shaun Kinghorn as a new co-editor. You will recognise that a number of the chapter titles remain the same but the content has been revised to ensure that the text maintains its relevance to clinical practice and the contemporary challenges within palliative nursing. We are delighted to include some new and significantly reconstructed chapters which we are confident will give added value to the text. These chapters include: the changing role of the nurse; sexuality in palliative care; care of the dying pathway; principles of symptom management; evidence-based practice; global issues in palliative care; spiritual care; complementary therapies and ethical issues at the end of life.

One major theme that is capturing the attention of those who commission and deliver palliative care services is the needs of those requiring palliative care who do not have cancer. You will note that a significant proportion of the chapters make specific reference to this issue. The result is a text that acknowledges that the principles that apply to the care of those with a malignant disease can be also applied to those who have a non-malignant life-limiting disease.

One thing that has not changed in this second edition is the focus on the development of palliative nursing. This text has consciously retained its emphasis on the philosophy of 'written by nurses for nurses', although it is important to point out that a significant proportion of this text is highly relevant to those staff that practise as professionals from different disciplines. This perspective is ably addressed by the contributions of our colleagues from other professions.

We do hope that this second edition makes for pleasurable reading but, more importantly, helps you deliver high-quality palliative care wherever you practise.

Shaun Kinghorn and Sandra Gaines
2007

Acknowledgements

The editors would like to thank all authors for taking the time to share their knowledge, experience and insights into the complex issues surrounding end-of-life care. We are particularly grateful for the ongoing support and enthusiasm of the commissioning and editorial teams at Elsevier in Edinburgh. Additionally we are mindful of the valuable contribution of our close colleague, Sharon Robson, who had the unenviable task of keeping us on track.

Personal acknowledgements

Thank you to those who make 'being at home' such a pleasure – my wife and best friend Melanie; Ashley, Anna, Joseph, Aaron and Jude, Melanie (junior) and Dave, and our lovely grandchildren Alastair, Layla and Beth – Happy Days.

Shaun Kinghorn

Thank you to David, Kameron, Jonathan and Simon. Without your belief in me I could not have aspired to complete this text; thank you also to April, George, Amy, Michael and Jacinta, our 'family' in New Zealand.

Sandra Gaines

Chapter **1**

Strategic and global issues in palliative care

Elizabeth Travers and David Mitchell

Palliative care is at the gateway to a process of considerable change as it moves beyond its traditional roots in cancer care to include non-malignant life-threatening illnesses and a projected ageing population. Hospices and palliative care teams are renowned for developing their services and expertise through a patient and carer focused approach, and for sharing that experience and expertise throughout the world. However, although the UK has a considerable influence on the development of palliative care services around the world, there are also lessons to be learned from looking at the global picture of palliative care and from other models of palliative care services in developed and developing countries.

Looking within the UK there is a genuine fear that the future will bring change that, while significantly increasing the availability for palliative care for vast numbers of patients, will result in a reduced service for cancer patients and their carers. This fear may be real, but hope lies in the national palliative care organisations that have a tradition of cooperation and consultation, and are already actively engaged in the debate.

This chapter explores the current and future development of palliative care services, nationally and globally, to address these strategic challenges. The chapter aims:

- to analyse the political, organisational and societal factors that have influenced the development of palliative care
- to evaluate the current issues that will influence the future development of palliative care.

THE DEVELOPMENT OF PALLIATIVE CARE

The World Health Organisation (WHO) first defined palliative care in the early 1990s. At that time the focus of palliative care was undoubtedly cancer; however, the WHO has updated the definition to encompass all life-limiting conditions:

Palliative care is an approach that improves the quality of life of patients and their families facing the problems associated with life threatening illness, through the prevention and relief of pain and suffering by means of early identification and impeccable assessment and treatment of pain and other problems, physical, psychosocial and spiritual.

Palliative care:
- provides relief from pain and other distressing symptoms

- affirms life and regards dying as a normal process

- intends neither to hasten nor postpone death

- integrates the psychological and spiritual aspects of patient care

- offers a support system to help patients live as actively as possible until death

- offers a support system to help the family cope during the patient's illness and in their own bereavement

- uses a team approach to address the needs of patients and their families, including bereavement counselling, if indicated

- will enhance quality of life, and may also positively influence the course of illness

- is applicable early in the course of illness, in conjunction with other therapies that are intended to prolong life, such as chemotherapy or radiation therapy, and includes those investigations needed to better understand and manage distressing clinical complications.
(World Health Organisation 2002)

Although the development of palliative care has a general focus of approach that 'should form the basis of good care for all people with life limiting illness and be provided by anyone in a caring role' (National Council for Palliative Care 2002), its modern roots are in the hospice movement. However, many hospices have gone on to develop as providers of specialist palliative care:

Specialist palliative care is the active total care of patients with progressive, far advanced disease and limited prognosis, and their families, by a multiprofessional team who have undergone recognised specialist palliative care training. It provides physical, psychological, social and spiritual support and will involve practitioners with a broad mix of skills.
(Clinical Standards Board for Scotland 2002)

This chapter will consider strategic issues in both generalist and specialist palliative care. Although specialist palliative care has evolved from a generalist palliative approach, there is also a clear sense in which they complement each other, and the boundaries between one and the other get blurred.

PALLIATIVE CARE IN THE UK

Throughout the 1990s and into the new millennium a number of key agencies have influenced the development and delivery of palliative care in the UK. Statutory bodies, including the National Health Service (NHS), NHSScotland, the National Institute for Health and Clinical Excellence (NICE) and NHS Quality Improvement Scotland (NHS QIS), together with the National Council for Palliative Care (NCPC), the Scottish Partnership for Palliative Care (SPPC), Help the Hospices and voluntary hospices, have all contributed to the strategic direction and implementation of palliative care in the UK.

It can be argued that much of this development has been shaped, coordinated and disseminated by the NCPC and the SPPC. These organisations were formed in 1991 and are national umbrella bodies for palliative care in the UK. They bring together NHS bodies and voluntary and professional organisations to promote better understanding of palliative care, to make it available to all those who need it, and to improve standards of care for patients and families.

Standards, guidelines and best practice

One important aspect of modern palliative care is its attempt to encourage the sharing of good practice through the setting of standards and guidelines and the publication of best practice statements.

The respective UK departments of health in England and Wales, and Scotland have chosen different methods by which palliative care services can be assessed. Scotland, through NHS QIS, has opted for clinical standards that are mandatory, whereas England and Wales focus on guidelines developed by NICE. Despite this different approach, the scope and rationale of both approaches are similar.

In Scotland the clinical standards are designed for specialist palliative care as it is delivered in hospices and hospital palliative care support teams. The standards seek to assess eight aspects of care (Clinical Standards Board for Scotland 2002):

1. Access to services
2. Key elements of specialist palliative care
3. Managing people and resources
4. Professional education
5. Inter-professional communication
6. Communication with patients
7. Therapeutic interventions
8. Patient activity.

Within the standards, the core members of the multidisciplinary team are defined, referral guidelines to related therapies and specialists are required, and the therapeutic interventions include the core elements of the WHO (2002) definition of palliative care: physical, psychological, social and spiritual with the addition of bereavement.

The guideline approach adopted by NICE (2004) follows a 13-topic format which includes:

- Coordination of care
- User involvement
- Face-to-face communication
- Information
- Psychological support services
- Social support services
- Spiritual support services
- General palliative care services
- Specialist palliative care services
- Rehabilitation services
- Complementary therapy services
- Services for families and carers including bereavement
- Research in supportive palliative care.

Although the guidelines seem more comprehensive, they apply only to adults with cancer and are not mandatory. However, the model has been adapted by other non-malignant disease-specific groups, such as the Coronary Heart Disease Collaborative, highlighting how easily the principles of palliative care can be adapted to diseases other than cancer (NHS Modernisation Agency 2004).

The effect of guidelines and clinical standards is to promote good practice. Local flexibility and varia-

tion can be maintained while at the same time ensuring that current practice is structured in a way that is effective and evidence based.

STRATEGIC ISSUES IN PALLIATIVE CARE

The National Council for Palliative Care policy document states (NCPC 2003):

> Every person with advanced, progressive and incurable illness should receive palliative care, appropriate to their assessed need.

This statement heralded a significant change of focus for the palliative care sector. Traditionally palliative care had its roots in cancer care and there is no doubt that the development of palliative care owes much to the voluntary sector, and in particular to the independent hospices and cancer charities that have driven the agenda, encouraged the recognition of palliative care as a specialty, and collaborated with the statutory bodies to formalise palliative care through guidelines, standards and best practice. The significant challenge is to take palliative care from its roots in cancer care and to move forward, recognising the palliative care needs of patients with other life-threatening non-malignant conditions.

This change in focus is further explored in the NCPC (2005) paper '20:20 Vision', which looks at the momentum behind palliative care and to the future of palliative care in 20 years' time. The paper considers the changing shape and culture of populations and the likelihood of an increasingly elderly population, the impact of non-malignant illnesses, economic and policy changes in health and social care, and the impact for specialist palliative care services of including palliative and supportive care in mainstream healthcare.

ACUTE ILLNESS, CHRONIC ILLNESS AND CO-MORBIDITY

It is widely recognised that life expectancy is increasing in the UK, and developments in healthcare technology, knowledge and skill clearly enhance that development. However, such advances are likely to have an impact on the need for palliative care. It is predicted that, as healthcare advances and people live longer, more people will survive acute life-threatening disease and the likelihood is that they will live longer with chronic life-limiting conditions (NCPC 2005). In addition, co-morbidity is also likely to increase, with older people living with multiple pathologies.

The resource implications for palliative care services are considerable. Increased patient numbers over a longer period of time, and the complexities of managing concurrent conditions, will create challenges that require additional resources and improved workforce planning, education and training.

THE CHALLENGE OF NON-MALIGNANCY

Although a number of existing palliative care services have traditionally embraced non-malignant neurological conditions, there is no doubt that the expertise and development of palliative care is firmly rooted in cancer care. It is clear that palliative care is an approach that is applicable to all healthcare, and should not be limited to those with cancer (WHO 2002); however, within specialist palliative care there is a legitimate concern that the current expertise is cancer focused and that the expertise required to meet the complexity of non-malignant conditions cannot simply be 'included in the service' without giving thought to the advanced knowledge and skills that would be required of healthcare professionals.

As with the ageing population, the resource implications of including non-malignant conditions in palliative care are considerable. In addition, given that the majority of specialist palliative care services are funded by voluntary organisations, some of which specifically raise money to provide cancer care, is it ethical or legal to raise money for cancer care and then spend it on something else? Clearly there are significant questions that need to be addressed before patients with non-malignant conditions receive the quality of palliative care services available to cancer patients. However, there is an added concern that simply by including non-malignant conditions in existing palliative care services the quality palliative care currently received by cancer patients might be diminished.

Palliative care has long been recognised for its understanding of the complexity of the challenges that patients, families/carers and staff experience in end-of-life care. Their particular expertise is in assessing and addressing these issues with openness and honesty. These issues regularly involve difficult conversations and complex ethical dilemmas.

PLACE OF CARE OR WHERE TO DIE

A comment regularly made is that, given a choice, most people would choose to die at home. However, the reality is that the majority die in hospital, hospice or care home. Marie Curie Cancer Care has commissioned market research in the area of choice for end-of-life care and its implications for health services and patients. The Delivering Choice Programme is an initiative to provide choice for place of care and death to terminally ill patients and to offer support to their carers (Marie Curie Cancer Care 2004). Clearly the focus is to develop processes and protocols that increase the number of patients who are able to have their wish to be cared for and to die at home. However, the 'choice' element needs to be maintained for those who will change their mind – those who decide that the care they need is more than can be provided in their home and elect for hospital or, where appropriate, hospice as their place to be cared for and die.

CARDIOPULMONARY RESUSCITATION

Cardiopulmonary resuscitation (CPR) for people who are terminally ill is a topic that engenders much debate. On the one hand, a number of professional bodies offer guidance that suggests that resuscitation should be discussed with all patients, yet, on the other hand, there is no need to discuss any treatment that is judged to be futile (Resuscitation Council [UK] 2001, National Council for Palliative Care and Association for Palliative Medicine 2002). Some professions advise that all deaths at home should involve an emergency call and resuscitation unless there is a signed Do Not Resuscitate Order (DNR) in the patient notes, yet many healthcare professionals find themselves in a quandary and exercising discretion where a death is expected. The issue for palliative care services is: should you discuss CPR with patients for whom you would not consider resuscitation, or do you exercise professional judgement and discuss it only with those patients for whom in your professional judgement it may be an issue?

The issue is perhaps clearer in inpatient services, where local protocols for discussing DNR and CPR can be developed. However, in the community, where patients will access different services, more thought is required. It may be that the Delivering Choice Programme (MCCC 2004) will enable discussion to take place across services, including the ambulance service, and a protocol can be agreed that advances good practice.

EUTHANASIA

Since the start of the millennium there has been considerable debate and discussion in the UK on euthanasia, although the debate has been framed in much softer terminology: The Assisted Dying for the Terminally Ill Bill debated in the House of Lords (Lord Joffe 2004) and the lesser known Dying with Dignity paper produced for the Scottish Parliament (Purvis 2005).

Palliative care is often held up as the alternative to euthanasia, and is often misrepresented as being wholly and unequivocally opposed to euthanasia. In their press statement in response to the Joffe Bill, the Association of Hospice and Palliative Care Chaplains (AHPCC 2003) might have been expected to focus on 'sanctity of life' arguments, yet many chaplains have empathy with those who are genuinely suffering and seek euthanasia; instead they chose to focus on the impracticalities of the bill and the practical and ethical implications for healthcare professionals should the Bill become law. How do you define 'unbearable suffering'? Are doctors the best professionals to decide on this issue? What about the multidisciplinary team? Although doctors will be not be prosecuted for prescribing the lethal dose of medication, what of the nurse who is likely to set up the equipment for the patient to self-administer or the pharmacist who knowingly makes up a lethal dose of medication?

Although the issue is not going forward to the UK parliaments in its present form, it is likely to return, given its popular appeal in the media.

As a relatively new specialism, palliative care has developed at a considerable pace. It has demonstrated a willingness to engage in open constructive political and professional debate, to work collaboratively across agencies and to extend its boundaries to include all individuals with palliative needs.

PALLIATIVE CARE: THE GLOBAL PERSPECTIVE

Arguably, the development of palliative care in the UK has had a profound impact on the development of palliative care throughout the world, and many hospices and palliative care services have links with services in other countries. Alongside this UK influence, a number of organisations, including the WHO and the International Observatory on End of Life Care (IOEOLC), have promoted and championed the development of palliative care throughout the world. A number of factors influence the strategic development of healthcare in general and of palliative care in particular, for instance economics, trade, new technologies, availability of drugs, changing populations, vulnerable groups (older people, children and adolescents), culture and ethnicity, equity of access, education and training, and the prevalence of HIV/AIDS.

The strategic and global advancement of palliative care varies considerably from nation to nation. A key factor is often whether the nation is considered to be developed or developing; for the latter, the issues are often related to availability of resources and expertise. Clark & Wright (2003), focusing on Eastern Europe and Central Asia, noted that often the development of palliative care rests with a few committed individuals and can be hampered by ideological, political and social factors. The difficult questions that need to be addressed in the developing world have been reported by Laughton & Becker (2004) and include: How do you get the medical profession to be interested in the dying if they are paid only for active treatments? Can you have palliative care without morphine? Should work on palliative care and AIDS be integrated?

The key resource providing comparison on hospice and palliative care in more than 60 countries is the International Observatory on End of Life Care website: http://www.eolc-observatory.net/ The reports include Africa, India, the Middle East and Eastern Europe. An additional resource, which includes the wider world, is the International Association for Hospice and Palliative Care website, which has a focus on individual palliative care services rather than national reports: http://www.hospicecare.com/ Help the Hospices also has an international focus, and its report 'Suffering at the End of Life' considers the inequality of suffering, the palliative care response to suffering at the end of life, and offers a detailed worldwide resource list to encourage readers to find 'a way ahead' (Help the Hospices 2005).

GLOBAL PALLIATIVE CARE ISSUES

Pain control

In the UK, a central focus in the development of palliative care has been the significant advances and successes in symptom control, and in particular pain. One anomaly in the global perspective is that the countries that produce the opiates, which are so effective in pain control, can often be the countries where opiates such as morphine are not available. Added to this picture can be the local healthcare system: if doctors are paid only for curative treatments, there is a disincentive to prescribe palliative medications.

It can be argued that without the availability of opioids palliative care is not possible, but the effect of this is to deny the other achievable and necessary aspects of palliative care outlined in the WHO principles of palliative care mentioned previously (WHO 2002). Although the availability of opioids should not be regarded as the only measure of palliative care, it is a significant factor. As opioids are cheap, safe and effective, their availability could be used as a measure of progress in countries developing their palliative care services (Help the Hospices 2005).

Non-malignancy

The challenge of non-malignancy takes a different form from that in the UK, particularly in countries where HIV/AIDS is a significant or common cause of death. The effect is to reduce rather than lengthen national life expectancy statistics. In sub-Saharan African countries such as Botswana, Ethiopia, Uganda and Zimbabwe, average life expectancy at birth is 40–50 years and deaths from HIV/AIDS are 4–10-fold those of cancer (WHO 2004). Many African countries are experiencing some stability in infection rates, but others, such as Swaziland and Botswana, have respective infection rates of 33.4% and 24.1%, with three females for every one male infected (WHO 2006).

Putting the worldwide statistics for cancer and HIV/AIDS together results in a significant shift that has implications for palliative care: more than 10 million people are diagnosed with cancer each year, but there are currently 42 million people living with HIV, 29 million of whom are in sub-Saharan Africa (Help the Hospices 2005).

Hospice care or community care?

Analysis of the International Observatory on End of Life Care reports shows that palliative care services vary in their models of delivery throughout the world. Often it is historical links that influence the development of services, or what external donors are prepared to fund and support. Services with Western and UK hospice links tend to frame themselves on the inpatient model with day hospice and outreach as the norm, yet in other areas services function with no inpatient facilities and are entirely community based.

In Africa, for example, there is considerable variety in services. In Tanzania, inpatient hospice services report large areas to cover, difficulty in patients travelling to services and patients simply 'turning up' without referrals as the main issues. In Swaziland, palliative services are home-care based; they are structured geographically and function with the

support of dedicated palliative care nurses and part-time parish nurses (retired), and work in cooperation with agencies such as the Salvation Army (IOEOLC 2005).

Clearly there is not one ideal palliative care model that suits all. Simply replicating the UK model in other situations may not be practical or desirable. Drug availability for symptom control, including pain, is a significant global issue. Patients with AIDS, with cancer trailing in second place, may be the main population group in need of palliative care services, and the type of service developed may be influenced as much by historical relationships and what outside agencies are prepared to fund as by local need.

CONCLUSION

In exploring the strategic and global issues in palliative care, it is clear that a period of significant change is on the horizon. The question is whether palliative care services will rise to the challenge or be swamped and retreat to their roots in cancer care.

Through the guidance and leadership of the National Council for Palliative Care, the Scottish Partnership for Palliative Care and Help the Hospices, palliative care in the UK has made great strides and provides standards, guidelines and best practice that are the envy of many other healthcare services. However, there are two significant issues that have the potential to pressurise or swamp existing services: the growth of an ageing population, which will result in much greater numbers and people with long-term chronic life-limiting illness, and the inclusion of non-malignant life-threatening conditions into what has until now been a cancer-focused specialty. The reality is that current issues and predicted future trends will bring change in palliative care.

When considering palliative care globally, attention is often focused on the experience and resources that the West, and the UK in particular, has to offer to others. This may be true in terms of access to expertise, education and training, and appropriate drugs. However, whether or not a UK inpatient-focused model with additional day and home care services is the best model is open to debate. It may be that in looking to develop choice for patients in their place of care and death we need to draw on the experience of countries where the community-based services are successful and working.

By recognising these strategic and global issues, the hope is that all of those affected by life-limiting conditions in need of palliative care will receive care at least to the level that existing cancer patients receive, and that existing services will continue to develop. The fear is that the pressures of increasing patient numbers, availability of resources, expertise, education and training could result in a compromise that offers an improvement on the current provision of palliative care for a substantial majority of patients at the cost of a reduced service for patients with cancer.

Hope is a key theme in palliative care, but it has to be a realistic and achievable hope – or people are simply being set up to fail. The hope for the future of palliative care is a realistic hope if palliative care can remain true to its definition: to take 'an approach that improves the quality of life of patients and their families facing the problems associated with life

threatening illness' (WHO 2002). As the following chapters in this book will show, palliative care is rooted in caring for patients and their families, and palliative care professionals have an expertise that they share openly and widely. Arguably the key to significant service developments in palliative care will be in its organisation and structure, in coordinating the NHS and the voluntary sector, and that work is already begun. The National Council for Palliative Care, the Scottish Partnership for Palliative Care and Help the Hospices have the strategic and global issues on their agenda. Experience shows that they will not compromise the principles of palliative care services; rather, they will seek to set them in place and earth them firmly in our healthcare systems.

References

Association of Hospice and Palliative Care Chaplains 2003 Response to the Assisted Dying for the Terminally Ill Bill. AHPCC, Swanwick

Clark D, Wright M 2003 Transitions in end of life care: hospice and related developments in Eastern Europe and Central Asia. Open University Press, Buckingham

Clinical Standards Board for Scotland 2002 Clinical standards: specialist palliative care. NHS Quality Improvement Scotland, Edinburgh

Help the Hospices 2005 Suffering at the end of life: the state of the world. Help the Hospices, London

International Observatory on End of Life Care 2005 Hospice and palliative care development in Africa: a review of services and experiences. Online. Available: http://www.eolc-observatory.net/global/africa.htm Aug 2006

Laughton R, Becker R 2004 UK forum annual conference: supporting palliative care around the world. International Journal of Palliative Nursing 10:554–555

Lord Joffe 2004 Assisted Dying for the Terminally Ill Bill. The House of Lords, London

Marie Curie Cancer Care 2004 Delivering choice programme. Online. Available: http://www.mariecurie.org.uk/deliveringchoice/ February 2005

National Council for Palliative Care 2002 Briefing Bulletin 11: Definitions of supportive and palliative care. NCPC London

National Council for Palliative Care 2003 Palliative care for adults with non-malignant diseases: developing a national policy. NCPC, London

National Council for Palliative Care 2005 20:20 Vision – the shape of the future for palliative care. NCPC, London

National Council for Palliative Care and Association for Palliative Medicine 2002 Ethical decision making in palliative care: cardiopulmonary resuscitation for people who are terminally ill. Journal of the Royal College of Physicians of Edinburgh 32:91–96

National Institute for Clinical Excellence 2004 Improving supportive and palliative care for adults with cancer manual. NICE, London

NHS Modernisation Agency 2004 Coronary Heart Disease Collaborative. NHS Modernisation Agency, Leicester

Purvis J 2005 Consultation Paper: Dying with dignity. The Scottish Parliament, Edinburgh

Resuscitation Council (UK) 2001 Decisions relating to cardiopulmonary resuscitation: a joint statement from the British Medical Association, the Resuscitation Council (UK) and the Royal College of Nursing. Resuscitation Council (UK), London

World Health Organisation 2002 WHO definition of palliative care. Online. Available: http://www.who.int/cancer/palliative/definition/en/ 6 July 2004

World Health Organisation 2004 Sub-Saharan report. WHO, Geneva

World Health Organisation 2006 Overview of the global AIDS epidemic. WHO, Geneva

Chapter **2**

Managing symptoms: what can nurses do? A principle-based approach

Alison Conner and Michelle Muir

For many patients with progressive disease, uncontrolled symptoms can affect their quality of life and their ability to cope with illness and subsequent death (Higginson 1997). Families and carers may find it hard to witness the person experiencing symptoms and this can affect their subsequent grieving process (Steinhauser et al 2000). For this reason, palliative care emphasises the need to control symptoms as well as supporting the family and carers. This is an essential role for all healthcare professionals in all settings, although access to specialists in palliative care may be needed for complex cases. The overall goal is to relieve suffering with due regard to self-esteem, maintenance of activity, independence and something of a normal life . . . in the place where the person wishes to be. This requires individualised care that takes account of the whole person, their circumstances and their wishes. The approach and skills needed to accomplish all this should be cultivated by all nurses.

> Diseases need medicine but human beings who suffer will always need a touch of magic.
> (Buckman & Sabbagh 1993)

The aim of this chapter is to examine the role of the nurse in palliative symptom management, specifically:

- the importance of assessment
- principles of symptom management
- the synergistic use of psychological and physical approaches
- managing symptoms at the end of life
- what can be done if symptoms remain.

The underlying premise of the chapter is that individual practitioners will reflect on the issues discussed, adapt and utilise information to apply to their own practice.

The authors recognise that palliative care is delivered by nurses in many different settings across the world, to patients with varying needs. They draw from their experience as clinical nurse specialists in the UK to describe a set of principles that can be adapted as necessary, and examine what can be done when symptoms remain. Palliative care is a relatively young specialty which is growing and changing quickly. The focus of published literature on symptom management appears to have moved on since the first edition of this book so that some things are now 'accepted practice'. From defining and describing elements of the specialty, multidisciplinary approaches and methods of quantifying symptoms, the focus now is on how to implement best practice in a methodical and equitable manner. The role of nurses has changed a lot in that time too; they have extended skills in, for example, prescribing. This chapter has been updated to reflect these changes, but the founding elements remain the same: the nature of suffering, holistic nursing assessment skills and the need for symptom management for all patients with life-threatening illnesses.

DEFINITIONS

A symptom has been defined as subjective evidence of disease, i.e. something perceived only by the patient. A sign is objective evidence of disease, i.e. something that is apparent to the patient, nurse and others (MedicineNet.com 2006).

This subjectivity means that assessment, measurement and treatment of symptoms depend on the descriptions of symptoms given by the patient. Twycross (1997) identified the most common symptoms in cancer patients as:

- *Physical* – lack of energy, pain, drowsiness, dry mouth, nausea and anorexia
- *Psychological* – worrying, feeling sad, feeling nervous, difficulty sleeping, feeling irritable and difficulty concentrating.

It is generally agreed that patients' symptoms vary and change as their disease progresses or their feelings and circumstances alter. In addition, the degree to which patients are distressed by these symptoms varies between individuals. Treatment of symptoms such as fatigue, confusion and breathlessness requires the patient to give detailed descriptions so that management is as specific as possible.

Physical symptoms can be entwined with emotions and may be associated with a sense of social isolation or spiritual abandonment (Stiefel & Guex 1996). For example, a breathless, anxious patient who is frightened and unable to get up and about may constantly seek attention by reporting lots of minor discomforts or, alternatively, withdraw into themselves with no mention of any problems (Gillis 1988). Because psychological reactions to illness in general and to symptoms in particular do differ and may affect the level of distress felt, the management of symptoms needs different approaches depending on the way the patient has reacted. The nurse will need to build a rapport and be flexible in the way in which the patient is approached.

Suffering

Suffering is a word commonly used when speaking of symptoms. It encompasses the meaning of the symptom to the patient or family and this meaning will affect the degree of distress felt and the choices made about treatments (Saunders 1993). Suffering is a unique experience that is not simply a physical, psychological or spiritual symptom but involves the whole person including their memory, intellect and insight. It is constantly changing and cannot be predicted by others – what would be an insignificant episode for one person may be extremely distressing for another. A patient's understanding of their suffering plays a significant part in their response to it. For example, if constant nausea and vomiting is seen as an undeserved punishment (divine or not), the patient may feel great distress. But if their nausea is caused by treatment in the pursuit of increased life expectancy, it may be seen as a tolerable event and distress may be less (Salt 1997). The key is to understand suffering as part of the patient's perspective on life and the world, and that the control of physical symptoms is only part of alleviating that suffering (Ohlen 2002).

A FEW STATISTICS

In the UK in 2004 (National Statistics 2006):

- 1.2 million people were living with a diagnosis of cancer.
- Some 610 000 people died (all causes).
- One in five of those people died at home.
- 85% were people aged 65 years and older.
- 25% died from cancer, 19% from heart disease, 14% from respiratory disease and 11% from stroke.
- Pain, dyspnoea and fatigue occur in 50% of patients with cancer, AIDS, heart disease, chronic obstructive pulmonary disease and renal disease (Solano et al 2006).

- By the year 2051 the number of annual deaths will be 800 000.

In essence there will be many people living with illnesses other than cancer that may cause distressing symptoms, and they are not all living at home. It is recognised that palliative care should be available to all people with progressive life-threatening illnesses and that, as people are living longer and the diseases listed above are most prevalent in the elderly, the need for palliative care will grow in the coming years. This seems to present a huge problem for such a small specialty, but it may be that provision of palliative care can be adapted in different areas. Thomas (2006) has suggested that there are three illness trajectories for patients with these diseases:

1. Cancer – ongoing treatment with relatively high function that overlaps with an increasing palliative focus as these patients decline in a fairly predictable manner.
2. Organ failure – slowly declining function and increasing morbidity with multiple crisis admissions and then a sudden 'unexpected death'.
3. Elderly frail – sometimes demented, who decline slowly and unpredictably with several co-morbid conditions, can be described as 'skating on thin ice'.

The challenge is to provide palliative care for patients with different diseases, on different trajectories, in different settings. The authors of this chapter argue that the model of palliative care for *cancer* patients may not be the right one for other disease trajectories, but the principles of managing symptoms effectively will remain the same.

The assessment and management of symptoms and symptom distress is a vital aspect of nursing patients with advanced and incurable diseases. It should be guided by a comprehensive, individual assessment that incorporates an understanding of the illness, the multidimensional nature of symptoms and the issue of quality of life for the individual.

WHAT ARE THE PRINCIPLES OF SYMPTOM MANAGEMENT?

Assessment is the first step in determining the health needs of any patient (Castledine 2004). The process starts as soon as a nurse comes in contact with a patient and, as nurses in whichever field we choose to work, we should be practised and skilled at it. Not only is the future care plan based upon good assessment, but much of the multiprofessional care plan is formulated around the information that nurses have

collected and recorded. Assessment of symptoms in patients with palliative care needs is therefore the role of every nurse, not just the specialist nurse.

The importance of assessment

Any assessment involves collecting two kinds of data: objective and subjective. Objective data are obtained through observation and questioning, and can be verified (Castledine 2004). Subjective data are much more difficult to record (e.g. patient's emotions), but if we do not shy away from this more difficult part of the assessment process the 'data' gathered can really contribute to our ability to make a difference to the palliative care patients we care for.

Assessment must be recorded as an ongoing process. It must not be the sole remit of the 'admitting' nurse, but must be revised constantly as the plan of care is revised. If time is limited, or a patient is very ill, focusing on current problems in order of priority to the patient (as their priority may differ from that of the professional) will provide the most valuable information.

The introduction to the assessment procedure must not be underestimated. All too often professionals do not formally introduce themselves and their purpose. Patients often relay their confusion at the numbers of professionals they meet along their 'journey'. If the patient knows your name and role they may feel more at ease answering your questions and giving you the information you seek. Patients should be given permission to disclose their concerns if they choose to, no matter how trivial *they* may think they are. They are never trivial if they are a concern.

Nurses are more confident in their ability to assess physical than psychological aspects of illness. This may be because nurses, like many other professionals, lack the skills needed to communicate effectively (Heaven & Maguire 1996). Many nurses fear upsetting their patients; others fear not being able to answer difficult questions or saying the wrong thing (Maguire 1985). The ability to assess and elicit patient concerns, symptoms and fears requires effective communication (Wilkinson 1991). Communication is of such importance that it will be covered in depth in a later chapter.

Symptoms are multidimensional experiences that may be evaluated in terms of their specific characteristics and impact on the patient and family. The impact of symptoms may be described in relation to functioning (family, social, financial or physical) or to wider concepts such as symptom distress or quality of life (Ingram & Portenoy 1996). The challenge of symptom measurement is to capture relevant symptoms as they evolve and perhaps to anticipate their possible evolution. When they do evolve, measures should be used that are simple and quick, so as not to burden the patient or the staff. The measures used should also generate information that is useful to inform care planning. It is considered by some that assessment of patients with advanced disease is burdensome and sometimes unfair on the patient; however, it is to be remembered that in order to try to achieve quality of life for the patient we must ask patients their wishes, desires, fears and opinions to inform our care provision.

Using tools for the assessment of symptoms

There is a wide range of tools that can be used to measure symptom distress and quality of life in palliative care patients. This chapter will briefly look at a small selection in order to signpost readers to their existence and use. Further reading is needed to find a tool appropriate to individual settings and practice.

- The Rotterdam Symptom Checklist (RSCL) (de Haes et al 1990) is a validated measure that can be used to evaluate a range of common symptoms in terms of patient-rated distress. It consists of 34 symptoms covering physical and psychosocial problems. It provides quantitative information about global symptom distress.

- The Support Team Assessment Schedule (STAS) (Higginson 1993) is a quick, comprehensive tool with multiple topics and its own scoring criteria (Carson et al 2000). It was originally designed in the UK in community settings, and consists of 17 items covering: pain and symptoms, psychosocial issues, insight, family needs, communication, home services and support of other professionals. This tool is used widely and can be useful as it takes on average 2–3 minutes to complete.

- The Palliative Care Outcome Scale (POS) consists of a 10-point questionnaire for both staff and patients (Hearn & Higginson 1999).

- The Palliative Care Assessment (PaCA) tool is a quick numerical scoring system (Box 2.1) that can be easily completed with the patient.

Over an 8-year period a specialist palliative care team in a large teaching hospital used the validated PaCA tool (Ellershaw et al 1995) to monitor their effectiveness in controlling a variety of symptoms. The symp-

toms included pain, confusion, low mood, nausea and breathlessness. These authors found that, although a simple tool, the PaCA allows a defined patient-focused scoring system to be applied to any symptom. This simple, quick tool allows rapid completion and gives valuable data for use in monitoring clinical effectiveness and, more importantly, patient symptom management. This is the tool currently being used by the authors of this chapter in their daily practice; it has proved to be very useful in day-to-day assessment.

Box 2.1   Scoring of the Palliative Care Assessment tool

Problem absent = 0
Problem present but not affecting the patient's day = 1
Problem present and having a moderate effect on patient's day = 2
Problem present and dominating the patient's day = 3

Where to begin?

Ask the patient to prioritise their symptoms; remember our priorities may not be theirs.

Case Study 2.1   The importance of individualised assessment

A young man had severe neuropathic pain down one leg from a spinal tumour. His priority was not for good pain control. Psychologically, he believed that if his pain was taken away he would find this point in his cancer journey more difficult to deal with, because the pain he was experiencing helped him to cope with the fact the cancer was real. He needed the pain to move forward in his journey. His actual priority at that point in time was financial worries, due to his inability to work.

All treatments for symptoms should be kept as simple as possible and should consider not just pharmacological interventions. Keep the balance between the goal of treatment and the patient's goal for improved quality of life, or even for things to be 'less bad'. Weigh up the benefits of treatment against side-effects and length of time needed to achieve any benefit.

Box 2.2 Principles of symptom management

- Talk to your patient and family, and remember the patient is central in all processes.
- Have a thorough knowledge of the pathophysiology and disease process of the disease you are managing, and any coexisting diseases. Synthesise this knowledge with that of current pharmacology and recognised disease treatment regimens when formulating plans for symptom management. Concentrate on close attention to detail.
- Consider the most appropriate routes of administration for all medications; for example, give antiemetics non-orally if nausea and vomiting are present.
- Consider quality of life and ethical issues.
- Think creatively and laterally in order to help formulate care plans.
- Do not change too many things at once, or it will be unclear what has helped. Leave things unchanged if the patient is comfortable.
- Constantly reassess by talking to your patient and family.
- Anticipate problems. A specialist knowledge and training along with experience allows nurses to consider the possibility of new problems before they happen, and to have a plan in place in case they do (e.g. anticipatory prescribing of analgesia and/or sedation in the event of a catastrophic bleed). Use an active problem-solving approach involving the multidisciplinary team.

The principles of symptom management listed in Box 2.2 are by no means exhaustive, but serve as an aide memoire of key areas for consideration. They also highlight that the essence of palliative care nursing can be seen as a creative and competent blend of the nurse, patient and family relationship together with knowledge and skills (Coyle 2001). There is a reading list at the end of the chapter giving texts that will provide more detailed discussion around principles of symptom management.

Case Study 2.2 Putting principles into practice

Case Study 2.2 and comments were supplied by Senior Staff Nurse Karen Wallace and Staff Nurse Cara Hubbuck, General Medical Ward, Newcastle upon Tyne, UK.

Case Study 2.2 Putting principles into practice — cont'd

Mr Brown, aged 68 years, was admitted with lung cancer and uncontrolled nausea and vomiting. He was distressed, thinking that his cancer had spread.

On admission, an assessment tool was used to explore this symptom. He reported that he usually felt bloated and vomited after meals, preceded by nausea, but that symptoms resolved after vomiting. Blood results did not indicate a chemical cause and Mr Brown was not constipated, although he had signs of reduced gut motility. A prokinetic agent, metoclopramide 30 mg as a 24-hour subcutaneous infusion, was prescribed, with a full explanation to the patient of the rationale.

After 4 days Mr Brown was able to eat small amounts without nausea or vomiting, so conversion to oral medication followed. He felt calm and able to manage at home again.

"When people are admitted with horrendous symptoms it's great to be able to apply these principles successfully. It's rewarding to get relief for them and gives you confidence that you know what you're doing ... that you're doing something well. You feel like you've achieved something."

Why is symptom management different at the end of life?

The principles of symptom management should be the same at the end of life as any other stage. However, the patient may not be capable of taking part in treatment and care decisions. Family may become more anxious about symptoms (e.g. pain, noisy breathing) than previously. There is evidence that psychological distress and morbidity in the bereaved can be reduced if quality of life in dying is maximised and carers are prepared (Parkes 1990).

For the patient, preparation time for death may be accelerated and too short. Symptom control can be lost or symptoms can remain inadequately controlled (Rogers et al 2000). As death approaches, issues of withdrawing or withholding medical treatments that are considered futile can be fraught with emotion on the part of the family and professionals. Owing to the ethical emphasis on the situation, such discussions need experienced skilled staff with time and sensitivity (Von Guten et al 2000) and effective interdisciplinary working.

Anxiety and distress in both the family and professionals can cloud their ability to assess and plan appropriate care unless it is recognised that death is approaching. This phase requires redefinition of goals and reappraisal of treatments and symptom control – a 'gear change' (National Council for Hospice and Specialist Palliative Care Services [NCHSPCS] 1997) is often needed. It is important to communicate and explain the patient's changing condition to the family so that they may understand changing approaches to care. This is prompted by several factors, including the patient's increasing difficulty taking oral medication, inability to cooperate with care, disinterest in activity, and increased need for rest and sleep (Ellershaw & Wilkinson 2003). Reassessment of symptoms is important at this stage as patients' tolerance of previous symptoms may be poor due to their debility and they may develop new symptoms (Conill et al 1997, NCHSPCS 1997).

MANAGING SYMPTOMS AT THE END OF LIFE

Diagnosing dying

Recognising the last days or hours of a patient's life is not always easy, not even for experienced professionals. A study by Oxenham & Cornbleet (1998) showed that a nursing auxiliary was able to predict imminent death more accurately than other health professionals. This is often still the case today. Shah et al (2006) undertook a study in patients with end-stage cancer and non-cancer diseases to compare, amongst other things, patients' and professionals' estimations of prognosis. Results showed that patients were well aware of their prognosis, perhaps more so than their doctors, and did not object to questions about end of life issues. We should be mindful of the value of asking our patients their views, needs and fears in order to be effective practitioners.

Physical and behavioural changes that occur over weeks or days may provide clues. For most patients, a gradual weakening occurs as the body's vital functions fail and the patient becomes less conscious, then unconscious, leading to respiratory and cardiac failure and death.

These changes may include some or all of the following:

- Altered appearance – translucency and faded colour of skin; cool cyanosed extremities; lank hair, greasy sweat; gaunt facial features; the cartilage of ears and nose pale and prominent; eyes become glazed, distant and hollow
- Decreased physical functioning – profound weakness; whispering voice; increased dependency; increased tiredness and longer periods of sleep; disinterest in food and fluids; continence problems
- Change in mental functioning – poor concentration; preoccupation or vagueness; reduced response to outside stimuli; disorientation; confusion; restlessness
- Altered vital signs – changes in pulse and breathing rate, rhythm and volume
- Other changes – losing interest or engagement in social interaction; focussing on memories of those who have already died; merging of night and day; knowledge of impending death; farewells with loved ones.

Sudden deterioration over a few days should prompt a search for potentially reversible causes, for example hypercalcaemia, infection or side-effects from changes in medication.

In the absence of reversible causes, the main aims of care are now the maintenance of comfort and dignity, continued palliation of symptoms, and quality of remaining time. It is important to remember at this stage to anticipate possible problems – to plan for changes; for example, medications being changed from an oral to a non-oral route and to have prescriptions *pro re nata* (prn) – or for new symptoms that may develop (e.g. terminal restlessness, respiratory secretions).

The patient who has been taking long-term medication for angina or hypertension is unlikely to benefit from this medication in the terminal phase and the treatment could be stopped. Similarly, hormone treatment for breast cancer is of no benefit at this stage. Other treatments that do need to be considered may also have to be given by a different route if the patient cannot swallow. If tolerance of existing symptoms is poor, current treatments may need to be changed. These changes need careful explanation, so that the family understands the reason. Misunderstandings about motives for changing therapy may lead to families feeling that professionals have given up on their loved one or are even attempting to hasten death.

A systematic approach to end-of-life care

Care of the dying is an area of healthcare in which one would hope to achieve excellence. However, inadequacies have been identified in the hospital setting around symptom control and psychological support (The Support Principal Investigators 1995), and in the community setting around lack of symptom control and poor experiences of services (Thomas 2003, Thorpe 1993). Guidance from the National Institute for Health and Clinical Excellence (NICE 2004) on supportive and palliative care confirms the need to develop all aspects of services relating to care for patients nearing the end of their life, and their practical recommendations provide a useful framework for developing services.

When multiprofessional treatment decisions are being considered, clinical guidelines based on up-to-date research findings, whether devised for use by specific units or for wider consumption, can be both helpful and necessary. Many such guidelines exist and this chapter will not discuss them in greater depth. However, nurses developing such guidelines should ensure that they are patient focused and, where appropriate, involve patients in their development.

It is unrealistic and unnecessary to expect palliative care teams to see every dying patient. Therefore, in recent years numerous guidelines and several national frameworks have been developed to help every practitioner to provide high-quality care at the end of life:

- *The Liverpool Care Pathway (LCP)*. This framework allows the caring team, either in hospital or in the community, to plan care using specific goals, guideline-based interventions and a flow sheet that outlines an expected course of a patient's care (Ellershaw & Wilkinson 2003). Whilst the nature of a pathway may seem to some to be quite prescriptive, the LCP allows for one of the care principles of palliative care (that of being patient focused) by allowing for frequent communication and assessment of patient care through the concept of variance recording. This framework has been shown to improve patient care in the end stage of life and to improve symptom control (Ellershaw & Wilkinson 2003, Liverpool Care Pathway 2006, Mirando 2005).

- *Gold Standards Framework (GSF)*. The GSF aims to improve community palliative care for primary care teams. It seeks to facilitate consistent, good-quality palliative care in the community setting through the use of guidelines, mechanisms and assessment tools (NICE 2004, Thomas 2003, 2006). The GSF proposes a three-step model of good practice in which practitioners: (1) identify palliative care patients, (2) assess their needs, including the needs of the carers, and (3) plan care and support to meet the needs. The framework centres on seven key areas: communication, coordination, control of symptoms, continuity, continued learning, carer support and care of the dying. King et al (2005) in a study of 15 general practices highlighted the ability of the GSF to help standardise care, making it more consistent. Practitioners felt more aware of the patient's needs. The GSF encourages regular meetings to discuss palliative care, and the use of a supportive care register plays a role in contributing to the success of the GSF. It particularly facilitates improved communication, anticipatory care and better patterns of working within teams (The Gold Standards Framework 2006, Thomas 2006).

- *Preferred Place of Care (PPC)* is an example of an advanced care planning tool. This is a patient-held document that can be taken into all care settings. It has space for information about family and significant people in the patient's life, and space to record the patient's thoughts and wishes – specifically allowing the patient to record their wishes about where they would like to be cared for at the end of their life. The patient is encouraged to keep the document up to date if any of their wishes should change as they go through their journey. The use of this document has already shown its transferability to diseases other than cancer (e.g. learning disability, motor neurone disease, and respiratory and heart failure). Initial evaluations of the use of this tool are positive, and indicate that by using it nurses gain confidence in their communication with dying patients and families (Lancashire & South Cumbria Cancer Network 2006, NHS End of Life Care Programme 2006).

HOW TO APPLY THE PRINCIPLES OF SYMPTOM MANAGEMENT

How do I know which symptom to treat first? Which is the most severe and troublesome symptom? What is the best treatment to try first? How can I anticipate what might happen next?

As discussed in the previous section of this chapter, answers to these questions require:

- *Knowledge* – of the symptoms that are likely to occur in that patient's illness; of the symptom management strategies that are useful in such cases, including surgical or oncological options and pharmacological or psychological approaches; of where to access assistance from other professionals or services; of sources of information, for example in medical textbooks or research journals such as those listed at the end of this chapter.

- *Skills* – communicating with the patient to assess the nature and severity of their symptoms and which ones bother them the most; judging which management approaches would be appropriate and that the patient would find acceptable; anticipating future events in order to plan for the worst whilst hoping for the best; collaborating with and coordinating other professionals in a team approach.

Symptom experience is subjective, leading to variation in the level of patients' distress. It is recognized that the interaction between physical and psychological symptoms works in the other direction as well (Mustapha 2005). Patients who are very distressed can lose their appetite, feel nauseated, be less tolerant of pain and have trouble sleeping. One way to understand this interaction has been described by Moorey & Greer (2002), who developed a cognitive model of the psychological effects of physical symptoms. In this model it is the personal meaning of thoughts about symptoms that is of key importance. These thoughts are affected by memories, experiences and the patient's adjustment to their illness, and there will be a mixture of realistic thoughts and distorted thinking.

There is evidence that other psychological and behavioural approaches can also be useful in reducing the severity of physical symptoms, and patients often find them empowering because they control the therapy to a large extent. For example, pain and

---

Case Study 2.3 Integrating psychological and physical approaches

A man with prostate cancer who has persistent nausea and vomiting reports feeling anxious and tearful and is having trouble sleeping. He thinks the sickness is a sign that his cancer is taking over his body and that he won't be able to eat any more. He knows that if he doesn't eat he will get thinner and thinner until he dies, and he has a picture in his mind of his body looking like a skeleton with skin hanging off it. He can remember seeing pictures of starving people on the television who looked like this.

It isn't surprising that this man has a high level of distress about his nausea and vomiting, and that this would be his top priority for treatment. He is found to have hypercalcaemia and is dehydrated. It would be appropriate to treat his metabolic problems with pharmacological approaches and to review any oncological treatments that may prevent this symptom from recurring. It would also be appropriate to examine his view of the meaning of these symptoms as these extreme images are likely to increase his anxiety and this can, in turn, cause nausea.

He may be able to balance his realistic and distorted thoughts about the effects of the illness by gaining an understanding of likely signs of disease progression. Then his vivid catastrophic thoughts and images about starving to death may fade and be less distressing.

---

nausea can be reduced for many patients using hypnotherapy or progressive muscle relaxation (Redd et al 2001, Taylor & Ingleton 2003).

How do I know which symptom is distressing?

As noted previously, it has been shown that carers' and professionals' assessments of patients' symptoms do not match those of the patient themselves (Hinton 1996), so we need to ask how it is for them. Palliative care patients are vulnerable and often have complex needs; gaining information from them can be difficult if they are physically, psychologically or emotionally incapacitated. A sensitive and flexible approach is needed which makes use of technical knowledge, advanced communication skills, and assessment tools (such as those mentioned previously) that can be adapted or shortened as needed.

In addition to asking individual patients how it is for them, it can be useful to have an idea of what other patients have said in similar circumstances. Research with palliative care patients who have a variety of illnesses, in different settings, opens a window on issues that may be important when trying to manage symptoms (Conner et al 2005, Seymour et al 2003). Researchers have sought patients' views on this by means of questionnaires, interviews or satisfaction surveys. However, this information should be interpreted with caution as, although it gives an indication, it does not give us an accurate picture: the views of 'users' will not be representative of the entire population of palliative care patients (Addington-Hall 2002).

The amount of patient research is small in palliative care generally, and in palliative nursing in particular, possibly because there is concern about causing extra stress for seriously ill people. In fact it has been said that 'to research at all into the needs and experiences of this client group could be said to be an affront to the dignity of those people' (De Raeve 1994). This view is held by many health professionals and has led to difficulty in recruiting patients from acute hospital and community caseloads (Addington-Hall 2002). In fact, the specialty of palliative care is no stranger to this research – Dame Cicely Saunders and John Hinton in the 1960s collated material from patient interviews that was then presented in newspapers and on radio to demonstrate the need for a different approach to caring for dying people (Saunders 2003).

Much of the available symptom research with patients has been carried out in hospices in the UK, so the issues that are important for such patients may not be the same in other settings. The influence of the environment and the particularities of different settings and cultures must be remembered in relation to symptom management as a whole. Gaining the patients' view will include an understanding of the needs of the specific population. For example, in the UK, South Asian people have a heavy disease burden in coronary heart disease but access palliative care services less frequently than other UK residents (Owens & Randhawa 2004). In addition, in Britain, patients over the age of 65 years are less likely to access palliative care than younger patients (Catt 2005).

An international example would be from South Africa where 90% of palliative care patients have diseases other than cancer (Doyle 2003). Research shows that elderly patients, those with heart disease and other life-threatening illnesses do experience distressing symptoms, so the key to knowing why they do not access services to manage those symptoms is to try to understand their wishes and provide services appropriately. It may be that a home visiting service or a telephone service would be most desirable for some patients who cannot travel easily, or that personnel need to be one of their social group if they are to be trusted.

In some cultures the role of women does not include positions of responsibility or authority, and it would cause offence if a female nurse questioned, or gave instructions to, a male patient. Even the way the patient is asked about symptoms may need to be tailored where speaking of bodily functions with a stranger is unacceptable (Doyle 2003). Palliative care is in its infancy in many countries around the world and in some places medicines are scarce. In others, patients have to pay for all medicine and treatment and this will affect their reporting of symptoms and their priorities.

In summary, applying the principles of symptom management relies upon knowledge and skills used flexibly to meet the individual patient's needs. This may be influenced by physical, psychological, environmental, social or cultural factors, but the patient must be at the centre when determining the right treatment for the right symptom in the right way at the right time.

What can I do when symptoms remain?

Sometimes symptoms remain in spite of skilled symptom management and approaches that address the patient's and family's concerns. This may be temporary and will most often be in the face of continuing efforts to improve the patient's experience. In many cases, the nurse is the one who is with the patient for longer periods of time than other health professionals. So it is common for nurses to feel uncomfortable, or even distressed, at witnessing the patient's continuing symptoms. The nurse's interpretation of events, their own perspective on suffering, as well as their personal beliefs about their role as a carer, contribute to this anguish. Despite knowing that the rest of the multidisciplinary team is making all efforts, there can be a strong desire to do something – anything – to help the patient.

This section of the chapter offers a few ideas and techniques that may help both patients and nurses in this situation.

When talking to patients about their experiences, researchers have found that hope plays an important part in the way they cope (Duggleby & Wright 2005). Patients describe the way they foster hope by acknowledging life the way it is and reappraising it. One of the greatest threats to hope is the loss of control over significant present circumstances (Flemming 1997).

It is important that these reappraisals are done by the patient and not provided by the nurse making assumptions about the patient's experience. Dialogue with patients about how physical symptoms affect their daily lives is only the beginning. If we know the effect that symptoms have on patients' view of themselves and how this makes them feel, we can facilitate the process of generating new ways of seeing things, fostering hope and so reduce distress.

Loss of function or role through continuing symptoms can erode patients' sense of control and

---

Case Study 2.4   Facilitating adjustment to persistent intractable symptoms

An elderly woman with heart failure may find that her breathlessness prevents her from washing herself in the mornings. She will need to rely on others for this, which she resents because it affects her independence, privacy and dignity, so she continues to struggle to do it alone. Her breathlessness distresses her and she feels resentful of it because she thinks it is forcing her to become an invalid.

If she were able to accept some limitations to her activity and view her need for help in a different way, she might feel less distressed and more hopeful, even though the symptom had not changed. Seeking positive outcomes in this situation would be difficult, but she might be able to find something. For example, making use of the help in the morning might preserve her energy for doing something that she enjoys later in the day.

self-esteem, and, in turn, leads to depression or anxiety (Moorey & Greer 2002). Finding ways in which patients can make changes for themselves will help. One example of this is mindfulness meditation, which is a technique that is growing in popularity in Britain. It has been shown to improve depression, anxiety and stress symptoms in cancer patients (Smith et al 2005), and to improve coping in patients with chronic pain. It involves learning to pay attention in a particular way: on purpose, in the present, and non-judgementally (Kabat-Zinn 2003). For patients with ongoing symptoms, mindfulness encourages acceptance that suffering is normal, a focus on what action is to be taken to get on with life and continue to attend to what is going on without trying to sort it out. It also teaches people to access soothing and caring feelings from memory or through imagery so that they can use these as a source of internal comfort when needed. Mindfulness techniques are useful for health professionals themselves as they deal with emotionally taxing and potentially stressful situations that they are not able to control on a daily basis. Sharing this approach with patients, even in a small way, may help both patient and nurse to get through difficult times.

Alleviating suffering is not just the management of physical symptoms; it encompasses comfort, human relationships and spirituality. Penson (2000) highlights the importance of providing comfort through simple techniques learned in childhood such as stroking a hand, plumping a pillow or applying lavender water to the forehead. It is important to convey that care will continue for as long as it is needed; that the patient will not be abandoned, however hard it is. Emotional and supportive care through humanistic and egalitarian interactions makes patients feel valued and can actually reduce the severity of physical symptoms (Conner et al 2005, Richardson 2002, Skilbeck & Payne 2003). But, often, being with patients who have persistent symptoms involves hearing them ask difficult questions like 'Why am I suffering?' and 'What is the purpose of living like this?' The experience of physical discomfort pushes people to search for the meaning of such events, and not reaching a sense of meaning can be associated with higher symptom distress (Taylor 1992).

The spiritual dimension of symptom management makes many healthcare professionals uncomfortable as it is nebulous, personal and, for some, linked with religion. It is hard to define, assess and measure but this should not give nurses permission to ignore it. When trying to capture what spirituality means, one useful description is that 'Spirituality gives us a sense of personhood and individuality. It is an inner, intangible dimension which motivates us to be connected with others and our surroundings. It drives us to search for meaning and purpose. It comes into focus at critical junctures in life when we face emotional stress, physical illness or death' (Narayanasamy 2004, p 1140). Attending to the spiritual needs of palliative patients with symptoms is vital to the process of alleviating suffering; they need to have involvement and control, a positive outlook, companionship, an opportunity to experience nature and religion (Hermann 2001). Spiritual care may not be a problem-solving exercise but more about showing concern, support, commitment, integrity and respect so that patients feel accompanied during their own search for meaning (Taylor 1992). The key to providing this kind of care is learning how to feel compassion while maintaining the delicate boundaries that preserve carers from being burned out emotionally. One small-scale study has shown that a 3-day training course in spirituality, based on Buddhist ideology, positively influenced healthcare professionals' level of compassion for their palliative patients whilst reducing work-related stress levels (Wasner et al 2005).

The ways in which nurses can help when symptoms remain are based on human interaction and presence. Patients say that it is not the things we do but the way we are while we do them that matters (Sparks 2002). As technology replaces human touch in healthcare, and the time spent with patients is reduced, the quality of our presence gains significance. Ohlen (2002) says that, in order to have the openness, sensitivity and courage to share suffering with another person, we need to examine our own understanding of what it means to be hurt, vulnerable and at the mercy of others for managing daily life. This requires personal reflection and self-nurture in order to have the strength to use oneself as a resource. Then, when symptoms remain, nurses can foster hope by being actively present, maintain their focus on the patient, and access theory about suffering, caring and comfort as well as using biomedical approaches to symptom management.

CHALLENGES FOR NURSES IN SYMPTOM MANAGEMENT

The essence of palliative care nursing is a *creative* and *competent* blend of the nurse, patient, and family relationship together with *knowledge* and *skills*.

(Coyle 2001)

This chapter will now go on to consider the significance of the nurse's role within the current UK healthcare agenda in relation to palliative care. As part of the UK government's modernisation agenda there is a focus on strengthening nursing leadership and further developing interprofessional collaboration. The role of nursing is constantly evolving; this is no different within the sphere of palliative care, and symptom management in particular. Nurses are currently facing many issues that they need to consider and formulate opinions on, such as nurse prescribing, with the aim of meeting users' needs more effectively (Ovretveit 1997, Pollard et al 2005). It is important for nurses in any field to have a voice to be able to articulate their skills, knowledge, attitudes and opinions to others, be it about the national agenda or the individual care of a single patient. Historically, as a body of professionals, and sometimes as individuals, we are not as skilled at this as we could be. Owing to the UK government's rapidly developing health service agenda, increasingly a broad range of non-cancer specialties are requesting palliative care inclusion in their multidisciplinary teams, in part to address symptom management. This is a positive development, which should be welcomed, but at the same time it is a challenge for many services to provide owing to limited resources. Within palliative care, the nurse's voice has traditionally been heard loudly and clearly; nurses working within palliative care are in a prime position at this time to be able to lend their voices to the choir and articulate their knowledge for the ultimate comfort of these patients.

To be able to develop palliative care nurses' contribution to the wider modernisation agenda and to the care of an increasingly broad spectrum of patients, we need to consider ways of articulating this knowledge to the wider interdisciplinary team and the patient (Edwards 2002). Nursing knowledge is the means by which we define nursing care. It is what defines us as nurses (Hall 2005). Describing nursing knowledge is very difficult (Benner 1984), and this difficulty has not helped the acceptance of nursing as a profession by other disciplines. However, palliative care nurses are in a prime position to communicate nursing knowledge to others to enable better symptom management, interdisciplinary working and improved patient care. This nursing knowledge has been described by Carper (1978) as consisting of four main elements:

- *Aesthetic knowledge* – the art of nursing, expert practice and understanding the human journey through illness.

- *Empirical knowledge* – empirical research, scientific enquiry and quantitative approaches to research will generate this type of knowledge.
- *Personal knowledge* – self-awareness: bringing self to caring through experience and/or intuition.
- *Ethical knowledge* – this includes the ability to question the withdrawal of treatments, and resuscitation decisions. It includes moral knowledge and decision making and prioritising. It includes the knowledge to make decisions where there is no easy answer to a dilemma.

Carper (1987) identified that no *single* type of knowledge was greater or lesser than another, or sufficient for all purposes (Edwards 2002). All branches of nursing may use these categories of nursing knowledge; however, nurses caring for palliative care patients use all four types of nursing knowledge on a daily basis, whilst dealing with patients and their families at their most vulnerable – a skill not to be underestimated.

> ... by a miraculous interplay of craft and wisdom, someone has had their suffering diminished.
>
> (Wright et al 2004)

An increasingly technical approach to care does influence palliative and terminal care (Clark 2002, George et al 2002). As technology strides on in medicine and nursing, palliative care nurses need to be able to 'see the wood for the trees'. Nurses must remember nursing (Castledine 2004) to prevent, in the words of Roy (2004) '... the unreflective use of technology rather than the careful mastery of technology in the service of patients' goals and aspirations'. Otherwise we may lose sight of the fundamental reasons why palliative care crawled from the mud in the first place. As nurses we can embrace extended skills such as nurse prescribing, clinical assessment skills and psychological therapies such as cognitive behavioural therapy for the benefit of our patients. By undertaking and utilising research, we are well placed to contribute in a major way to the wider national health agenda whilst helping to strengthen the position of palliative care nursing at the same time.

WHAT NEXT?

This chapter has explored the importance of assessment, ways of applying principles in symptom management, and the interplay between psychological and physical elements of symptoms. It has also looked at any differences when managing symptoms at the end of life and dealing with intractable problems. As stated at the beginning of the chapter, the underlying premise has been that individual practitioners will need to interpret and adapt the information in this chapter to be able to apply it appropriately for the benefit of their patients.

With this in mind, the authors decline to reach conclusions on the readers' behalf, providing instead some guiding questions to assist the reader in their task.

How do I keep the momentum going? It's time for reflection

As this chapter draws to an end, we ask you to reflect on its content and consider how you, as professionals, can synthesise these ideas to inform your practice. In order to do this we pose a number of questions for you to consider.

REFLECTION POINT

- How do you assess your patients' symptoms?
- How do you document your assessment?
- In what ways could you improve your ability to assess your patients?
- Could an assessment tool be adapted for your area?
- How do you feel as a nurse when symptoms remain uncontrolled?
- If you do not use an end-of-life care pathway or framework, could one be adapted for use in your area?
- How can you develop your practice using patients' views?
- Which issues from this chapter do you want to explore in more depth?
- Can you identify one thing that you can do straight away to improve symptom control for your patients?
- How can *you* keep momentum going?

References

Addington-Hall J 2002 Research sensitivities to a palliative care patient. European Journal of Cancer Care 11:220–224

Benner P 1984 From novice to expert. Addison-Wesley, Menlo Park, California

Buckman R, Sabbagh K 1993 Magic or medicine? An investigation into healing. Macmillan, London

Carper B 1978 Fundamental patterns of knowing in nursing. Advances in Nursing Science 1(1):13–23

Carson M G, Fitch M I, Vachon M L 2000 Measuring patient outcomes in palliative care; a reliability and validity study of the Support Team Assessment Schedule. Palliative Medicine 14(1):25–36

Castledine G 2004 Patient assessment: a key requirement of nursing care. British Journal of Nursing 13(20):1233

Catt S 2005 Older adults attitudes to death, palliative treatment and hospice care. Palliative Medicine 19:402–410

Clark D 2002 Between hope and acceptance; the medicalisation of dying. British Medical Journal 324:905–907

Conill C, Verger E, Henriquez I et al 1997 Symptom prevalence in the last week of life. Journal of Pain and Symptom Management 14:328–331

Conner A, Allport S, Dixon J, Somerville A M 2005 Newcastle Palliative Care Users Project, Newcastle upon Tyne (unpublished report)

Coyle N 2001 Introduction to palliative nursing care. In: Ferrel B, Coyle N (eds) Textbook of palliative nursing. Oxford, Oxford University Press, p 3–6

De Haes J, van Knippenberg F C, Neijt J P 1990 Measuring psychological and physical distress in cancer patients: structure and application of the Rotterdam Symptom Checklist. British Journal of Cancer 62:1034–1038

De Raeve L 1994 Ethical issues in palliative care research. Palliative Medicine 8:298–305

Doyle D 2003 The world of palliative care: one man's view. Journal of Palliative Care 19(3):149–160

Duggleby W, Wright K 2005 Elderly palliative care patients' descriptions of hope fostering strategies. Palliative Nursing 10(7):352–359

Edwards S 2002 Nursing knowledge: defining new boundaries. Nursing Standard 17(2):40–44

Ellershaw J, Wilkinson S 2003 Care of the dying. A pathway to excellence. Oxford University Press, Oxford

Ellershaw J E, Peat S J, Boys L C 1995 Assessing the effectiveness of a hospital palliative care team. Palliative Medicine 9(2):145–152

Flemming K A 1997 An exploration of the meaning of hope to palliative care cancer patients. International Journal of Palliative Nursing 3(1):14–18

George J, Grypdonk M, Dierokx de Casterle B 2002 Being a palliative care nurse in an academic hospital: a qualitative study about nurses' perceptions of palliative care nursing. Journal of Clinical Nursing 11:785–793

Gillis L 1988 Human behaviour in illness, 4th edn. Faber and Faber, London

Hall A 2005 Defining nursing knowledge. Nursing Times 101(48):34–35

Hearn J, Higginson I J 1999 Development and validation of a care outcome measure for palliative care; the Palliative Care Outcome Scale. Palliative Care Audit Project Advisory Group. Quality in Health Care 8(4):219–227

Heaven C, Maguire P 1996 Training hospice nurses to elicit patient concerns. Journal of Advanced Nursing 23:280–286

Hermann C 2001 Spiritual needs of dying patients: a qualitative study. Oncology Nursing Forum 28(1):67–72

Higginson I 1993 A community schedule. In: Higginson I (ed.) Clinical audit in palliative care. Radcliffe Medical Press, Oxford

Higginson I 1997 Palliative and terminal health care needs assessment, 2nd series. Radcliffe Medical Press, Oxford

Hinton J 1996 How reliable are relatives' retrospective reports of terminal illness? Patients' and relatives' accounts compared. Social Science & Medicine 43:1229–1236

Ingham J, Portenoy R 1996 Symptom assessment. Haematology/Oncology Clinics of North America 10:21–39

Kabat-Zinn J 2003 Mindfulness-based interventions in context: past, present, future. Clinical Psychology: Science & Practice 10:144–156

King N, Thomas K, Martin N, Bell D, Farrell S 2005 'Now nobody falls through the net': practitioners' perspectives on the Gold Standards Framework for community palliative care. Palliative Medicine 19:619–627

Lancashire & South Cumbria Cancer Network 2006. Online. Available:http://www.cancerlancashire.org.uk/ppc 24 July 2006

Liverpool Care Pathway 2006 Promoting best practice for care of the dying. Online. Available: http://www.lcp-mariecurie.org 24 July 2006

Maguire P 1985 Improving the detection of psychiatric problems in cancer patients. Social Science and Medicine 20(8):815–823

MedicineNet.com 2006 MedTerms Medical Dictionary. Online. Available: http://www.midterms.com 30 June 2006

Mirando S 2005 Introducing an integrated care pathway for the last days of life. Palliative Medicine 19:33–39

Moorey S, Greer S 2002 Cognitive behaviour therapy for people with cancer. Oxford University Press, Oxford

Mustapha A 2005 Depression can cause severe physical symptoms. British Journal of Nursing 14:482

Narayanasamy A 2004 The puzzle of spirituality for nursing: a guide to practical assessment. British Journal of Nursing 13(19):1140–1144

National Council for Hospice and Specialist Palliative Care Services 1997 Changing gear – guidelines for managing the last days of life in adults. NCHSPCS, London

National Institute for Health and Clinical Excellence 2004 Guidance on cancer services: improving supportive and palliative care for adults with cancer. NICE, London

National Statistics 2006 Home of official UK statistics. Online. Available: http://www.statistics.gov.uk 30 June 2006

NHS End of Life Care Programme 2006 Online. Available: http://www.endoflifecare.nhs.uk 29 July 2006

Ohlen J 2002 Practical wisdom: competencies required in alleviating suffering in palliative care. Journal of Palliative Care 18(4):293–299

Ovretveit J 1997 How to describe interprofessional working. In: Ovretveit J, Mathias P, Thompson T (eds) Interprofessional working for health and social care. Palgrave, London, p 9–33

Owens A, Randhawa G 2004 'It's different from my culture; they're very different.' Providing community based culturally competent palliative care for South Asian people in the UK. Health and Social Care in the Community 12(5):414–421

Oxenham D, Cornbleet M 1998 Accuracy of prediction of survival by different professional groups in a hospice. Palliative Medicine 12:117–118

Parkes C M 1990 Risk factors in bereavement: implications for the prevention and treatment of pathological grief. Psychiatric Annals 20:307–313

Penson J 2000 A hope is not a promise: fostering hope in palliative care. International Journal of Palliative Nursing 6(2):94–98

Pollard K C, Ross K, Means R 2005 Nurse leadership, interprofessionalism and the modernization agenda. British Journal of Nursing 14(6):339–344

Redd W, Montgomery G, Duhamel K 2001 Behavioural interventions for cancer treatment side effects. Journal of the National Cancer Institute 93:810–823

Regnard C, Dixon J, Besford S et al 2005 Monitoring a hospital palliative care team using the PaCA tool. European Journal of Palliative Care 13(2):82–84

Richardson A 2002 Health promotion in palliative care: the patient's perception of therapeutic interaction with the palliative nurse in primary care setting. Journal of Advanced Nursing 40(4):432–440

Rogers A, Karlsen S, Addington-Hall J M 2000 Dying for care: the experiences of terminally ill cancer patients in hospital in an inner city health district. Palliative Medicine 14:53–54

Roy D 2004 Palliative care in a technological age. Journal of Palliative Care 20(4):267

Salt S 1997 Towards a definition of suffering. European Journal of Palliative Care 4:58–60

Saunders C 1993 Introduction – 'history and challenge'. In: Saunders C, Sykes N (eds) The management of terminal malignant disease, 3rd edn. Edward Arnold, London, p 1–14

Saunders C 2003 A voice for the voiceless. In: Monroe B, Oliviere D (eds) Patient participation in palliative care – a voice for the voiceless. Oxford University Press, Oxford, p 3–8

Seymour J, Ingleton C, Payne S, Beddow V 2003 Specialist palliative care: patients' experiences. Journal of Advanced Nursing 44(1):24–33

Shah S, Blanchard M, Tookman A et al 2006 Estimating needs in life threatening illness: a feasibility study to assess the views of patients and doctors. Palliative Medicine 20:205–210

Skilbeck J, Payne S 2003 Emotional support and the role of clinical nurse specialists in palliative care. Advanced Nursing 43(5):521–530

Smith A, Richardson J, Hoffman C 2005 Mindfulness-based stress reduction as supportive therapy in cancer care: a systematic review. Journal of Advanced Nursing 52(3):3–5

Solano J Gomes B Higginson I 2006 A comparison of symptom prevalence in far advanced cancer, AIDS, heart disease, COPD and renal disease. Journal of Pain and Symptom Management 31(1):58–69

Sparks B 2002 Being there: there is no greater personal experience for a nurse to re-evaluate core nursing values of presence, caring and connection, than as a client. Are you making a difference, or are you going that extra mile? The Canadian Nurse 98(4):8

Steinhauser K E, Christakis N A, Clipp E C et al 2000 Factors considered important at the end of life by patients, family, physicians, and other care providers. Journal of the American Medical Association 284(19):2476–2482

Stiefel F, Guex P 1996 Palliative and supportive care: at the frontier of medical omnipotence. Annals of Oncology 7:135–138

Taylor E 1992 The search for meaning among persons living with recurrent cancer. PhD thesis, University of Pennsylvania

Taylor E, Ingleton C 2003 Hypnotherapy and cognitive behaviour therapy in cancer care: the patients' view. European Journal of Cancer Care 12:137–142

The Gold Standards Framework 2006 A programme for community palliative care. Online. Available: http://www.goldstandardsframework.nhs.uk 24 July 2006

The Support Principal Investigators 1995 A controlled trial to improve care for seriously ill hospitalised patients.

The Study to Understand Prognoses and Preferences for Outcomes and Risks of Treatment (SUPPORT). Journal of the American Medical Association 274:1591–1598

Thomas K 2003 The Gold Standards Framework in community palliative care. European Journal of Palliative Care 10:113–115

Thomas K 2006 Palliative care. Geriatric Medicine 36(6):9–13

Thorpe G 1993 Enabling more dying people to remain at home. British Medical Journal 307:915–918

Twycross R 1997 Symptom management in advanced cancer. Radcliffe Medical Press, Oxford

Von Guten C F, Ferris F D, Emanual L L 2000 Ensuring competency in end of life care: communication and relational skills. Journal of the American Medical Association 284:3051–3057

Wasner M, Longaker C, Fegg M J, Borasio G D 2005 Effects of spiritual care training for palliative care professionals. Palliative Medicine 19:99–104

Wilkinson S 1991 Factors which influence how nurses communicate with cancer patients. Journal of Advanced Nursing 16:177–188

Wright S, Benton D, Clark J, Heath H 2004 Deconstructing nursing: from practice to theory. Nursing Standard 18(52):14–19

Further reading

Back I N 2001 Palliative medicine handbook, 3rd edn. BPM Books, Cardiff

Dickman A, Schneider J, Varga J 2005 The syringe driver: continuous subcutaneous infusions in palliative care, 2nd edn. Oxford University Press, Oxford

Doyle D, Hanks G, Cherny N, Calman K 2005 Oxford textbook of palliative medicine, 3rd edn. Oxford University Press, Oxford

Ellershaw J, Wilkinson S 2003 Care of the dying: a pathway to excellence. Oxford University Press, Oxford

Kaye P 2003 A–Z pocketbook of symptom control. EPL Publications, Northampton

palliativedrugs.com 2006 Providing drug information to healthcare professionals worldwide. Online. Available: http://www.palliativedrugs.com

Regnard C F B, Tempest S 1998 A guide to symptom relief in advanced disease, 4th edn. Hochland and Hochland, Hale, UK

Twycross R, Wilcock A 2002 Symptom management in advanced cancer, 3rd edn. Radcliffe Medical Press, Oxford

Twycross R, Wilcock A, Charlesworth S, Dickman A 2002 Palliative care formulary, 2nd edn. Radcliffe Medical Press, Oxford

Watson M, Lucas C, Hoy A, Back I 2005 Oxford handbook of palliative care. Oxford University Press, Oxford

Chapter 3

Pain control

Keith Farrer

Improving the management of pain and distress in patients with palliative care needs is now more than ever on the healthcare agenda across the UK. The National Institute for Clinical Excellence (NICE), in its guidance on supportive and palliative care, highlights how improving the knowledge and skills of healthcare staff will produce improved outcomes in the management of cancer pain (NICE 2004). Similarly, the organisation tasked with improving and monitoring healthcare in Scotland, Quality Improvement Scotland, has in recent years published standards for palliative care services that underline the importance of evidence-based local guidelines for pain control (Clinical Standards Board for Scotland 2002). Across the UK, the Gold Standards Framework for palliative care (Thomas 2003) is being rolled out in primary care settings; central to this is having systems in place to ensure the systematic assessment of pain and other symptoms in end-of-life care. There is also recognition that within the health services across the UK healthcare professionals have not always been following the national and international guidance for pain management in palliative care (NICE 2004).

The difficulties in managing pain adequately are not just issues for the UK: Foley (2005) paints a similar picture in the US, stating:

> Despite advances in resource rich countries, undertreatment of cancer pain continues to remain a quality care issue in the United States with reports demonstrating undertreatment in dying adults, children, the elderly, and minorities.

This is despite the evidence cited by the World Health Organisation (WHO 1996) that adherence to its guidelines results in good pain control in the majority of patients with cancer pain. Studies that have systematically applied the WHO (1996) guidelines for cancer pain management have achieved adequate pain management in up to 90% of patients (Grond et al 1996, Ventafridda et al 1987). However, outside such studies, reports of cancer pain management in clinical areas highlight that this level of pain management is not achieved. Recent studies (Bonica 1990, Cleeland 1994, Farrer et al 2004) still reveal that approximately one-third to one-half of cancer patients needlessly experience moderate to severe pain (McCaffery & Ferrell 1997).

WHY IS CANCER PAIN STILL POORLY MANAGED?

The reasons for not achieving adequate pain control for cancer patients are multifaceted and multidisciplinary. Recent literature in nursing and medicine points to a multitude of factors that impinge on our ability to deal with cancer pain adequately (McCaffery & Ferrell 1997, Paice et al 1998, Twycross 1994). These include:

- poor knowledge of cancer pain management
- inappropriate attitudes (i.e. cancer pain is inevitable)
- poor clinical skills (particularly in the assessment of pain)
- inappropriate beliefs regarding the management of cancer pain (fears of addiction and tolerance to opiates)
- a lack of appreciation of the non-physical manifestations of cancer pain.

Despite the best efforts of those providing education and training around this area, there is little evidence that this has been effective (Scottish Intercollegiate Guidelines Network [SIGN] 2000).

Both the attitudes, knowledge and skills of healthcare professionals and patient behaviours are crucial to successful pain management. Klepstad et al (2000) cite patient barriers towards the use of opioids as contributing towards the problem. Specifically, these barriers may stem from one or more of the following:

- low expectations of pain management and a belief that pain is inevitable
- inappropriate beliefs regarding pain management strategies (i.e. fear of addiction and tolerance)
- beliefs that side-effects of medications are inevitable (i.e. sedation).

These difficulties may lead to patients under-reporting pain and result in difficulties with drug compliance.

This chapter focuses on two areas that need to be addressed to ensure better pain management in palliative care. These are:

1. Strategies to improve pain management in the clinical areas
2. Effective educational interventions in pain management in palliative care.

It is hoped that the introduction of strategies and processes supported by effective education will improve patient outcomes across the different care settings. More than ever, particularly with the advent of initiatives such as nurse prescribing, the core skills for managing pain are transferable across the different healthcare professionals. Therefore, much of this chapter is relevant and transferable to other health professionals (i.e. medical staff or pharmacists); most importantly, effective teamwork is required to improve care consistently for patients in this area.

It is not the intention to provide an authoritative text in all areas relating to cancer pain management in nursing. Rather, the emphasis will be on strategies that are most likely to produce positive outcomes and, at the same time, be achievable within clinical settings.

In recognition that different clinical contexts require differing levels of skills within nursing, the chapter has been split into the following two parts:

1. Standard practice – what every nurse needs to know
2. Higher level of practice.

This structure is based on the premise that all nurses should achieve a core level of knowledge and skill in pain management for patients requiring palliative care. However, in specific clinical areas (such as in oncology and specialist palliative care settings) where a major component of nursing is pain management, there is a requirement for a higher level of practice (UK Central Council for Nursing, Midwifery and Health Visiting [UKCC] 1999). This higher level of practice equates to level 3 and 4 as outlined in the Royal College of Nursing's framework for nurses working in palliative care (RCN 2002).

PART 1: STANDARD PRACTICE – WHAT EVERY NURSE NEEDS TO KNOW

UNDERSTANDING PAIN

An initial function of pain is to protect and warn that something is not as it should be. Pain undoubtedly protects us from serious injury (such as touching something that is hot), and in the context of illness is often a presenting feature that leads a person to seek medical advice. However, beyond this function, pain becomes less useful, and in chronic illness becomes debilitating and a source of constant distress. The focus of this chapter is on pain that has long since ceased to serve as a protective mechanism for a person with an illness that is life-threatening (such as cancer) and not amenable to curative treatment.

There have been several attempts, none of which is completely satisfactory, to explain and define pain. Perhaps the most recognised definition of pain, is that it is:

> an unpleasant sensory and emotional experience associated with actual or potential tissue damage, or described in terms of such damage.
>
> (International Association for the Study of Pain [IASP] 1986)

This definition, arrived at by a multidisciplinary expert committee, begins to hint at the possibility of pain being more than just a physical experience, but does not go far enough in encapsulating the total experience or the consequences of unrelieved pain. Pain, associated with an underlying life-threatening and chronic illness, has emotional and spiritual components, and often limits the social functioning of the patient, family and friends.

It is not uncommon to hear both the healthcare professional and the lay person discussing a person's pain in terms of a low or high pain threshold. In a clinical situation this is not a useful discussion, as it is unhelpful in the management of the person's pain. Moreover, a patient's supposedly low pain threshold may be used to excuse poor pain management.

Contrary to popular beliefs, pain thresholds, defined as 'the least experience of pain a person can recognise' (IASP 1986), are remarkably similar amongst healthy volunteers and across different cultures (Bowsher 1993, Twycross 1994). A more important concept is that of pain tolerance: the greatest level of pain that a person is prepared to put up with in a given circumstance or context; Box 3.1 gives definitions related to this area. This pain tolerance is influenced by a number of factors that, if present, can amplify the perception of pain – rather like turning up the volume button on a radio. These include the following (Hemming & Maher 2005):

- insomnia
- fatigue
- anxiety and fear

Box 3.1 Definitions of pain and related concepts (IASP 1986)

DEFINITION OF PAIN
Pain is an unpleasant sensory and emotional experience associated with actual or potential damage.

PAIN THRESHOLD
The least experience of pain which a subject can recognise.

PAIN TOLERANCE LEVEL
The greatest level of pain which a subject is prepared to tolerate.

- sadness
- boredom
- isolation
- lack of stimulation
- lack of interaction
- poor communication
- family stress and trauma
- unknown – not knowing.

It is also suggested (particularly in chronic non-cancer pain) that tolerance levels are reduced the longer the pain remains unrelieved. The consequences of unrelieved pain are far reaching and, as would be expected, have a negative effect on all aspects of a person's life. Additionally, Strang (1998) argues that physical pain provokes emotional, social and existential distress in the patient with cancer. He outlines the negative impact of pain affecting:

- mood
- social activities
- activities of daily living
- sleep
- cognitive functions
- the existential domain.

It is also recognised that unrelieved pain can be a precursor to other clinical problems such as depression and severe anxiety. Clearly, if the aim of palliative care nursing is to address the social, emotional and spiritual aspects of suffering, then it is inherent in the nurse's role in managing pain to develop strategies to assess and manage these issues. Interventions for dealing with these, along with guidelines on the pharmacological management, are outlined in the following sections.

PAIN ASSESSMENT

Pain assessment is the foundation of the nursing management of cancer pain. Nurses, by virtue of the time they spend with patients, and their role in administering analgesia, have a pivotal role to play in this assessment. However, it must be remembered that pain assessment is a multidisciplinary responsibility and must go 'hand in hand' with a thorough medical examination and investigations into the possible causes of pain.

Pain assessment does not stop with the identification of pain, but needs to be ongoing throughout any treatment – failure to do this results in the under-treatment (and sometimes over-treatment) of a patient in pain.

A common misconception is that pain assessment starts and finishes with a pain assessment tool or chart. Although these are extremely useful (if not essential), pain assessment in the context of a life-threatening illness is much broader than an assessment chart. Brant (2003) suggests the following 'ABCDE' approach to pain assessment and treatment:

- **A**sk the patient, and assess regularly, and systematically
- **B**elieve the patient: the patient is the expert about their own pain
- **C**hoose interventions and treatments that suit the patient
- **D**eliver treatment on time
- **E**mpower the patient so that they, or the person they choose, has control of the situation.

Asking the patient about their pain is the first step in obtaining a detailed pain assessment, and should include the history of the pain as well as its intensity and severity. This step is particularly relevant when the pain is being assessed for the first time. Although pain charts and pain assessments are important, no pain assessment is complete without obtaining a history or 'pain story'. Asking the patient to tell you about the pain, almost as if telling a story, will give clues as to when the pain started, what makes it better or worse, and how the person feels about the pain (Box 3.2).

Active listening and the use of empathy during this process (as outlined in Chapter 7) will help convey to the individual that you believe their account of the pain and that you are serious about helping to alleviate it.

Allowing the person to tell their 'pain story' will reveal much of the information needed to determine the treatment options. However, it is almost always necessary to ask additional questions regarding the exact physical nature of the pain. Assessing the physical component of the pain is something that is not limited to nursing practice but can be done equally by medical staff – good interdisciplinary communication is necessary to prevent the patient being subjected to a duplicated pain assessment.

The assessments of the physical components of pain are covered in well designed pain assessment tools and charts, and usually include the following two areas.

> ### Box 3.2   The 'Pain Story'
>
> - What, if anything, does the patient think is causing the pain?
> - When did they first notice this pain?
> - What else was happening at this time? (i.e. had their drugs been altered, had they recently had any treatment for the underlying illness, etc.)
> - Has the pain remained constant since they noticed it, or is it getting worse?

Initial assessment

This includes determining the following:

- Site or sites of the pain – patients with cancer often have more than one site of pain (Twycross et al 1996)
- Pattern of the pain – is the pain worse at any time of the day or night, continuous or spasmodic?
- Aggravating factors – does movement or position affect the pain?
- Relieving factors – concentrating on previous medications or interventions
- The patient's description of the pain – what does the pain feel like? (i.e. aching, dull, shooting, burning, etc.).

Ongoing assessment

Once the above has been performed it is necessary formally to determine the response to treatment. There is still good evidence that nurses continue to underestimate pain (McCaffery & Ferrell 1997), and therefore patients should be involved in any assessment. This can be done by asking them to complete a pain assessment tool or by questioning them directly about the severity of the pain and their response to treatment.

Although assessment of the *severity of the pain* can be done simply by enquiring about whether the pain is better or worse, this does not provide sufficient information on which to base future treatment strategies. In an effort to be consistent, it is recommended that a rating scale be used, such as a 0–10 numerical scale or a verbal rating scale, discussed in more detail in Part 2 below. For patients with multiple pains it is necessary to rate each pain separately. This is more easily achieved using a body chart, to illustrate clearly, with the patient, which pain is being rated.

One of the most neglected aspects in pain assessment relates to *response to treatment.* Failure to do this results in the administration of ineffective drugs and, at worst, increases distress through unwanted side-effects. This is particularly problematic in the case of opioids, when rapid escalation of the dose, without attention to assessment of effectiveness, results in patients experiencing sedation, hallucinations and myoclonic jerks (muscle twitching). This is discussed in more detail in the management of pain in Part 2. When a patient has started taking a new analgesic it is important to determine whether this is being effective. As different types of pain (e.g. bone pain, nerve pain) are unlikely to respond equally to the same analgesic drug (e.g. morphine), each pain should be assessed independently. To achieve this, the effectiveness of the analgesic administered must be evaluated by asking the patient to rate the severity of their pain(s) at a time when you expect the drug to have reached its maximum potential benefit. If the patient still reports pain, answers to the following questions need to be determined:

- Has there been any improvement in the patient's rating of the severity of the pain?
- If the analgesic helps, for how long does the benefit last?

The answers to these questions will determine whether to modify or change the analgesic regimen (see section on the pharmacological management of cancer pain).

In addition to the above physiological aspects, assessment must cover the effects of the pain on other areas of the patient's life.

It is well documented that unrelieved pain is strongly associated with feelings of anxiety, depression and uncertainty (Strang 1998). Moreover, Arathuzich (1991) showed in a sample of patients in pain from breast cancer that more than 50% experienced difficulties with daily activities, disrupted sleep, dependency and helplessness, which contributed to spiritual distress. Clearly, successful pain management requires attention to these issues, and needs to start with assessment.

There is no simple formula for doing this, but good communication and assessment skills are a starting point. Often active listening and empathy are sufficient to help alleviate the distress related to these issues. Although not suitable for every patient and situation, the probes highlighted in Box 3.3 can be a good starting point in the assessment of these difficulties.

Pain assessment tools

Pain assessment tools are needed primarily for the following reasons:

1. To encourage patient involvement
2. To provide an accurate and reliable measure of the person's pain over a period of time (i.e. when new interventions are introduced)
3. To provide a consistent and accurate record of the patient's pain experience amongst the healthcare team.

Although it may be possible to perform a good assessment (based on the previous discussion)

Box 3.3   Assessment of non-physical aspects of pain

ANXIETY (ABOUT THE MEANING OF THE PAIN)
Do you worry about the possible cause of the pain?
Do you worry about what is going to happen in the future?
Do you get a frightened feeling, as if something awful is about to happen?

HELPLESSNESS AND DEPRESSION
Are you able to sleep at night?
Are you able to concentrate?
Do you find it difficult to make decisions?
Are you able to enjoy the things you normally enjoy?

ANXIETY (ABOUT THE TREATMENT OF THE PAIN)
Are you concerned about the treatment of the pain?
Do you worry about having to take the pain-killers?

SOCIAL WORRIES
Is the pain stopping you from doing the things you like to do?
How is your family managing at home?
Do you have any money worries?

without an assessment tool, it is unlikely that this will be communicated consistently and sustained over any period of time.

Even though pain assessment tools have been advocated for over a decade (Latham 1990, Walker et al 1987), good evidence remains that they still do not feature in the routine nursing care of patients with pain (Clarke et al 1996). Moreover, often when assessment tools are used, they do not inform subsequent pain management strategies (Carr 1997).

Promoting comfort should be the foundation of nursing practice, and pain assessment is pivotal in the drive to alleviate pain and distress. Without a formalised approach to pain assessment, it is doubtful that good pain management can be sustained.

There are many published examples of good pain assessment tools. The core components of the pain assessment tool for patients with chronic/cancer pain should include:

- a body chart – to illustrate multiple pains
- a method of rating the severity of pain
- an area to detail aggravating and relieving factors – particularly whether the pain is worse on movement (incident pain)
- the diurnal variation of pain – noting whether pain is worse during the night
- the patient's description of the pain.

The clinical specialty governs the choice of the pain assessment tool. A diary may be more feasible for patients to use in the community (de Wit et al 1999), compared with a chart which may be appropriate for hospital use. Where possible, the pain assessment tool needs to be valid and reliable in the population and setting for which it is intended. However, as valid and reliable pain assessment tools are not available for every setting, a certain degree of compromise is needed (Part 2 of this chapter discusses the area of pain measurement in more detail). If in doubt, contacting a pain management or palliative care specialist is recommended.

Although measuring pain intensity has only limited value as a pain assessment tool, it can be used to screen for pain and to highlight patients for whom a more detailed and formal pain assessment is needed. Figure 3.1 gives an example of a pain assessment tool incorporated into an existing blood pressure chart.

THE PHARMACOLOGICAL MANAGEMENT OF CANCER PAIN

The management of cancer pain was the subject of the WHO Working Party in 1996 and their subsequent guidance is the basis for the following paragraphs on the drug management of cancer pain (WHO 1996).

Drug treatment remains the main approach to managing cancer pain and includes a detailed assessment and adherence to the WHO (1996) guidance for cancer pain management. The following paragraphs briefly overview this guidance, but it is strongly recommended that those new to these concepts visit the following website for a more detailed overview: http://www.whocancerpain.wisc.edu/

BASIC PRINCIPLES OF CANCER PAIN MANAGEMENT

By mouth

Where possible, analgesics should be given by the oral route. It is a common misconception amongst healthcare staff that systemic routes (intravenous, intramuscular, subcutaneous) of the equivalent oral dose are more efficacious in relieving pain. Systemic routes should be reserved for situations where the patient is unable to take oral medications or when there are doubts about drug absorption in the gastrointestinal tract.

By the clock

Analgesics should be given by the clock (at fixed times) and not on an *ad hoc,* or p.r.n. (as required), basis. The dose of the analgesic must be titrated against the patient's pain until either a ceiling dose is reached (the maximum recommended dose of the drug) or the pain is relieved effectively, or until the patient begins to experience intolerable side-effects. Extra (p.r.n.) doses should be given as required, *in addition* to the fixed-interval doses.

By the ladder

The principles of the analgesic ladder are key features of pain management in palliative care. Analgesics should be prescribed and administered according to both the severity of the pain and the response to the drug(s) prescribed (Fig. 3.2). These are outlined below.

Step 1: mild pain

Step 1 of the ladder is appropriate for patients with mild pain and involves the use of a non-opioid analgesic such as paracetamol or a non-steroidal anti-inflammatory drug (NSAID). If this fails to alleviate

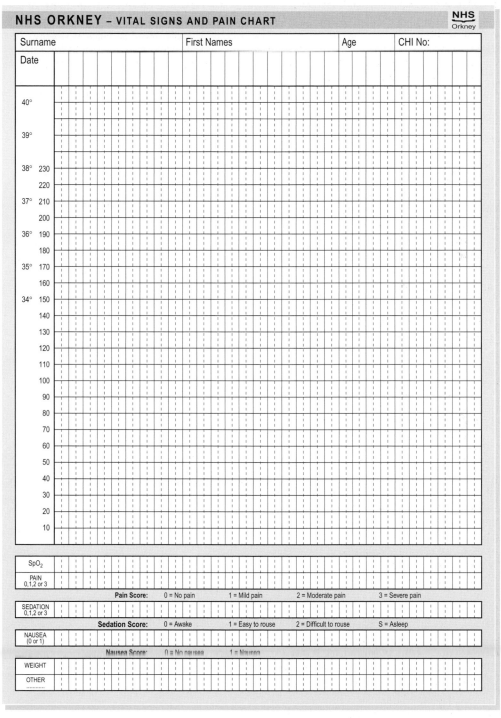

Figure 3.1   Vital signs and pain chart.

The following information details the general principles and guidelines useful in the choice of analgesics for pain in patients with advanced cancer. It is essential that before any analgesics are chosen a detailed assessment of the patient's pain is performed. This must include details on the exact site of the pain, the possible cause of the pain, the type of pain, and its severity.
The World Health Organisation recommends that to achieve optimal pain relief analgesia must be given as follows:

- by the mouth
- by the clock (regularly and not on a p.r.n. basis)
- by the ladder (see below).

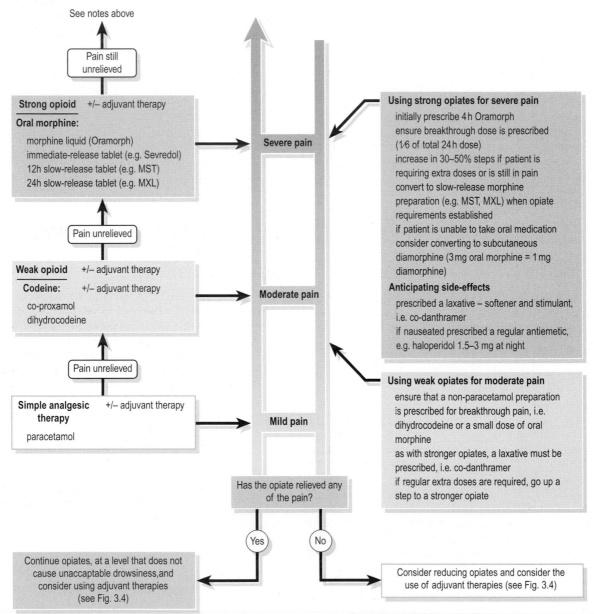

Figure 3.2   Guidelines on the use of analgesics for the patient with advanced cancer. (From Western General Hospitals NHS Trust, Edinburgh, with permission.)

the pain (when given 'by the clock'), the prescribing of analgesics should be guided by step 2.

Step 2: moderate pain

This step should be used to treat pain that is mild to moderate or when step 1 has been unsuccessful. There are numerous step 2 analgesics, with most of these drugs containing codeine or similar preparations (i.e. dihydrocodeine). Step 2 analgesics are weak opioids and to be effective should have at least 30 mg codeine per tablet or capsule. Clinical evidence suggests that opioids work better when co-prescribed with a non-opioid such as paracetamol and/or a NSAID (SIGN 2000).

Tramadol is a step 2 weak opioid but is not recommended for routine use in cancer pain, owing to a high prevalence of side-effects in this patient population (SIGN 2000).

Step 3: moderate or severe pain

Drugs in step 3 are those most commonly associated with cancer pain management (frequently morphine in the UK). The choice of a strong opioid should be governed by the severity of the pain (as reported by the patient) and/or failure of step 2 of the ladder.

The effective dose is whatever relieves the pain; the dose must be increased gradually, until either pain relief is achieved or side-effects become problematic. The presence of side-effects (such as drowsiness, hallucinations and muscle twitching) are an indication that the dose has been increased too rapidly and/or that the pain is not completely opioid-responsive. The principles of administering strong opioids are the same as those in step 2, namely given 'by mouth' and 'by the clock'. As with weak opioids (step 2), a non-opioid drug such as paracetamol and/or a NSAID should be co-prescribed. An appropriate breakthrough drug (p.r.n.) must be prescribed, normally approximately one-sixth of the total 24-hour opioid dose. If patients are unable to take oral medication then other strong opioids are given by other routes (e.g. subcutaneous or transdermal).

Some pains, such as bone and nerve pain, do not respond completely to opioids and therefore co-analgesic drugs may need to be prescribed alongside non-opioid and opioid analgesics. Co-analgesics include steroids, tricyclic antidepressants and anti-epileptic drugs; a detailed discussion of these drugs is beyond the scope of this chapter and interested readers should consult other texts (e.g. Twycross 1994). Oncological treatments, particularly radiotherapy for bone pain, should always be considered.

Other important notes on the pharmacological management of cancer pain

There are many different types of analgesic drugs, particularly weak (step 2) and strong (step 3) opioids. However, it is important to point out that most of these within each group offer no better pain relief than similar drugs at an equivalent dose. For example, codeine is no better or worse an analgesic than dihydrocodeine at an equivalent dose. However, an expert working group (Hanks et al 2001) recommended that morphine should remain the opioid of first choice for moderate to severe pain. The rationale for this is that it is widely available in a variety of formulations (tablet and liquid) and that no other alternative opioid has been shown to have a significant advantage over morphine. Nevertheless, there are instances when an alternative opioid is recommended; this is discussed in more detail in Part 2 of this chapter.

OTHER STRATEGIES FOR ENHANCING PAIN MANAGEMENT

Anticipating side-effects

Many of the side-effects commonly associated with analgesics can be anticipated and managed effectively. Constipation is a side-effect of all opioids and can be prevented with regular prescriptions of stimulant and softening laxatives. Nausea is normally a transient side-effect of opioids; it settles in most patients within a few days and can be alleviated with a regular antiemetic. Similarly, transient drowsiness associated with opioids that are titrated gradually against pain usually settles within a short period of time. When possible, other drugs that have sedative side-effects should be rationalised when opioids are prescribed. If these symptoms do not settle with appropriate treatment, it may be worth trying a different opioid (see Part 2), but before doing this, advice should be sought from local palliative care services.

Managing anxieties and fears

The provision of timely and appropriate information will help to ensure compliance with drug regimens and allay anxieties and misconceptions surrounding drug management. Frequently, particularly with recent media reporting surrounding opioid prescribing in terminal care, patients and their families harbour misconceptions about drug treatments.

These misconceptions are almost always unfounded and only increase anxiety and distress for the patient and family.

Addiction

Characterised by a craving for the drug and an overwhelming preoccupation with obtaining it (McCaffery & Ferrell 1997), addiction is perhaps the most common fear and misconception, and yet is almost never an issue in clinical practice (WHO 1996). Many patients also worry about developing tolerance to the analgesic properties of opioids, but this is rarely a serious clinical issue. In the small group of patients who develop clinically significant tolerance, this can be managed by changing to a different opioid. There are many good booklets available from cancer charities (e.g. BACUP – British Association of Cancer United Patients) and pharmaceutical companies that help in providing clear information for patients.

Reassess and seek advice

Pain management based on a meticulous assessment and a structured approach to administering analgesia (using established guidelines) will achieve effective pain control for the majority of patients. A small minority of patients will sometimes experience intractable pain. In these situations it is first necessary to reassess and evaluate the pain and treatments instigated. The patient may have developed a new pain, or the pain may not be completely opioid-responsive. Lack of attention to the non-physical manifestations and interventions for these will hamper effective pain management.

NON-PHARMACOLOGICAL STRATEGIES FOR THE MANAGEMENT OF CANCER PAIN

There are a number of strategies available to nurses that have been demonstrated to help alleviate pain associated with cancer. Issues relevant to practice are:

- providing relevant and accurate information to the patient and family
- dealing with common myths and misconceptions about cancer pain management
- maximising compliance with analgesic drug regimens.

Although there is a growing body of literature on other non-pharmacological methods for pain management, they are not included in this section because of contradictory evidence about effectiveness. Part 2 addresses some of these issues in more detail.

Providing relevant and accurate information to the patient and family

The provision of accurate verbal and written material has been shown to improve patients' knowledge of pain and to decrease pain intensity (de Wit et al 1999, Walker et al 1987). The pain management strategies outlined previously may seem straightforward to healthcare professionals but, for patients and families who are unclear about the aims and purposes of the interventions, it can only exacerbate their anxiety. Some drugs are not expected to provide immediate relief, such as antidepressants for nerve pain. This must be explained.

Some patients struggle with the number of drugs used initially to establish pain control. Where this is the case reassurance that the drug regimen can be simplified should be stressed for example with slow-release analgesic preparations. When good pain control is achieved, the drug regimen should be simplified and rationalised to avoid confusion about dose intervals and the number of drugs to take. Compliance can also be improved by consistent communication; it is good practice to write the drug regimen on paper for patients and families. This should include clear instructions of:

- the drug name (as on the bottle!)
- the purpose of the drug
- the dosage and interval to be taken.

Many pharmacy departments have specific guidelines and existing resources for providing written information to patients.

Dealing with common myths and misconceptions about cancer pain management

Patients and families often have anxieties about the drug management of pain – particularly morphine (Thomason et al 1998). It is important that healthcare workers are clear about their beliefs and values regarding cancer pain management, before attempting to address patient concerns. Although McCaffery & Ferrell (1997) and Elliott et al (1995), in the USA, have indicated that beliefs about addiction are less prevalent in nursing and medical staff than in previous years, there are still common misconceptions about the related concepts of tolerance and physical dependence (Farrer et al 2004, Wells et al 2001); see Box 3.4 for definitions.

Box 3.4 Addiction, tolerance and physical dependence

Addiction – craving for the drug and an overall preoccupation with obtaining it.

Tolerance – characterised by decreased efficacy and duration of action with each repeated dose.

Neither tolerance nor addiction is a clinical problem for patients receiving opioids for cancer pain.

Physical dependence – characterised by withdrawal symptoms if the drug is stopped suddenly.

Withdrawal symptoms may arise if the opioid is suddenly stopped – can be avoided by gradual reduction in 25% steps.

Adapted from WHO (1996).

Addiction in settings where pain relief is the primary aim is not an issue. A large survey of 12 000 patients taking strong opiates after surgery revealed possible problems with addiction in only four patients (Porter & Jick 1980).

Tolerance to opioids is a related but more prevalent misconception amongst patients and healthcare workers (Elliott et al 1995, Thomason et al 1998). This is not surprising given conflicting views presented in the literature and inaccurate 'media hype' concerning opioid use in terminal care. McCaffery & Ferrell (1997) describe tolerance as being a potential problem in up to 75% of patients taking opioids for longer than 3 months. However, it is unclear what evidence this assumption is based on – patients with progressive illnesses are as likely to need increases in analgesia due to increasing disease progression. This view is supported by Elliott et al (1995) who state: 'clinically relevant tolerance rarely develops to the analgesic effect of morphine'.

Nevertheless it is clear that a few patients develop tolerance, particularly those with unrelieved nerve pain. Strategies for managing tolerance do exist and are outlined in Part 2 of this chapter.

Nurses involved in administering opioids to patients for the first time need to address these misconceptions. Failure to do this may compound anxieties and reduce compliance. The probes, outlined in Box 3.2, are a good starting point. Additionally, a short screening tool has been designed (for the American population) that may be worth further exploration for use in the clinical setting (Ward et al 1993).

CONCLUSION

Although managing cancer pain necessarily involves structured drug interventions, nurses must consider the person behind the pain, including issues surrounding the meaning of pain, the person's social life and the impact of pain on emotional well-being.

Although such an integrated and holistic approach to pain management will achieve pain relief for the majority, there will always be instances when pain relief is difficult to achieve. For this minority it may be necessary to obtain advice from local specialist palliative care services.

Part 2 of this chapter deals in more detail with some of the issues surrounding the more complex and intractable pains.

PART 2: PAIN MANAGEMENT AT A HIGHER LEVEL OF NURSING PRACTICE

INTRODUCTION

Continuing changes in healthcare delivery are providing nurses with exciting and challenging opportunities. These have 'increased the skills and decision making capacity required of all practitioners' (UKCC 1999). More recently the advent of nurse prescribing is opening up exciting opportunities for developing advanced nursing practice. However, this brings with it a responsibility to ensure that new skills are underpinned by sound knowledge and understanding of the areas concerned. This chapter seeks to provide readers with the additional knowledge and understanding required to manage more complex pain.

It is anticipated that readers interested in the following paragraphs will be from a variety of areas and backgrounds, including:

- specialist clinical areas – hospice/palliative care, oncology
- community or hospital specialist palliative care services
- nurse prescribers, keen to extend their knowledge base.

It is important to point out that the skills and interventions at an advanced level should be undertaken only once the practitioner is satisfied that they are competent to practise at this level and according to local practice and policies.

The core principles (outlined in Part 1) will make the biggest impact in alleviating cancer pain. Readers should be competent with these skills before considering the following discussions.

The skills required to practise at a 'higher level' within this area are difficult to articulate (Benner 1984) and will develop through extensive clinical practice and exposure to the more complex issues surrounding cancer pain management. Specialist practice in this field is broader than the following discussions on managing complex pain, and necessarily involves a commitment to developing practice through audit, research and education (Humphris 1994, UKCC 1997). The remit of this chapter limits the discussions to the clinical aspects of higher-level practice and specifically addresses the following issues:

- assessment of complex pain
- recognition and management of opioid toxicity
- developments in the management of complex pain
- managing anxiety associated with pain and suffering.

For clarity, complex pain is defined as pain that is not easily alleviated by the guidelines set out in Part 1 – based on the WHO (1996) guidelines.

ASSESSMENT OF COMPLEX PAIN

The importance of a thorough and meticulous pain assessment cannot be underestimated. An incomplete assessment may be responsible for a pain that is 'seemingly' difficult to alleviate. The first step in the nursing management of a complex pain is to go 'back to basics' by reassessing the pain and surrounding issues. In many instances this will provide enough information to manage the pain. Nurses working at a higher level may need to obtain the necessary knowledge and skills in the following areas.

Physical examination

A physical examination should always be performed as part of any pain assessment, and must be carried out in conjunction with medical staff. This will give clues to possible causes of pain (e.g. constipation, nerve damage, bone involvement) and will guide treatment. Medical staff experienced in palliative care will look for pain syndromes to help identify the aetiology of the pain (e.g. lumbar plexopathy, vertebral syndromes or spinal cord compression) (Portenoy & Lesage 1999).

Nurses may need to perform a physical examination, to obtain clues to the possible causes of the pain.

This typically will involve looking for obvious sources of pain, such as pressure sores or open wounds, and an examination by light pressure and touch of areas surrounding the pain.

Many pains that are difficult and complex to manage are neuropathic in origin (discussed below) and commonly exhibit peculiar sensations on the skin innervated by the damaged nerve. These sensations have been usefully defined and classified, and form the basis of diagnosing neuropathic pain (Box 3.5).

Physical examination around the distribution of the pain may reveal one or more of these problems, and should be documented and reported. The creative use of a pain chart to document these is recommended.

Reassess analgesic response to previous treatments

Patients often receive complex drug therapies – often concurrently! It may be difficult to find out what helps, but detailed questioning about the pain and the effectiveness of current and previous interventions is essential for planning future treatments. In the case of opioids it is always beneficial to enquire whether an immediate opioid preparation helps (almost always some benefit from opioids is derived). If at all possible, patients should be asked to rate the severity of their pain following administration of an analgesic.

Assessment of other related physical and non-physical problems

Pain does not exist in isolation from the whole person, and, as mentioned, the impact of other possible

---

Box 3.5   Definitions of altered skin sensations common in neuropathic pain

Dysaesthesia – an unpleasant abnormal sensation
Allodynia – pain due to a stimulus that does not normally evoke pain (e.g. light touch)
Hyperalgesia – an increased response to a stimulus that is normally painful (i.e. a painful perception lasts longer than expected)
Hyperpathia – an increased pain response with an increased pain perception

Adapted from Twycross (1994) and IASP (1986).

sources of distress must be considered within any assessment. Patients with life-threatening and progressive diseases experience many symptoms and problems that will have a direct bearing on their experience of pain. These problems may be attributed to the global distress and suffering experienced in the context of their illness or related to problems associated with the treatment of the pain.

Pain as a component of suffering

In Part 1 of this chapter the concepts of pain thresholds and tolerance were outlined, and these principles remain important in considering the assessment of complex pain. Saunders (1967), using a model called 'total pain', highlighted the many areas of potential suffering that influence pain perception. This model is widely recognised as important for conceptualising the plight of suffering in terminally ill patients (Fig. 3.3). Similarly, a paper by Cassel (1982) highlighted that pain is experienced by the whole person, is linked to suffering, and is intensely personal and different between individuals. Any assessment must reflect the complexity of pain and its link with suffering.

Pain that is difficult to alleviate is something that some patients find intolerable, particularly in the context of failing health and loss of independence. Unrelieved pain is one common cause of prolonged suffering that Mystakidou et al (2006) argue is a predictor of a desire to hasten death. This, they argue, under-

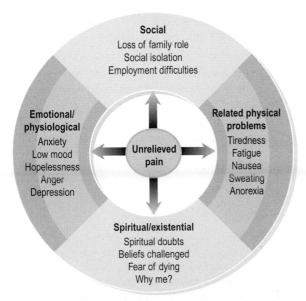

Figure 3.3 The multifaceted nature of pain in palliative care.

lines the importance of a 'supportive therapeutic relationship that conveys the attitude that much can be done to alleviate emotional and physical pain'.

In specialist palliative care, it is accepted practice that assessment should be 'problem-based', from the patients' perspective, enabling discussion of *their* most pertinent worries and difficulties. A problem-based assessment will give clues to other treatable causes of distress and enables support to be focused on areas of difficulties identified by the patient. A problem-based assessment simply involves asking a patient: 'What are your main worries or problems?' This assessment strategy often highlights that pain, although often severe, is not the main problem. Subsequent attention and support that is directed towards the main problem might help reduce pain perception.

Other clinical problems, not always easily articulated by the patient and family, such as uncertainty, anxiety and depression, may affect pain perception and therefore must be considered in the assessment of complex pain problems.

Assessing side–effects and opioid toxicity

The majority of patients can achieve good pain control, and suffer few side-effects. Analgesics for the treatment of pain, particularly opioids, are not without potential problems. Hanks et al (2001) explain that daytime drowsiness, dizziness or mental clouding commonly occur at the start of treatment but resolve when patients are stabilized (usually within a few days). When patients have settled on a strong opioid (i.e. are alert and pain-free) there is good evidence to suggest that the ability to drive a car is not compromised (Vainio et al 1995).

Opioids are a major cause of constipation, dry mouth, nausea and transient drowsiness, particularly when these are not anticipated and treated.

Tolerance to sedation and nausea/vomiting usually occurs within 1 week; however, dry mouth and constipation invariably persist and require ongoing nursing attention. Many other drugs used as co-analgesics and adjuvants for pain relief have potentially problematic side-effects, which if undetected will further compound the misery of a patient with complex pain.

However, a small proportion of patients display signs of toxicity to morphine. This is more common in patients with:

- renal impairment
- complex pain that requires higher doses of opioids (e.g. nerve pain or pain on movement)

- rapid escalation of the opioid dose without regard to its effectiveness
- opioids prescribed to sedate a patient.

Recently, a better understanding of the pharmaco-kinetics and neurophysiology of opioids has emerged and is changing how we manage opioid side-effects. It is postulated that many of the problems associated with 'opioid toxicity' are due to opioid metabolites (a byproduct of opioid metabolism) causing unaccept-able side-effects in some individuals. Although it seems that a small proportion of patients are very sen-sitive to these metabolites, more frequently this toxicity is the result of the overzealous use of opioids for pain that is only partially opioid-responsive. Concurrent physical problems such as renal failure and/or dehy-dration can lead to the accumulation of some metabo-lites (which are primarily excreted by the kidneys).

It is thought that two opioid metabolites (mor-phine-6-glucuronide and morphine-3-glucuronide) are responsible for some of the problems associated with opioid toxicity. These side-effects include cogni-tive impairment (drowsiness and reduced concen-tration), nausea/vomiting, and, in severe cases, myoclonus (muscle twitching), hallucinations and delirium. It is postulated that severe opioid toxicity may be associated with hyperalgesia and allodynia in neuropathic pain (Dickenson 1994).

Opioid toxicity is a common feature in difficult pain problems and is common in the terminal stage of a person's illness, where either the need for opioids has decreased and/or they have developed renal failure or dehydration. In some patients this can lead to the vicious cycle described by O'Neill & Fallon (1998) where opioid toxicity is interpreted as pain, resulting in increased opioids and sedation, and leading to further distress from symptoms of toxicity. It is important that nurses learn to recognise these scenarios for which the management is discussed below.

Involve family/carer(s) in the assessment

It is good practice to involve the family in all aspects of palliative care provision, enabling a more detailed account of the background to the patient's experi-ences to be gained. The family may have concerns and worries about the pain and its treatment. A close family member may confirm any worries about issues such as compliance and confusion over drug regimens. Failure to involve and support rela-tives is postulated by Meittinen et al (1998) as one indicator of the probability of inappropriate pain control.

THE MANAGEMENT OF COMPLEX PAIN

The management of complex pain requires the full attention of the multidisciplinary team. Although many interventions revolve around drug therapies, this should not be at the expense of other non-pharmacological methods. The following discussions presume that the approaches covered in Part 1 have been exhausted.

Pharmacological interventions

Complex pains are almost always opioid-responsive, but the degree of relief obtained may vary consider-ably between individuals. As in some cases it is undesirable side-effects that limit the use of appro-priate doses of opioids, the following questions need to be explored:

1. Does the opioid relieve the pain but side-effects prevent required increase in the opioid?
2. Is the pain only partially relieved by the opioid despite incremental increases in the dose?

Rapid escalation of the opioid in the presence of side-effects and/or the absence of an analgesic res-ponse will produce the symptoms of opioid toxicity described above. Management of opioid toxicity is directed at treating the causes and palliating side-effects. This involves:

- reducing the opioids gradually
- treating dehydration and reversible causes of renal failure
- stopping or reducing other drugs that may be con-tributing to the problem
- treating delirium and hallucinations (with drugs such as haloperidol/droperidol).

If pain remains a problem and side-effects prevent increases in the dose, trial of a different strong opioid is indicated.

Alternative opioids

A better understanding of opioid side-effects (includ-ing the role of morphine metabolites) has enabled the development of a clearer strategy in the management of pain that is opioid-responsive but limited by side-effects. These strategies focus on changing to a dif-ferent opioid ('opioid switching' or 'rotation') in the hope that the patient will experience fewer side-effects and therefore tolerate a higher dose (Olson & Sjogren 1996). For many years morphine and diamor-phine have been the only strong opioids used in pal-liative and terminal care, but more recently other options have become available. These include oxyco-done, hydromorphone, fentanyl, methadone and buprenorphine.

Each of these opioids has different properties and differing potencies compared with morphine. Guidance by the European Association for Palliative Care suggests that second-line opioids should be either oxycodone or hydromorphone (Hanks et al 2001). Both of these are synthetic derivatives of morphine and when used at equi-analgesic doses are similar in terms of efficacy and side-effects. Crucially, however, both of these opioids are more suitable for patients with renal impairment, as excretion of the metabolites is not as dependent on renal function compared with morphine and diamorphine.

Other alternatives (including fentanyl and buprenorphine) are available via other routes such as buccal and transdermal, but are not recommended for treating unrelieved complex pain (Hanks et al 2001).

Table 3.1 outlines the conversion ratios from one opioid to another, but this needs to be treated with caution as considerable variability exists between individuals. Switching opioids requires careful monitoring and supervision.

Pain poorly responsive to opioids

Complex pain that is not alleviated by opioids is treated, in the first instance, by adjuvant analgesics. The choice of drug is dependent on the cause of the pain, as illustrated in Figure 3.4. A discussion of all of these is beyond the scope of the chapter and therefore readers are encouraged to consult other authoritative texts (Twycross 1994). When appropriate it may be necessary to treat the cause of the pain. This may involve radiotherapy, chemotherapy and, in some instances, surgery. The possible benefits of these treatments for each individual must be balanced against risks and possible side-effects.

As pain from nerve damage disproportionately represents causes of complex pain, the following discussion will outline some of the available treatment options.

Neuropathic pain

Pain due to nerve damage (neuropathic pain) can arise from a multitude of factors and in the case of cancer pain may be tumour- or treatment-related. There is a wide variety of other causes of neuropathic pain not related to cancer, often evident in chronic pain syndromes (e.g. phantom limb pain, post-stroke pain or diabetic peripheral neuropathy).

The first step in managing neuropathic pain in palliative care is to apply the previously outlined analgesic ladder. In some instances neuropathic pain may be very opioid-responsive, but in other cases strategies warrant the use of co-analgesics (see Fig. 3.4). Numerous co-analgesics are reported to help nerve pain, but the evidence in cancer pain is sparse. The following drug classes are those with evidence of effectiveness in the chronic pain (non-cancer) population or from clinical consensus (not proven in clinical trials):

- anticonvulsant drugs (McQuay et al 1995)
- tricyclic antidepressants (McQuay & Moore 1997)
- steroids.

If these co-analgesics, along with opioids, do not produce adequate analgesia, other drug and non-drug methods must be considered.

There is growing interest in drugs that dampen down excitatory neural activity, postulated to be one of the causes of neuropathic pain (Ventafridda et al 1996). This phenomenon of abnormal neural activity in the spinal cord is commonly called *wind-up*, and may occur in the absence of a painful stimulus. It has been shown (in animal models) that certain drugs block the N-methyl-D-aspartate (NMDA)

Table 3.1   Approximate analgesic equivalence to oral morphine for oxycodone and hydromorphone

Analgesic	Ratio with oral morphine[a]	Duration of action (h)	Example
Oxycodone (oral)	2	3	Morphine 20 mg (oral) = oxycodone 10 mg (oral)
Hydromorphone (oral)	7.5	4	Hydromorphone 1.3 mg (oral) = morphine 10 mg (oral)

[a]The conversion ratios shown are *approximate* and should be used only as a guide. Patients vary in their response to individual opioids. Dose conversions should be conservative and doses rounded down. It is safer to give the patient a lower regular dose initially and to use breakthrough medication as needed until the dose requirements are clear.
Adapted from Lothian Palliative Care Guidelines (2006).

The choice of co-analgesic depends on the likely cause of the pain, so that making a detailed reassessment of the patient's pain is crucial. Below are some of the common pains that do not always respond totally to the use of opioids, and suggestions for their management.

Co-analgesic drugs		Non-drug methods
• NSAIDs (e.g. diclofenac) • Steroids (e.g. e) • Bisphosphonates (specialist use only)	**Bone metastasis**	• Radiotherapy • Nerve blocks • Hot/cold pads • Immobilisation or surgery if impending fracture or fractured
• Trial of steroids • Tricyclic antidepressants (amitriptyline 10–50 mg at night) • Anticonvulsants (gabapentin–see below. Start at 300 mg at night and then increase daily up to a maximum dose of 600 mg t.d.s.)	**Nerve pain**	• Nerve • Heat/cold pads • TENS • Acupuncture • Cordotomy
• Antispasmodics (e.g. hyoscine butylbromide 20 mg q.d.s.)	**Colic**	• Hot/cold pads • Relaxation techniques • TENS
• Trial of steroids • NSAIDs (e.g. diclofenac)	**Liver capsular pain**	• Coeliac plexus block
• Paracetamol/codeine phosphate • Steroids (if due to raised intracranial pressure • NSAIDs (if severe and unrelieved by the above)	**Headaches**	• Radiotherapy (if cause is metastasis/brain primary) • Relaxation techniques – if due in part to tension/anxiety
• Opioids • Entonox • IV sedation (midazolam)	**Painful procedures**	• Nerve blocks • Distraction techniques
• NSAIDs • Muscle relaxant (e.g. diazepam 2 mg)	**Muscular pain**	• Heat pad • Massage • Relaxation

Note: These are only guidelines – please contact the Team for further advice

Figure 3.4 Adjuvant therapies and co-analgesics for pain management. (From Western General Hospitals NHS Trust, Edinburgh, with permission.)

receptor thought to be important in the development of 'wind-up' (Dickenson 1994). The common drugs used for this purpose include ketamine and methadone:

• Ketamine does not have analgesic properties *per se*, but can alleviate neuropathic pain by blocking NMDA receptors in the spinal cord (Mercadante 1996).

• Methadone, a strong opioid, has a potential to block this receptor (Morley & Makin 1998).

As with the discussion of alternative opioids, use of these drugs requires a specialist knowledge and experience, and careful monitoring of potential side-effects is necessary.

Finally, neuropathic pain and other complex pains of different origin may not always be completely amenable to drug treatment and therefore non-drug interventions may be necessary (see Fig. 3.4). The complexity and difficulties in managing these pains highlight the need for good links with other disciplines, including palliative medicine, oncology and chronic pain management.

NON-PHARMACOLOGICAL MANAGEMENT OF DISTRESS ASSOCIATED WITH PAIN

The importance of conceptualising pain as a multi-faceted concept, as outlined in Figure 3.3, has been discussed previously. In recognising the multifaceted experience of pain in palliative care, attention to non-physical distress needs intervention alongside the management of the physical component of the pain. For this to occur it is necessary for open and honest communication to take place in all stages of palliative care provision. Such communication must constantly assess for possible non-physical causes of distress that impact on the patient's pain perception. The possible causes of such distress have been thoroughly documented in the palliative care literature (Cassel 1982, Saunders 1967), and in many instances can be addressed through good communication and active steps to support the patient and family during the illness. Nurses working at a higher level of clinical practice need to use well developed communication skills to ensure that patients are constantly informed and involved in the decision-making process that is required to manage pain. Encouraging patients who are able to take an active role in the management of their pain has been clearly demonstrated to produce positive outcomes (de Wit et al 1995) and is particularly important when pain is not easily alleviated by the more straightforward strategies outlined in Part 1 of this chapter. Involving patients and families in the management of the pain is not always easy, as their decisions may not always be what we would choose on their behalf. Healthcare professionals need to remain flexible and open minded in their willingness to engage individuals in their care, while at the same time ensuring that they have correct and accurate information to enable informed decision making.

For some patients, the active role that they adopt may involve trying non-pharmacological interventions that are not traditionally associated with the medical management of pain in palliative care. These may include interventions such as:

- imagery
- music therapy or art therapy
- acupuncture

- transcutaneous electrical nerve stimulation (TENS)
- aromatherapy
- relaxation
- hypnotherapy.

Although there may be little scientific evidence of the benefits of some of these therapies for pain management in palliative care (Sindhu 1996), patients who choose to try these therapies should be supported – at the very least because it encourages them to take an active role in the management of their pain.

It is necessary to ensure that these therapies are practised safely and are not contraindicated by other treatments. Any nurses offering such interventions must ensure that they operate within professional guidelines (UKCC 1997) and according to local policies.

The role of relaxation techniques in cancer pain management deserves further investigation and discussion. Relaxation techniques are commonly used within chronic pain management programmes and there is emerging evidence that some patients in the palliative care population will benefit from some form of relaxation training (Syrjala & Donaldson 1995). More research is needed to demonstrate its effectiveness (Wallace 1997), in particular to determine which groups will derive the most benefit. The relationship between pain and anxiety is suggested by Montes-Sandoval (1999) to be reciprocal and interconnected at both the physical and non-physical level. Although this relationship is not fully understood, it is clear that for some individuals relaxation therapies will reduce pain. Nurses working at an advanced level in palliative care must develop the skills needed to offer relaxation training to patients. Teaching patients relaxation invariably opens up opportunities to discuss other worries and anxieties that they may be experiencing. There are many forms of relaxation therapies, but whatever is offered must be simple and practical in the clinical area it is being used in. Most community and hospital services have liaison psychiatry services that will be able to advise and teach nurses practical relaxation techniques.

CONCLUSION

Part 2 of this chapter aimed to introduce readers to some of the newer developments in pain management in palliative care and outline the importance of good communication for patients and their families. Evidence of the effectiveness of some interventions (such as relaxation) exists; there is a need for nurses practising at a higher level to engage in further research to evaluate their effectiveness and develop methods of introducing them into clinical practice. Nurses must participate and initiate programmes of clinical audit to determine what areas within their practice need improvement; see Farrer (1999) for a full discussion of research and audit in palliative care nursing.

Additionally, Part 2 has discussed some of the developments in cancer pain management, in particular in relation to neuropathic pain. Although our understanding of neuropathic pain is increasing, this is a rapidly evolving area that will hopefully lead to improved treatments.

Current developments in the treatment of intractable cancer pain are important, but it must be remembered that the core principles outlined in Part 1 of this chapter will bring the most benefit to the majority of patients. The responsibility of nurses working at a higher level of practice must extend beyond the application of the more specialist pain management strategies, to ensuring through educational initiatives that all colleagues within the multidisciplinary team are conversant with the core principles of cancer pain management.

References

Arathuzich D 1991 Pain experience for metastatic breast cancer patients. Cancer Nursing 14:41–48

Benner P 1984 From novice to expert: excellence and power in clinical nursing practice. Addison Wesley, London

Bonica J J 1990 Cancer pain: current status and future needs: In: Bonica J J (ed.) The management of pain. Lea & Febiger, Philadelphia, p 400–445

Bowsher D 1993 Pain management in nursing: In: Carroll D, Bowsher D (eds) Pain management and nursing care. Butterworth Heinemann, Oxford, p 5–15

Brant J 2003 Pain management. In: O'Connor M, Aranda S (eds) Palliative care nursing: a guide to practice, 2nd edn. Radcliffe Medical Press, Melbourne, p 123–158

Carr E C J 1997 Evaluating the use of a pain assessment tool and care plan: a pilot study. Journal of Advanced Nursing 26:1073–1079

Cassel E J 1982 The nature of suffering and the goals of medicine. New England Journal of Medicine 306(11):639–645

Clarke E B, French B, Bilodeau M L, Caapasso V C, Edwards A, Empoliti J 1996 Pain management, knowledge, attitudes and clinical practice: the impact of nurses' characteristics and education. Journal of Pain and Symptom Management 11(1):18–31

Cleeland C S, Gonin R, Hatfield A K et al 1994 Pain and its treatment in outpatients with metastatic cancer. New England Journal of Medicine 330(9):592–596

Clinical Standards Board for Scotland 2002 Clinical Standards: Specialist palliative care. Online. Available: http://www.qualityimprovementscotland.com 9 Jan 2007

de Wit R, van Dam F S, van Buuren A et al 1995 Pain counselling for chronic cancer pain patients: a nursing intervention study. Seventh International Symposium on Supportive Care in Cancer, September 1995 (meeting abstract)

de Wit R, van Dam F, Hanneman M et al 1999 Evaluation of the use of a pain diary in chronic cancer pain patients at home. Pain 79(1):89–99

Dickenson A H 1994 Neurophysiology of opioid poorly responsive pain. In: Hanks G W (ed.) Palliative medicine: problem areas in pain and symptom management. CSHL Press, New York, p 21

Elliott B A, Murray D M, Elliott T E et al 1995 Physicians' knowledge and attitudes about cancer pain management: a survey from the Minnesota Cancer Pain Management Project. Journal of Pain and Symptom Management 19(7):494–504

Farrer K 1999 Research and audit: demonstrating quality. In: Lugton J, Kindlen M (eds) Palliative care: the nursing role. Churchill Livingstone, Edinburgh, p 83–127

Farrer K, Hockley J, Sandridge A et al 2004 Focus on Research: An evaluation of a multidisciplinary hospital based palliative care team (HPCT). Scottish Executive Health Department Chief Scientist Office. Online. Available: http://www.sehd.scot.nhs.uk/cso/Publications/ExecSumms/OctNov04/farrer.pdf 9 Jan 2007

Foley K M 2005 Advances in cancer pain management in 2005. Gynecologic Oncology page 126

Hanks G W, Forbes K 1997 Opioid responsiveness. Acta Anaesthesiologica Scandinavica 41(Part 2):154–158

Hanks G W, de Conno F, Cherny N et al 2001 Morphine and alternative opioids in cancer pain: the EAPC recommendations. British Journal of Cancer 84(5):587

Hemming L, Maher D 2005 Cancer pain in palliative care: why is management so difficult. British Journal of Community Nursing 10(8):362–367

Humphris D 1994 The clinical nurse specialist – issues in practice. Macmillan, Basingstoke

International Association for the Study of Pain 1986 Subcommittee on taxonomy. Pain 3(Suppl):216–221

Klepstad P, Kaasa S, Cherny N, Hanks G, de Conno F, Research Steering Committee of the European Association for Palliative Care 2005 Pain and pain treatments in European palliative care units. A cross sectional survey from the European Association for Palliative Care Research Network. Palliative Medicine 19(6):477–484

Latham J 1990 Pain control. Austin Cornish, London

Lothian Palliative Care Guidelines 2006 Equivalent analgesic doses/changing opioid. Online. Available:

http://www.scan.scot.nhs.uk/scan/Documents/1600/Display/PDF/LPCG2004_ChangingOpioids.pdf 9 Jan 2007

McCaffery M, Ferrell B R 1997 Nurses' knowledge of pain assessment and management: how much progress have we made? Journal of Pain and Symptom Management 14(3):175–188

McQuay H C, Moore A 1997 Bibliography and systematic reviews in cancer pain: a report to the NHS National Cancer Research and Development Programme, Oxford

McQuay H, Carroll D, Jadad A R, Wiffen P, Moore A 1995 Anticonvulsant drugs for management of pain: a systematic review. British Medical Journal 311:1047–1052

Meittinen T, Tilvis R, Karppi P, Arve S 1998 Why is pain relief of dying patients often unsuccessful? The relatives' perspectives. Palliative Medicine 12(6):429–453

Mercadante S 1996 Ketamine in cancer pain: an update. Palliative Medicine 10:225–230

Montes-Sandoval L 1999 An analysis of the concept of pain. Journal of Advanced Nursing 29(4):935–941

Morley J S, Makin M K 1998 The use of methadone in cancer pain poorly responsive to other opioids. Pain Reviews 5:51–58

Mystakidou K, Parpa E, Katsouda E, Galanos A, Vlahos L 2006 The role of physical and psychological symptoms in desire for death: a study of terminally ill cancer patients. Psycho-Oncology 15(4):355–360

National Institute for Clinical Excellence 2004 Guidance on Cancer Services: Improving supportive and palliative care for adults with cancer. Online. Available: http://www.nice.org.uk/pdf/csgspmanual.pdf 9 Jan 2007

Olson A K, Sjogren P 1996 Neurotoxic effects of opioids. European Journal of Palliative Care 3(4):139–142

O'Neill B, Fallon M 1997 ABC of palliative care: principles of palliative care and pain control. British Medical Journal 315:801–804

Paice J P, Toy C, Shott S 1998 Barriers to cancer pain relief: fear of tolerance and addiction. Journal of Pain and Symptom Management 16(1):1–9

Portenoy R L, Lesage P 1999 Management of cancer pain. Lancet 353:1695–1700

Porter J, Jick H 1980 Addiction rare in patients treated with narcotics. New England Journal of Medicine 302:123

Royal College of Nursing 2002 A framework for nurses working in specialist palliative care: competencies project. RCN, London

Saunders C M 1967 The management of terminal illness. Hospital Medicine Publications, London

Scottish Intercollegiate Guidelines Network 2000 Control of pain in patients with cancer. SIGN Publication No. 44.

Online. Available: http://www.sign.ac.uk/guidelines/published/index.html 9 Jan 2007

Sindhu F 1996 Are non-pharmacological nursing interventions for the management of pain effective? – a meta-analysis. Journal of Advanced Nursing 24:1152–1159

Strang P 1998 Cancer pain – a provoker of emotional, social and existential distress. Acta Oncologica 37(7/8):641–644

Syrjala K L, Donaldson G W 1995 Relaxation and imagery and cognitive behaviour training reduce pain during cancer treatment: a controlled trial. Pain 63:189–198

Thomas K 2003 The Gold Standards Framework in community palliative care. European Journal of Palliative Care 10:113–115

Thomason T E, McCune J S, Bernard S A, Winer E P, Tremont S, Lindley C M 1998 Cancer pain survey: patient-centered issues in control. Journal of Pain and Symptom Management 15(5):275–284

Twycross R 1994 Pain relief in advanced cancer. Churchill Livingstone, London

Twycross R, Harcourt J, Bergl S 1996 A survey of pain in patients with advanced cancer. Journal of Pain and Symptom Management 12(5):273–282

UK Central Council for Nursing, Midwifery and Health Visiting 1997 Prep – the nature of advanced practice. UKCC, London

UK Central Council for Nursing, Midwifery and Health Visiting 1999 A higher level of practice. UKCC, London

Vainio A, Ollila J, Matikainen E, Rosenberg P, Kalso E 1995 Driving ability in cancer patients receiving long-term morphine analgesia. Lancet 346:667–670

Ventafridda V, Tamburini M, Caraceni A, de Conno F, Naldi F 1987 A validation study of the WHO method for cancer pain relief. Cancer 59(4):850–856

Ventafridda V, Caraceni A, Sbanotto A 1996 Cancer pain management. Pain Reviews 3(3):153–179

Walker V A, Dicks B, Webb P 1987 Pain assessment charts in the management of chronic cancer pain. Palliative Medicine 1:111–116

Wallace K G 1997 Analysis of recent literature concerning relaxation and imagery interventions for cancer pain. Cancer Nursing 20:87–97

Ward S, Goldberg N, Millar-McCauley V 1993 Patient related barriers to management of cancer pain. Pain 52:319–324

Wells M, Dryden H, Guild P, Levack P, Farrer K, Mowat P 2001 The knowledge and attitudes of surgical staff towards the use of opioids in cancer pain management: can the Hospital Palliative Care Team make a difference? European Journal of Cancer Care 10:201–211

World Health Organisation 1996 Cancer pain relief. WHO, Geneva

Chapter **4**

Promoting comfort through radiotherapy, chemotherapy and surgery

Philippa Green and James Youll

INTRODUCTION

This chapter focuses on supporting patients while they are receiving palliative treatments. The management and possible side-effects experienced by patients undergoing palliative radiotherapy and chemotherapy are discussed. The indications for the use of palliative surgery and radiological interventions including use of stents are also explored. Case examples are used to illustrate the value of the latest stenting techniques where traditional palliative surgery may be difficult or impossible.

It is often difficult to imagine radiotherapy or chemotherapy being used in palliative care, especially if we have experience of caring for patients who have undergone these treatments when used with curative intent. These patients may experience side-effects that are often severe but tolerated because of the overall aim of treatment. When considering the use of chemotherapy and radiotherapy with palliative intent, thorough assessment must take place before and throughout treatment. Nurses are often in the best position to identify symptoms and aid diagnosis, as well as assess the overall effects of treatment, in conjunction with the patient and family.

Downing (2001, p 449) mentions that there are 'many individuals living with advanced cancer and many symptoms of advanced disease can be controlled, enhancing their quality of life'. Palliative treatment should be delivered with the intention of achieving control of local symptoms in a setting where cure is no longer possible, utilising treatment that should give minimal disturbance to the lifestyle of the patient (Hoskin 1994).

WHAT IS RADIOTHERAPY?

Radiotherapy is the use of ionising radiation to interfere with the replication of cancer cells within the body. Radiotherapy cannot differentiate between normal cells and cancer cells, so normal cells will be affected within the path of the radiation beam, causing the patient to experience side-effects (Green & Kinghorn 1995, Holmes 1996a, Hoskin & Makin 2003a, Kirkbride 1995, Munro 2003, Robinson & Coleman 1996).

The principles and practice of radiotherapy have changed very little in the last few decades. The main advances have come from the development of improved technology and a greater understanding of the effect radiotherapy has on tissue – radiobiology – and detailed descriptions of this have been given by Adamson (2003) and Faithfull (2001). If we are able to understand how the treatment works and why side-effects develop then we are better placed to support our patients undergoing these treatments.

Most radiotherapy departments use machines called linear accelerators, which generate radiation using electricity; this treatment is sometimes referred to as teletherapy. Radiotherapy can be given using linear accelerators or by placing radioactive material into the tissue or into a cavity close to the site of the cancer; this treatment is known as brachytherapy. Radioactive isotopes can be administered by either mouth or intravenous injection to carry out investigations or to treat certain cancers. All of these techniques can be used to treat cancer curatively or palliatively. As Kirkbride (1995) pointed out, despite the different applications the effects of the treatment will be the same.

SIDE-EFFECTS OF RADIOTHERAPY

The nursing care of patients with cancer is not focused solely on the disease but also on identifying and treating the side-effects that patients might experience as a result of their treatment (Oliver 1988). The side-effects produced by radiotherapy occur because of the damage caused to normal cells within the path of the radiation beam. It is always helpful to find out about any previous experience or ideas the patient may have about radiotherapy as misconceptions can easily occur, resulting in unnecessary worry. Accurate honest information has been shown to help patients cope with the potential side-effects and to give them a sense of control. Webb (1987) discusses the importance of patient teaching and how it can help the patient to be more involved with self-care. It could be argued that information-giving is the role of the medical staff, but nurses and other healthcare professionals are well equipped and should be able to support the patient by giving information about treatment effects, side-effects and coping strategies. Patients need to understand the potential for side-effects and, together with nurses, be alert for early detection. Prompt treatment of side-effects by the caring team is essential (Whale 1991).

Normal cells are more able to repair damage, whereas cancer cells are more limited in their ability to repair (Blows 2005, Faithfull 2001, Holmes 1996b, Kirkbride 1995); through radiobiological understanding we have been able to identify normal tissues that are more sensitive to radiotherapy. In some tissues, such as the skin, bone marrow and the lining of the gastrointestinal tract, the cells have a rapid rate of replication (Holmes 1996b, Needham 1997, Souhami & Tobias 2003). Side-effects in these tissues may occur early on in treatment and are sometimes referred to as acute effects. Cells that divide at a slower rate will be affected by radiotherapy, but this may not become evident for some time after treatment when the cells start to replicate. These side-effects are classed as late or chronic effects (Alison & Sarraf 1997, Rice 1997). Some of these late effects are irreversible, and patients should be made aware of them. Prompt recognition and treatment can prevent serious complications (Faithfull 2001, Holmes 1996b).

Palliative radiotherapy

The decision to treat curatively or palliatively is well thought out by the consultant clinical oncologist, usually together with the multidisciplinary team, which will include a surgeon or physician, taking into account the extent of the disease, the physical and personal circumstances of patients and their wishes.

Sometimes, at diagnosis, it may be evident that the disease is so extensive that cure may not be possible. It may seem strange to be considering radiotherapy as a palliative treatment because of side-effects, but it has been shown to be useful in managing patients who experience distressing symptoms and for whom cure is no longer possible. It has been estimated that approximately 45% of patients with cancer will receive radiotherapy at some time during their illness (Robinson & Coleman 1996) and that approximately half of radiotherapy treatments are given with palliative intent (Blyth 2001 in Colyer 2003, Hoskin & Makin 2003a, Kirkbride 1995).

The overall doses of radiotherapy used for palliative treatments are lower than those given with curative intent, but the daily dose may be higher; because of this the side-effects from treatment may initially be more intense. The delivery can range from a single exposure to several fractions spread over a period of up to 2 weeks. The aim of palliative treatment is to maintain or enhance quality of life.

Continuous monitoring of the effects of the treatment on the patient and their carers is important.

Nursing staff within hospital, community and nursing homes are relied upon to report any adverse effects to medical staff directly involved with the patient or to the radiographers within the department who can relay information to the appropriate staff.

Symptoms that may be alleviated by radiotherapy, side-effects and their management

Brain metastases

Brain metastases account for one-third of all brain tumours (Souhami & Tobias 2003). Breast cancer, small-cell lung cancer, melanoma and renal cancer commonly metastasise to the brain, as well as AIDS-related cerebral lymphoma. In these cases palliative radiotherapy produces a reasonable response (Neal & Hoskin 1997). Presenting symptoms of brain metastases may include headache, blurred vision, ataxia and possible seizures (Waller & Caroline 1996).

Patients initially start high doses of corticosteroids to reduce intracranial pressure and relieve cerebral oedema (Souhami & Tobias 2003) and other symptoms such as headache (Hoskin & Makin 2003b). Radiotherapy is a useful mode of treatment in patients with brain metastases and the response to treatment relates to the radiosensitivity of the primary cancer and to the response to corticosteroids.

Radiotherapy can be given to the whole brain if multiple deposits are present, or treatment can be directed towards a single deposit. Where there is a solitary metastasis, surgical excision may be an option (Hoskin & Makin 2003b). Choice of dosage and fractionation of radiotherapy remains contentious (Souhami & Tobias 2003).

Possible side-effects of radiotherapy to the brain

If the brain is being irradiated, the patient may experience side-effects, including headaches and nausea due to raised intracranial pressure as a result of cerebral oedema caused by the tumour and the inflammatory response of the brain tissue to the radiation.

Patients are generally given corticosteroids to reduce this response. Steroid-related complications can occur such as oral candida, oedema, diabetes, dyspepsia and insomnia (Kaye 2003, Regnard & Hockley 2004). These complications generally respond to a dose reduction. Analgesics and antiemetics may be administered to enhance patient comfort.

Hair loss will be a problem for the patient receiving radiotherapy to the brain; unfortunately, there is nothing that can be done to prevent this, so the patient will need support. If the treatment is targeted towards a specific area to treat a solitary metastasis then only the hair in that area may be affected, but if the whole brain is being irradiated then hair loss will be total. Wigs and hairpieces may help and have a positive influence on body image, but they serve as a constant reminder of the illness. Patients should be advised that their hair will grow back after treatment (Kaye 2003).

Chemotherapy may also produce a response in metastases where the primary cancer is chemosensitive, such as small-cell lung cancer or lymphoma (Hoskin & Makin 2003b, Kaye 2003).

Bone metastases

The development of bone metastases is common in cancers such as breast, prostate, thyroid and lung (O'Brien 1993). Waller & Caroline (1996) state that there is a 30–70% incidence of bone metastasis in all patients with cancer. Faull & Barton (1998) and Downing (2001) give a concise description of the pathophysiology behind bone metastasis.

Assessment and prompt identification are important as the patient can experience severe bone pain and, untreated, there is an increased risk of pathological fracture. Common presenting signs of bone metastases are pain, hypercalcaemia and pathological fracture (Blows 2005).

Bone metastases and associated pain are generally very responsive to radiotherapy (O'Brien 1993, Wells 2003), although the rate and duration of response can vary. Radiotherapy can be given as a single exposure. The dose is fairly high and any side-effects may be intense for a short period of time. Alternatively the radiotherapy may be given over 5–10 days. There may be a flare-up of pain following radiotherapy (Hoskin & Makin 2003c, Wells 2003). Patients should be informed of this and appropriate analgesia prescribed to help manage the pain.

Because of the increased risk of pathological fracture in long bones an orthopaedic consultation may be sought with a view to internal fixation. The patient will benefit from pain relief as a result of the internal fixation, and mobility will be maintained or regained. Postoperative radiotherapy can be given after pinning to aid healing and prevent tumour progression (Hoskin & Makin 2003c, Smith 1993). Some patients may present with widespread bone metastases; if this occurs, they can be treated with hemi-body radiation, as a single exposure (Copp 1991, Hoskin & Makin 2003c, Wells 2003). Again, the effects will depend on which half of the body has been treated. A premedication of an antiemetic and a corticosteroid is usually given. Once a patient has completed a course of radiotherapy to manage pain, the analgesic regimen should be reviewed to ensure that the patient is not taking more analgesia than is needed. This review may be carried out by either the hospital-based team or the primary healthcare team (PHCT) in the community.

Radioisotopes can also be used to treat bone metastases. Strontium-89 is a β-emitting isotope that works by following the biochemical pathways of calcium. Given by injection, it targets bony deposits and delivers radiotherapy locally, causing little damage to surrounding normal tissue (Day 1998, Needham 1997, Wells 2003).

With both hemi-body irradiation and strontium, bone marrow suppression can be a problem. Patient and carer education is important, with particular reference to control of infection.

Spinal cord compression (SCC)

Spinal cord compression is considered an oncological emergency. Downing (2001) stated it can be the most devastating complication of cancer metastases for cancer patients and their carers to experience. Rapid diagnosis, assessment and treatment are essential if neurological damage is not to become permanent (Coleman 1996, Faull & Barton 1998). Metastatic spread from breast cancer, cancer of the bronchus, lymphoma, prostate cancer, melanoma and unknown primary to the spinal cord is common (Souhami & Tobias 2003, Waller & Caroline 1996). SCC can be caused by bone metastases eroding the vertebral prominences or by tumour development in the spinal cord itself. Presenting symptoms include altered sensation, pain and muscular weakness. Loss of sphincter control is a late symptom (Downing 2001, Faull & Barton 1998). SCC may be treated by radiotherapy alone or surgical decompression followed by radiotherapy (Souhami & Tobias 2003).

As with other metastatic disease, response to radiotherapy may be determined by the radiosensitivity of the primary tumour. It is also dependent on the progression of the cord compression at the time of diagnosis. The earlier treatment can be initiated, the better the chance of the patient retaining mobility. The side-effects caused by the radiotherapy will depend on the area being treated. If the thoracic spine is being treated then side-effects such as dysphagia or oesophagitis may occur and should be treated in the same way as if the chest were being irradiated, as discussed later in this chapter. In addition, nausea and vomiting may occur; the management of this is also discussed below.

If the lumbar or sacral spine is being treated, diarrhoea could be a problem. Patients need to be made aware of this. Increased fluid intake should be encouraged to prevent dehydration. Chemotherapy may be of benefit but only if the primary tumour is known to be responsive to chemotherapy.

Superior vena cava obstruction

Another oncological emergency is superior vena cava obstruction (SVCO), which results from pressure on the vessels from a tumour in the chest or mediastinum, or secondary to thrombosis. Carcinoma of the bronchus is the commonest primary cancer causing SVCO; some 75% of cases of SVCO are associated with lung cancer (Hoskin & Makin 2003d). Lymphomas are also implicated, and metastases from breast cancer (Downing 2001). The presenting signs are swelling of the face, neck and arms, engorgement of the jugular vein and dilatation of superficial skin veins, breathlessness, headaches and blurred vision (Coleman 1996, Hoskin & Makin 2003d, Neal & Hoskin 1997, Souhami & Tobias 2003).

Treatment usually consists of radiotherapy combined with high-dose corticosteroids that are aimed at preventing an inflammatory reaction to the radiotherapy, as this will exacerbate the symptoms. The high-dose corticosteroids need to be reduced carefully and quickly to prevent complications. The radiotherapy may be given as a short course, depending on the primary diagnosis (Souhami & Tobias 2003). Chemotherapy may be considered if the primary tumour is chemosensitive, such as lymphoma or small-cell lung cancer (Hoskin & Makin 2003d).

Radiological stenting of the superior vena cava vessels has become possible and offers a valuable alternative to radiotherapy. It is a useful option if the problem recurs (Neal & Hoskin 1997).

Side-effects of radiotherapy to the chest

Oesophagitis, which can be troublesome for patients having treatment to the chest, occurs because of the rapid replication rate of the gastrointestinal mucosa. Pain can be a particular problem following intraluminal brachytherapy, because the radioactive source is close to the oesophagus. High fluid intake and an oral local anaesthetic with an alkaline or aspirin suspension will relieve pain by acting locally on the oesophageal mucosa. In severe cases morphine, together with sucralfate suspension, may offer relief from pain.

Pneumonitis may occur after radiotherapy to the chest if the lungs are in the treatment field. It has an acute phase, beginning from 6 weeks to 3 months after radiotherapy. Mild cases resolve but more serious cases require antibiotic treatment and steroids (Neal & Hoskin 1997). Pulmonary fibrosis and permanent respiratory compromise may result.

Oesophageal stricture

This is caused by a cancerous growth obstructing the oesophagus and can be treated palliatively in a number of ways. Surgical bypass may be an option, or the placement of a tube or a stent to allow the patient to maintain some oral intake of fluids (Souhami & Tobias 2003). Stenting is covered in more depth later in the chapter. Laser therapy can be used in conjunction with radiotherapy, although long-term evaluation is still awaited (Souhami & Tobias 2003).

Modest doses of radiotherapy can produce worthwhile results. The radiotherapy can be given externally over 1–2 weeks or it can be given as brachytherapy. Some patients may experience oesophagitis; the management of this was discussed above.

Fungating tumours

A fungating cancer is a primary or secondary malignant growth in the skin that has ulcerated, resulting in pain, exudate, bleeding, infection and malodour (Twycross 1997, Walding 1998). These tumours are common in patients with breast, vulval or penile cancers, and some head and neck cancers. The wound may have the appearance of a raised nodule or an ulcerated crater with a distinct margin (Moody & Grocott 1993). Because of the extent of the growth, treatment will be only palliative, but surgery may be considered, depending upon the site involved. Often a combined approach using a topical antibiotic agent such as metronidazole gel and radiotherapy is used. Metronidazole helps to reduce malodour and treats infection caused by anaerobic bacteria. Radiotherapy reduces tumour bulk and the amount of exudate produced.

Sucralfate gel can also be used in the management of both fungating tumours and surface bleeding (Regnard & Hockley 2004, Twycross 1997, Waller & Caroline 1996).

Haemorrhage

Non-acute bleeding can occur with some cancers as the growth erodes through smaller blood vessels. This can be seen as haemoptysis, vaginal bleeding, haematuria and rectal bleeding (Kaye 2003). Hoy (1993) describes radiotherapy as the most useful oncological treatment for tumour-related haemorrhage.

Radiotherapy can be given externally or by using brachytherapy techniques. Brachytherapy techniques can also be used to treat vaginal bleeding from gynaecological cancer. Whale (1991) believes that radiotherapy has an important role in palliating symptoms such as vaginal bleeding and pain. An applicator is placed into the vagina and uterus, into which radioactive sources are placed – brachytherapy. This is often an effective way of delivering radiotherapy treatment, but because of the close proximity of the bladder and bowel to the radioactive sources the patient may experience some short-term side-effects.

Diathermy or laser therapy may be of some use in the management of haemoptysis or haematuria (Neal & Hoskin 1997). Sucralfate can be given orally or used topically to treat superficial bleeding (Hoy 1993, Regnard & Hockley 2004, Waller & Caroline 1996). Some side-effects are common to radiotherapy and chemotherapy, and are discussed at the end of the section relating to side-effects from chemotherapy.

Care of site-specific side–effects

Skin care

Because the epithelial cells replicate rapidly they are more sensitive to damage caused by radiation (Campbell & Lane 1996, Holmes 1996b). In their paper on developing a skin care protocol, Campbell & Lane (1996) suggested that the use of research-based skin care would remove some of the outdated practices in use. One controversial area is whether patients can wash the area being treated or not. A study conducted by Campbell & Illingworth (1992) demonstrated that there was little difference in the incidence of skin reactions between patients who washed and those who did not. Webb (1979) pointed out that not washing can be distressing for patients and may be socially unacceptable.

Patients receiving chemotherapy and radiotherapy may be more prone to developing reactions, because chemotherapy can make the skin more prone to radiation damage. If a reaction does develop, the area may become reddened, like mild sunburn. This can progress from dry to moist desquamation (Campbell & Lane 1996). The skin will not repair until the treatment is complete, but prompt identification can prevent the reaction from progressing.

In patients receiving palliative radiotherapy, one would not expect to see anything more than a mild reaction, except in those having treatment over a 4-week period, in some head and neck cancers.

Oral care

Oral care is especially important for patients receiving radiotherapy to the head and neck area because the oral mucosa is prone to damage. Palliative radiotherapy may be considered in this group of patients to relieve obstructive symptoms (Neal & Hoskin 1997). The problems related to treatment in this area include mucositis, pain, dry mouth, infection, anorexia, altered taste and psychological problems (Feber 1995). These problems often develop early in treatment due to the fast replication rate of cells in this area (Faithfull 2001). Good oral hygiene should include using a soft toothbrush and regular mouthwashes (Turner 1996). Some over-the-counter mouthwashes contain alcohol, which can dry the oral mucosa, making it more susceptible to damage. Saliva substitutes can be used to lubricate the mucous membranes (Heals 1993). The use of bio-adherent gels may also help promote comfort, and should be considered as a dry mouth can have a detrimental impact on quality of life. Mouth dryness following radiotherapy can persist for some weeks after treatment is complete. High fluid intake will help to maintain lubrication. Good pain management is essential, and the prompt detection and treatment of oral infections will increase comfort.

Adequate nutritional intake is important to provide the body with sufficient protein to enable cellular repair. This can be compromised if the patient is experiencing altered taste, anorexia or dysphagia. Effective nursing and early involvement of a dietician can help with the management of these problems. Some patients may require enteral feeding during treatment, via a percutaneous endoscopic gastrostomy (PEG) tube, which can be managed by the patient or carer at home. This ensures adequate nutritional and fluid intake, thereby helping the body to cope with the effect of treatment, and can also have a positive impact on the recovery process.

Case Study 4.1

Mr Wright, a 74-year-old man, was diagnosed with lung cancer. His disease was locally advanced and he was not well enough to tolerate chemotherapy. He had a course of palliative radiotherapy to his chest. He had severe dyspnoea before treatment and found this worsened after his treatment. He was bed-bound, being frightened to move as any exertion worsened his breathlessness. He developed oesophagitis, had no appetite and was losing weight. He was not sleeping well and had a troublesome cough, which was worse at night. He had lost interest in his family and in things around him, and was feeling fairly hopeless. The treatment had made him feel worse than he did before he had it.

Mr Wright was prescribed a 2-week course of steroids to reduce the possible inflammatory response within the lung tissue, and it was hoped that they might also increase his appetite. He was prescribed oral morphine solution to take as required for his troublesome cough. He was referred to a community Macmillan physiotherapist in relation to managing his breathlessness. A stair-lift was provided to encourage him to go downstairs during the day, and a Zimmer frame to provide support when he was walking. The steroids had the desired effect and, despite taking a number of months, Mr Wright is now able to get out and about, and has regained a quality of life that he thought was no longer possible. He does not use the oral morphine now and is contemplating driving again. He is followed up by the chest physician and his disease is stable at present.

WHAT IS CHEMOTHERAPY?

Chemotherapy is the use of chemical agents that are toxic to cells (cytotoxic), aimed at eradicating or reducing the overall population of cancer cells. Unfortunately, as with radiotherapy, the drugs presently available do not act on cancer cells alone. Normal cells are also affected, causing the patient to experience side-effects. Cells that replicate rapidly are more readily affected by cytotoxic drugs (Blows 2005, Burton 1988, Dougherty & Bailey 2001, Holmes 1997). This applies to both malignant and normal cells.

There are currently 40 to 50 cytotoxic drugs licensed to treat cancer. Combinations of drugs may be used to increase the number of cancer cells damaged, but hopefully without producing more side-effects (Hoskin & Makin 2003e). Pharmacology and drug administration are not covered in this chapter, but have been discussed in depth by Dougherty & Bailey (2001), Holmes (1997), Luken & Middleton (1995) and Neal & Hoskin (1997).

Chemotherapy has proved successful in managing some childhood cancers, testicular teratoma, some lymphomas and leukaemias. There has been an increase in the use of chemotherapy as an adjuvant treatment together with surgery and/or radiotherapy, particularly in patients with breast cancer, colorectal cancer, and some head and neck cancers. Studies have shown this can improve disease-free survival time in some patients (Curt & Chabner 1987 in Holmes 1997).

Palliative chemotherapy

Chemotherapy is able to destroy both the primary tumour and distant metastases (Holmes 1996c). Kaye & Levy (1997, p 39) state: 'Palliative chemotherapy may be given to patients with locally advanced or metastatic disease in order to prolong life, control symptoms or improve quality of life'. They see palliative chemotherapy as a partnership between the patient and the professionals, and not focused just on the cancer. The aim of the treatment is to relieve symptoms while causing minimal side-effects. Oliver et al (1997) agree with this, stating: 'It is therefore essential to involve the patient and family in a therapeutic relationship. It is not sufficient merely to make information available: health professionals must be certain that the information is understood'. Hoskin & Makin (2003e) set out a list of indications for palliative chemotherapy.

Archer et al (1999) concluded that the evidence for palliative chemotherapy was growing because of the positive effect chemotherapy can have on quality of life. They examined a number of studies in a range of diseases.

Souhami & Tobias (2003) offer a salutary note that the potential benefits of palliative chemotherapy must be weighed carefully against unwanted effects. Many drugs developed to treat advanced cancer are given on a day case basis or as an oral preparation, if available, aiming to keep the patient at home while maintaining quality of life.

Kaye & Levy (1997) list the cancers commonly treated with palliative chemotherapy. Secondary deposits may respond to chemotherapy if the primary disease did initially. Palliative chemotherapy is frequently given to patients for whom there is little chance of response to other treatments and no chance of cure (Calvert & McElwain 1988). Patient information and education about the disease and treatment are vital as the patient must be able to have a sense of control and make informed choices.

Development of new drugs

Ling (1997) suggests that research in palliative care can meet with resistance, yet this is valuable work.

Calvert & McElwain (1988, p 300) point out: 'there are a large number of cancer patients for whom the chemotherapy drugs presently available have little or nothing to offer. Whether the research is studying new cytotoxic drugs, biological products, antibody-targeted drugs or non-cytotoxic anticancer agents they still need to be tested so that their role may be established'. Even though this was written over 10 years ago, it is still applicable today. Since 1988 we have seen the introduction and licensing of the taxanes, raltitrexed, epirubicin and carboplatin, to name but a few.

There is no way of knowing how effective the treatment will be, as Calvert & McElwain (1988, p 300) have stated: 'drugs which show remarkable and curative activity when given to animals may be completely inactive in humans'.

Some of the drugs developed are analogues of drugs previously available, the new drugs being developed in order to reduce the toxicity profile. Drugs are also developed to manage the side-effects caused by treatment such as antiemetics and colony-stimulating factors. All of these drugs go through a similar research development programme. To satisfy strict ethical guidelines, new anticancer drugs have to be tested in patients who have no prospect of benefiting from other treatment (Kaye & Levy 1997).

It is more relevant in palliative care to consider what happens to the patient not what happens to the tumour (Oliver et al 1997). Quality of life is an important issue within oncology and palliative care, and more often today clinical trials conducted with new drugs examine the clinical effectiveness of the drugs and the effects on the patient's quality of life. There is no value in developing a drug that leaves the patient debilitated. Conversely, some drugs/regimens have been shown to improve patients' quality of life while not having a dramatic clinical impact (Hardy et al 1989 in Oliver et al 1997).

Neal & Hoskin (1997) point out: 'measurement of quality of life has become an increasingly sophisticated exercise'. There are tools available such as the Rotterdam Symptom Checklist or the Hospital Anxiety and Depression scale. Clinical trials often incorporate the European Organisation for the Research and Treatment of Cancer (EORTC) questionnaire QLQ-C 30. This has supplements specific to certain cancer sites, for example breast cancer.

Clinical trials are strictly governed, requiring approval from multi-regional ethical committees (MRECs) and local ethical committees (LECs) before proceeding. Documentation has to be thorough, as data collection is usually overseen by the drug company or the group coordinating the research.

There are four stages or phases of clinical trials relating to the stage of use of the drug. At all phases the patient has to give written informed consent, having been given a full verbal and written explanation about the trial (Ling 1997). The patient has the right to withdraw from the trial at any time without giving a reason and without compromising future treatment and support (Oliver et al 1997).

In phase I studies the drugs are being given to humans for the first time. It is not known what clinical benefit will be seen, if any, at this stage (Holmes 1997). The aim of these studies is to identify a safe maximum dose to study at phase II, and to identify the drug's toxicity profile. Phase I studies are offered to patients for whom there is no recognised treatment (Neal & Hoskin 1997); they may have widespread disease, and be resistant to a variety of chemotherapy drugs (Souhami & Tobias 2003).

In phase II studies the drug is given to groups of patients with a specific cancer, in whom a response is expected. Patients in these studies may have had conventional treatment but have subsequently relapsed.

Phase III studies are often called randomised controlled trials (RCTs), where the new drug or regimen will be compared against the existing 'gold standard' treatment. One difficulty with phase III studies is that patients have to be given information about both treatments, and often hope that they will receive the new treatment, sometimes equating 'new' with 'best'.

Phase IV studies are post-marketing studies, usually with the new drug funded by the drug company (Coleman & Hancock 1996, Neal & Hoskin 1997).

Hoskin & Makin (2003f) point out that only a small number of patients who are eligible for clinical trials will be entered into them. In an attempt to improve this situation, a clinical trials network has been established to run alongside the already established Cancer Networks to try to ensure that those patients who are eligible are considered and offered the opportunity to take part in a clinical trial.

Liver metastases

Hoskin & Makin (2003g) point out that up to a half of patients dying with cancer will have liver metastases, the most common primary cancers being those of breast, lung and colon, with the cancer spreading to the liver via the bloodstream. The presentation may initially be vague but the patient may present with jaundice and an itch, due to bile salts being excreted on to the skin. Depending on the fitness of the patient and the extent of the disease, surgical resection may be an option if a solitary deposit is present. If jaundice has developed because of tumour obstructing the bile duct then insertion of a stent may give some relief. In colorectal cancer, 25% of relapses are confined to metastases in the liver (Hoskin & Makin 2003g). Chemotherapy may be offered depending on the overall clinical picture, often using drugs specific to the primary tumour type; a response is seen in 50–60% of patients with chemoresponsive primary tumours, such as breast or small-cell lung cancer (Souhami & Tobias 2003). In some cases this can produce a good response with resolution of symptoms occurring quickly. Unfortunately, symptoms often recur within a few months of completing chemotherapy (Hoskin & Makin 2003g).

Hypercalcaemia

Hypercalcaemia is a common problem occurring in approximately 10% of all cancer patients (Hoskin & Makin 2003h). It is associated with lung cancer, breast and prostate cancer, oesophageal cancer, and head and neck cancers. Presenting symptoms can be constipation, nausea, confusion and dehydration of varying degrees. Patients with the aforementioned cancers who present with these symptoms should have blood taken to check calcium levels.

Downing (2001) describes the physiology of hypercalcaemia as well as the treatment of this often distressing symptom. Intravenous fluids are often the initial treatment followed by the use of bisphosphonates which may be prescribed in the management of malignant hypercalcaemia (Fleisch 1995). Hoskin & Makin (2003c) identified that bisphosphonates are being used increasingly in the management of bone metastases in both breast cancer and myeloma. Bisphosphonates can be given intravenously or orally. They work by inhibiting bone resorption (Needham 1997, Souhami & Tobias 2003) and can also reduce pain, the risk of fractures and the need for analgesia, while enhancing quality of life (O'Brien 1993). There is an increase in the use of oral bisphosphonates; from a quality of life perspective, it reduces the frequency of hospital attendances.

Malignant effusions

Malignant effusions can develop within the pleural cavity, pericardial cavity and the peritoneal cavity. Pleural and pericardial effusion are most commonly associated with cancer of the lung or breast. Peritoneal effusion, or ascites, is associated with ovarian cancer or secondary liver disease from colorectal cancer.

These effusions can be drained, giving instant relief to the patient. However, as mentioned by Hoskin & Makin (2003d), repeated paracentesis or pleural aspiration can result in loculation of the fluid, which can reduce the efficacy of subsequent attempts to aspirate the fluid. However, if the effusions recur then, after drainage of the pleural effusion, pleurodesis can be performed. This involves instilling sterile talcum powder, and in some cases chemotherapeutic drugs or a radioactive isotope, into the pleural cavity. The aim of this is to encourage the development of adhesions between the pleural linings, thereby preventing recurrent build-up of pleural fluid (Hoskin & Makin 2003d, Kaye 2004). Similarly, after drainage of ascitic fluid, cytotoxic agents or a radioactive isotope can be instilled in an attempt to slow down the recurrent build-up of ascitic fluid. The careful use of diuretics can also be considered as a non-invasive way to manage ascites (Regnard & Hockley 2004).

SIDE-EFFECTS OF PALLIATIVE CHEMOTHERAPY

This section focuses on side-effects related to the administration of palliative chemotherapy. There are other side-effects, which are covered in depth in texts such as Dougherty & Bailey (2001), Holmes (1997), Luken & Middleton (1995) and Stein (1996).

Hair loss

Hair loss is a concern to all patients who need chemotherapy. It is therefore important to find out for the patient whether the drugs they are to receive will cause hair loss. Drugs that commonly cause hair loss are anthracyclines, vinca alkaloids, and other drugs such as ifosfamide, docetaxel, paclitaxel and etoposide.

Hair loss is a psychologically distressing side-effect of chemotherapy. It offers a constant reminder to the patient of the situation they are in. Patients and their carers may find it difficult to address the issue of their hair loss with their children or grandchildren. Whenery-Tedder (1997) talks of the social and psychological impact of chemotherapy-induced hair loss because of the patient's altered body image.

Reassurance should be given that hair will return after completion of the chemotherapy, but that its texture and colour might be different because of the effects of the drug on hair follicles. A hairpiece should be provided before hair loss occurs. Turbans and head scarves are a popular alternative.

Scalp cooling is a technique used to prevent hair loss by reducing the amount of drugs reaching the scalp (Dougherty 1996, Holmes 1997, Hoskin & Makin 2003e).

Peripheral neuropathy

This side-effect has been seen with cisplatin and the vinca alkaloids. Although it is a late effect, presenting months after completion of treatment, it is irreversible.

Since the introduction of the taxanes, patients have been known to develop mild to moderate neuropathy with early onset. The extent of the neuropathy ranges from pins and needles to reduced mobility. This effect does appear to improve on completion of the treatment, and patients should be made aware of its possibility before treatment. Aston (1997) suggests that patients need to be told how to cope with this distressing symptom.

Altered bowel habits

Diarrhoea or constipation may be experienced by patients receiving chemotherapy; they are equally distressing, often causing abdominal pain and discomfort. Diarrhoea often results from the effect that chemotherapy drugs have on the gastrointestinal mucosa (Dougherty & Bailey 2001).

The patient may be given antidiarrhoeal medication and dietary advice, such as to have a bland low-fibre diet and high fluid intake – up to 3 litres of fluid a day to prevent dehydration and electrolyte imbalance.

Constipation may be a problem, particularly in patients treated with vinca alkaloids, as these drugs reduce gut motility (Dougherty & Bailey 2001, Holmes 1997). There may be other factors that can compound the problem, such as the use of opioid analgesics, lack of exercise and alteration in diet. Prophylactic aperients can be prescribed, together with a high-fibre diet (Holmes 1997).

Giving information to the patient at an early stage will ease some distress and anxiety caused by lack of information. It also aids early recognition of problems and enables prompt treatment, although it may cause some patients concern.

SIDE-EFFECTS COMMON TO RADIOTHERAPY AND CHEMOTHERAPY
Nausea and vomiting

Nausea and vomiting are two distressing side-effects related to radiotherapy and chemotherapy. With radiotherapy they may be related to the area or the

Case Study 4.2

Freda, a 68-year-old woman, was diagnosed with cancer of the ovary. She also suffered from arthritis and had had two knee replacements and one hip replaced. Freda's main problem was hip pain. She saw an orthopaedic surgeon for consideration of another hip replacement. After diagnosis she received treatment with curative intent. Freda had surgery followed by eight cycles of chemotherapy, which she tolerated well. She was now on 3-monthly follow-up by the oncologist. Freda had her hip replacement and in the intervening time was referred to the physiotherapist as her mobility was worsening and she was developing back pain.

Freda was prescribed morphine to help control the pain she was experiencing in her hip and back. She had a bone scan prior to her hip replacement and made a good recovery in the immediate postoperative period. At follow-up it was identified that the levels of tumour markers were raised, and 18 months after her initial diagnosis she was found to have disease progression.

Freda had a different combination of chemotherapy drugs this time. She was aware of the possible side-effects. With her first course of chemotherapy, she had difficulty with her blood count but knew the signs to look out for. Freda had some nausea after her first cycle of chemotherapy so was prescribed metoclopramide 10 mg three times daily, but this was changed to domperidone as she started to feel agitated and restless. Freda was not sure whether this was due to the steroid that she was taking as part of her antiemetic regimen. Her hair fell out before the second cycle of chemotherapy; she had good support from her hairdresser and family. Freda had an anaphylactic

reaction when she was having her second cycle of chemotherapy; although this was very frightening for her, she was still keen to continue chemotherapy, so the carboplatin was changed to cisplatin which she received as an inpatient. After three cycles of chemotherapy a computed tomographic (CT) scan showed good response so Freda continued on chemotherapy and had six cycles in total. A CT scan after chemotherapy showed a good response, and Freda, despite knowing that she could not be cured, hoped to have a similar length of time, disease free, before needing more treatment. In the meantime Freda attended the day hospice to ensure that she did not become socially isolated as a result of her illness and treatment.

Freda recovered well after chemotherapy and it was possible to discontinue the morphine. Six months later disease progression was identified again as the levels of tumour markers were rising; a CT scan confirmed what was happening. Freda was keen to accept chemotherapy, if it was offered, her hope being to live a little longer. During this round of chemotherapy Freda lost her hair, had one or two treatments postponed because of a low neutrophil count, and had problems with nausea and vomiting. Peripheral neuropathy was also problematic; Freda loved to crochet and knit but found she was unable to do these activities because of the neuropathy; Fatigue proved to be frustrating for Freda as she liked to be as active as possible.

Freda has now completed her third course of chemotherapy and is well at the moment.

---

duration of treatment. The byproducts of cell breakdown, urea and creatinine, are normally toxic in large amounts. Large numbers of cells are being broken down as a result of treatment. The toxins produced will be detected in the blood by the chemoreceptor trigger zone and a response initiated. These mechanisms have been discussed more fully by Williams (1994) and Holmes (1997).

Quinton (1998) says that 'maintaining adequate control of nausea and vomiting can preserve the quality of an individual's life and enable patients and their families to endure what can be a demanding course of chemotherapy'. There is a number of factors that can induce nausea and vomiting (Williams 1994), and others that can predispose a person to be more likely to develop nausea and vomiting, such as motion sickness (Adams 1993). Good patient assessment will help to ensure the appropriate prescribing of antiemetic drugs and reduce the incidence of this

side-effect. It is helpful to understand the mechanisms involved in producing this response, as this will aid in more appropriate prescribing of antiemetics (Williams 1994). Williams (1994) states: 'Psychologically, uncontrolled nausea and vomiting may well cause anxiety and distress to patients, their relatives and friends'. Patients who have had chemotherapy previously, possibly intense or aggressive regimens, may experience anticipatory nausea and vomiting, which is difficult to manage because it is psychologically driven. An anxiolytic such as lorazepam can be useful because it helps patients forget the experience of vomiting.

Hypnotherapy can be used to help in the management of anticipatory nausea and vomiting by offering the patient a sense of control (Stein 1996). Other complementary measures such as pressure bands are described by Stannard (1989). Distraction and acupuncture have also been used with some success.

Bone marrow depression

This can present as anaemia, leucopenia and thrombocytopenia. Myelosuppression can be caused by both radiotherapy and chemotherapy; the presenting signs and care of the patient are similar, regardless of the cause. If patients have had a number of courses of chemotherapy, they may be at greater risk of developing myelosuppression.

With radiotherapy the development and extent of myelosuppression depends on the extent of bone marrow in the treatment field (Holmes 1996a). The structure of the bone marrow may be permanently altered, leaving the patient compromised (Holmes 1996a).

Dougherty & Bailey (2001), Luken & Middleton (1995) and Stein (1996) have pointed out that the myelosuppression caused by chemotherapy is the most common dose-limiting toxicity and is potentially fatal. A degree of myelosuppression is produced by all chemotherapeutic drugs, and the effect may increase if a combination of drugs is given or if the patient is receiving concurrent radiotherapy and chemotherapy.

The blood count is monitored before each pulse or cycle of chemotherapy. Treating a patient with a low neutrophil count can result in the patient becoming neutropenic, leading to an increased risk of developing septicaemia. The patient needs to be taught the signs and symptoms of all of these effects, and advised about home management and when to contact the hospital for further advice. Holmes (1997) noted that chemotherapy does not affect mature blood cells but damages the stem cells responsible for the replacement of depleted blood cells. Red blood cells are stored within the body; white blood cells and platelets are not stored but produced as needed. Anaemia is easily corrected by blood transfusion. Thrombocytopenia can be treated with a platelet transfusion.

Leucopenia is a significant problem in patients receiving chemotherapy, and is often the dose-limiting factor. A low neutrophil count leaves the patient susceptible to infection or septicaemia. Studies have shown that 85% of infections in neutropenic patients are caused by their own natural flora (Holmes 1997).

Leucopenia may present as a fever, rigor, redness and pus at a central catheter access site. Patients who do have a low white cell count and are without symptoms may be sent home to wait for the count to recover before the next cycle of chemotherapy. They may receive a course of prophylactic antibiotics. Patients who present with symptoms as well as a low white cell count may be admitted and receive intravenous antibiotics. They may require nursing in protective isolation until the bone marrow starts to recover.

The development and use of haematopoietic growth factors has had an impact on the management of chemotherapy-induced neutropenia, reducing the duration of neutropenia and reducing antibiotic use (Dougherty & Bailey 2001). These factors are not used routinely for all patients, but are often used to support patients having high-dose chemotherapy or those whose bone marrow is compromised as a result of previous treatment.

Fatigue

Fatigue can be experienced by patients having radiotherapy or chemotherapy. Fatigue is often associated with anaemia, especially that caused by chemotherapy. With radiotherapy the fatigue may be made worse by travelling to and from the treatment department. Patients often report that fatigue is a serious side-effect that has a detrimental effect on their quality of life. They are affected to varying degrees, both physically and psychologically (Snape & Robinson 1996), ranging from feeling tired, lethargic and anorexic to loss of social function and loss of libido. Fatigue can have a dramatic impact on a person's ability to carry out activities of daily living and can lead to a sense of frustration, emotional distress and low mood; often a lack of understanding can lead to problems between patients and their carers. Faithfull (2003) gives a detailed description of the aetiology of fatigue and reviews articles on the subject of fatigue and radiotherapy. The recommendations for clinical practice made by Faithfull (2003) can be applied equally well to patients being treated with chemotherapy.

A number of factors are thought to contribute to the development of fatigue: an increase in metabolic rate caused by the cancer; an increased demand on the body's resources to repair normal cells damaged by treatment; and an increase in cell breakdown and excretion of toxic byproducts (Snape & Robinson 1996). Fatigue may not develop immediately and can persist for months after treatment. It is valuable to find out what fatigue means to patients, as they may believe the symptoms to be caused by disease progression rather than fatigue or anaemia (Holmes 1996a). Patients should be informed of this possible effect of treatment and given support and advice about how to minimise its impact. Planning the day, resting before becoming tired and eating well can help. Two very useful reviews about fatigue in cancer patients have been written by Richardson (1995) and Stone et al (1998).

Stomatitis

A sore mouth can be caused by some chemotherapeutic drugs or radiotherapy to the head and neck. There is a dramatic shift towards administering oral chemotherapy drugs. This can range from general soreness, loss of taste and loss of papillae from the tongue, to severe painful ulceration. Stomatitis is produced because the oral mucosa replicates rapidly, making it more susceptible to the effects of chemotherapy.

Patient education about oral hygiene is important, as discussed earlier in the chapter. An oral hygiene regimen using a soft toothbrush and regular mouthwashes can help to keep the mouth moist and clean. In addition, mouthwashes containing a topical analgesic can reduce pain. Oral assessment tools can be beneficial. Patients receiving chemotherapy may be prone to oral infections, and the mouth can be an ideal entry point for bacteria. Corticosteroids may increase the susceptibility of the patient to the development of oral *Candida*, which can be treated with an antifungal or antibacterial preparation.

Taste alteration may occur and some patients develop an aversion to certain drinks or food. Some patients also experience a metallic taste in their mouth during administration of some drugs; sucking mints or sweets may help. This can be constant or intermittent and is often distressing, so mentioning the possibility of this sensation developing can ease some of the distress experienced. The taste generally reverts to normal when chemotherapy is completed (Speechley 1989).

Hormone therapy

The development of some cancers depends in part on certain hormones (Holmes 1997, Hoskin & Makin 2003e). Hormone manipulation is known to be of value in the management of some cancers, such as breast, prostate and endometrium (Hancock et al 1996, Kaye & Levy 1997, Moore 1995, Neal & Hoskin 1997). Hormones will not cure a patient but they can help to slow down the rate of growth (Hancock et al 1996). The aim of this treatment is either to block the action of hormones, modify the release of certain hormones or alter the hormonal environment (Hoskin & Makin 2003e). Most hormones can be taken orally which proves beneficial especially when using drugs in the palliative arena. Oestrogens, antioestrogens, androgens, progestogens and aromatase inhibitors are used. These drugs produce side-effects, which have been discussed by Fenlon (2001), Hancock et al (1996), Holmes (1997) and Moore (1995).

Case Study 4.3

Jen, a 51-year-old woman, completed a lengthy process of diagnosis which ended with her being diagnosed with mediastinal metastases from an unknown primary. It was initially thought that the metastases might be from a lung primary, but because Jen had a family history of breast cancer it was decided to treat Jen with a regimen of breast cancer chemotherapy.

Initially Jen had palliative radiotherapy to her chest to reduce the size of the metastases. Jen's partner was having radiotherapy for cancer of the prostate at the same time as Jen was receiving her treatment.

WHAT SIDE-EFFECTS MIGHT SHE HAVE EXPERIENCED FROM RADIOTHERAPY?
Jen completed her radiotherapy with few problems but 1 week after completion she developed oesophagitis, which was treated with sucralfate. She commenced chemotherapy a few weeks after completing radiotherapy, receiving six cycles of chemotherapy at 3-week intervals.

WHAT SIDE-EFFECTS MIGHT SHE HAVE EXPERIENCED FROM CHEMOTHERAPY?
Jen had a very pragmatic approach to the situation, but was also determined to fight as hard as possible. She tolerated the chemotherapy very well. The nausea and vomiting were treated with standard antiemetic medication.

When chemotherapy was completed, Jen's mood became quite low; she found not having treatment difficult to deal with psychologically. Jen does still have a degree of dyspnoea, possibly due to the development of pulmonary fibrosis in the areas of her lungs that were in the radiotherapy treatment field. She is waiting for a bone scan and CT at present as she has developed a new back pain.

RADIOLOGICAL INTERVENTION IN PALLIATIVE CARE

Silicone or metal stents are used widely in the palliation of cancer. Advantages have to be carefully balanced against the disadvantages and discomfort the patient may experience. Biliary and bronchial stents (Fig. 4.1) can alleviate symptoms from cholangiocarcinoma and lung cancer respectively, and compressed or compromised blood vessels such as the superior and inferior vena cavae can be managed by stenting. Stents can also be used in the management of oesophageal and renal obstruction (Watkinson & Adam 1996). The use of rectal stents is now accepted in some centres for advanced carcinoma of the rectum (Fig. 4.2). Usually these patients are not fit for surgical procedures owing to advanced disease, but require immediate symptom relief from rectal

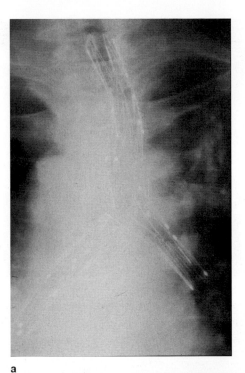

a

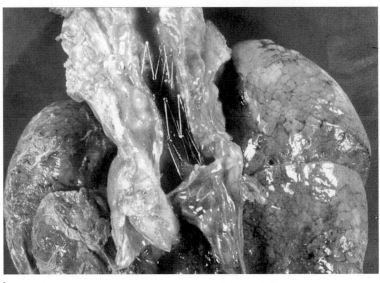

b

Figure 4.1   (a) Radiograph showing bronchial stents in position to maintain patient's airway which is severely compressed externally by tumour. (b) Position of the stents after autopsy. Note surrounding tumour compressing the bronchus. (By kind permission of South Tyneside NHS Foundation Trust.)

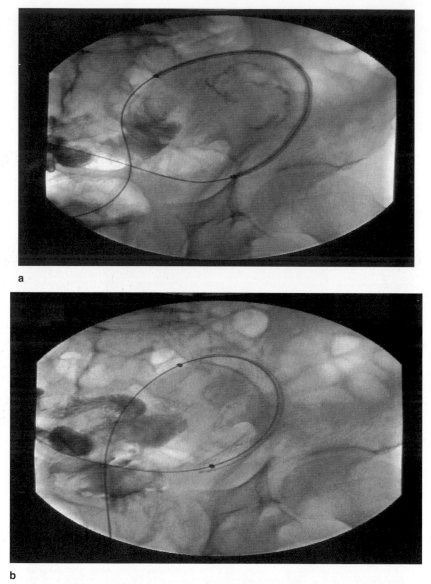

Figure 4.2   Radiographs showing a rectal stent **(a)** in position prior to deployment for rectal carcinoma and **(b)** fully deployed and open inside the rectum and maintaining a full lumen. (By kind permission of South Tyneside NHS Foundation Trust.)

obstruction by radiological interventions. Other reasons may include anaesthetic risk due to a poor health performance status, for example chronic obstructive airway disease, chronic heart failure or other cardiac-associated morbidities. Newer, covered oesophageal stents have an antireflux valve incorporated inside the stent body, including an 'antimigration' design – the Hanarostent or do stents, as they are referred to by some centres (Fig. 4.3).

The design prevents migration of the stent and, more importantly, the difficult symptoms that may follow oesophageal stent insertion, especially acid reflux, which is often distressing and painful for these patients. The main purpose of the stents is to maintain the natural lumen of the organ or vessel compromised (Fig. 4.4). Stents are usually made from an expensive material called nitinol. The expense of the stents must be considered in the light of the improvement in quality of life that they facilitate. A case study featuring a patient with recurrent oesophageal and pyloric carcinoma illustrates the benefits of stents. The patient's name is fictitious.

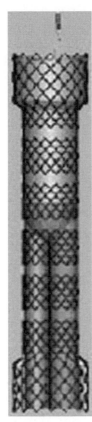

Figure 4.3 Covered oesophageal antireflux and antimigratory stent (Hanarostent or do stent). (By kind permission of M.I. Tech, c/o Diagmed, Thirsk, UK.)

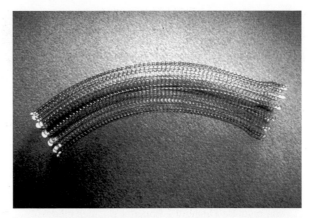

a

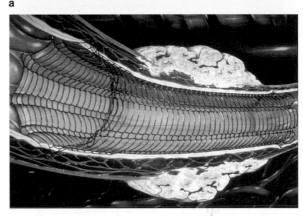

b

Figure 4.4 (a) The Boston Scientific Microvasive Ultraflex Stent; (b) stent *in situ*. (By kind permission of Boston Scientific, St Albans, UK.)

Case Study 4.4

INTRODUCTION

Palliative care is a programme of active, compassionate care that is directed primarily towards improving the quality of life. It is a discipline with its own growing research and knowledge base, and a specific set of skills aimed at symptom control and psychological support. Palliative care allows explicit goals for therapy and informed choices for patients. All of the family is affected by the chronic illness of one member and so palliative care services involve the whole family as the unit of care. Holistic care for both patient and family is delivered by an interdisciplinary team (Hanson & Cullihall 1996). This case study is unusual because of the palliative measures taken to alleviate difficult symptoms of oesophageal and secondary pyloric carcinoma, using modern invasive techniques. The team faced many difficulties, supporting the patient and his family through many disappointments. This time was also emotionally and physically demanding for those who cared for the patient. The study will make clear

why modern techniques to prolong and sustain life in the terminally ill should be used despite negative attitudes expressed by others. A combination of team effort and minimally invasive techniques brought comfort and dignity to the patient and his family.

PATIENT HISTORY

Dave, a 56-year-old man, was diagnosed with oesophageal carcinoma. He lived with his loving wife, Sylvia. His only daughter was married but remained close to her father. Seven months previously an oesophagectomy had been performed. The stomach had been pulled into the right thoracic cavity and the upper part of the oesophagus joined to the immobilised stomach and duodenum. A node dissection was performed at surgery. Dave received a course of radiotherapy soon after his surgical recovery. He was readmitted 4 months later because of epigastric pain and occasional nausea and vomiting. An oesophagogastroduodenostomy (OGD) examination 2

Case Study 4.4 – cont'd

days later revealed recurrent cancer obstructing the gastric pylorus. Abdominal ultrasonography showed liver metastases, and chest radiography demonstrated chest abnormalities.

On admission Dave was told about the possible recurrence and advancement of his disease and that the cancer was incurable. Dave and Sylvia were extremely anxious. Dave had not retired and they had made many plans, thinking the initial surgery had been successful. Their first grandchild was soon to be born.

Primary nursing was used to ensure continuity in nursing care throughout Dave's stay. His nursing care was organised using the Roper et al (1980) model of nursing. The surgical and palliative care teams worked together to care for Dave and his family. The primary nurse ensured that Sylvia was an integral part of Dave's care. Care was planned around a usual daily routine, while Dave was in hospital. Most of his subsequent care took place in a hospice, which helped ease the family's distress. Dave's initial aim was to 'get over this setback'. He wanted to live at home within the surroundings he and Sylvia had worked hard for over the years. Dave had never suffered from ill-health until he complained of difficulty in swallowing 4 months before his operation. Sadly, his disease had now spread, and Dave and Sylvia knew that time together was the only valuable thing during this difficult journey towards death.

OESOPHAGEAL CANCER

Oesophageal cancer is commoner in males, with a male:female ratio of about 2:1, and usually occurs in individuals over 50 years of age (Belcher 1992). In the UK, it has become more prevalent in the past 10 years. There is much evidence to indicate that oesophageal cancer is related to excessive alcohol and tobacco smoking, as well as to nutritional deficiencies and environmental carcinogens (Souhami & Tobias 1995).

Dysphagia is the commonest symptom and is almost always accompanied by weight loss, often amounting to 10% or more of body-weight. Recent evidence strongly supports the view that the incidence of adenocarcinoma of the oesophagus is increasing (Powel & McConkey 1990). Excision is the treatment of choice in patients who are generally fit and have no evidence of distant metastases. It is important to determine the extent of the lesion before definitive surgery. There is no evidence that preoperative radiotherapy influences recovery from the resection, operative mortality or overall survival (Earlam & Cunha-Melo 1980).

Dave's operation employed a technique using mobilised stomach above the diaphragm (Fig. 4.5) as a means of reconstruction. This is an extensive operation associated with a high risk of death. Surgical complications such as oesophageal stricture and anastomotic leak – resulting in mediastinitis, pneumonitis and septicaemia – can be fatal (Souhami & Tobias 1995).

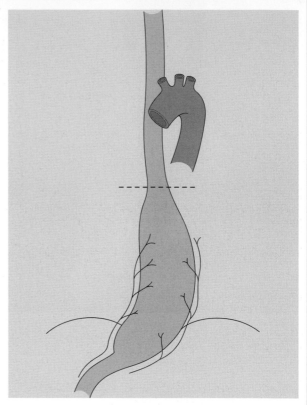

Figure 4.5 Surgery for oesophageal cancer, showing gastric mobilisation and pull-through for carcinoma of the lower third. (Reprinted with kind permission of Blackwell Science Ltd.)

With intensive nursing, Dave's surgery and recovery were successful, with no complications. He was discharged home until his present readmission with new symptoms and pain.

ISSUES REQUIRING CARE

Pain

Dave was experiencing epigastric pain, which became worse with episodes of nausea. It was difficult to know whether it was tumour pain or discomfort caused by the nausea. For most patients, physical pain is one of the greatest fears associated with cancer. Dave was afraid of morphine because of his experience when recovering from surgery. He had experienced hallucinations and was reluctant to take any medication. Although this is understandable, especially in responding as a nurse to a particular pain problem, the temptation may be to focus on that symptom alone. The patient must be allowed to identify his problems, and interventions should honour the value of the patient's perceptions (Davies & Oberle 1990).

Case Study 4.4 — cont'd

Pain assessment

Dave was allowed to talk about his fears about pain and to tell his story as a means of assessment. He looked pale and anxious. He talked about his original diagnosis and of his own and his family's hopes following the surgery. The pain seemed to indicate to Dave and his wife that the cancer had returned and they were frightened. They felt the possibility of metastatic spread had not been made clear to them at the time of the first operation. They both had ambivalent feelings towards medical staff and healthcare professionals. These feelings faded with careful handling, honesty and truth. Although Dave's general practitioner had asked for an urgent referral to the consultant, Dave had had to wait 4 weeks for admission. Despite the informality of the information gathering, the responses were sorted into pain concepts, so that appropriate resources could be utilised. Dave loved life and was looking forward to having grandchildren. He now felt he would never work again or drive a car and that, ultimately, this was the end.

It was decided to discuss Dave's fears of morphine with medical staff before choosing an appropriate analgesic. At this point a pain and symptom chart was introduced, using a new chart piloted by the ward, combining pain and associated symptoms on one chart. This was used to record when Dave admitted to having pain or was observed and assessed as having pain, and when analgesics were administered. There is a need for simple, efficient and valid assessment tools that can provide rapid evaluation in clinical settings of the major aspects of pain experienced by cancer patients (Foley 1982).

In view of Dave's nausea and the unsuitability of oral analgesics, it was decided to use 150 mg tramadol administered subcutaneously via a 24-hour syringe driver. Tramadol is a safe and effective agent introduced in the late 1970s to alleviate cancer pain. Its efficacy appears to be equivalent to that of morphine but is dose-dependent. It causes less constipation or respiratory depression. It causes weak activation of both central pain and inhibitory mechanisms in the opioid receptors, as well as the descending monoaminergic system (Budd 1995). Initially, tramadol did not control Dave's pain, so the dose was increased.

Dave experienced anxiety and depression as a result of his illness and altered body image. Both of these emotions are likely to exacerbate pain symptoms. Saunders (1990) described somatic and psychological experience of pain as 'total pain'. It is also directly related to the pain gate theory (Melzack & Wall 1965), and the role of the limbic system in which anxiety and depression serve to open the gate to varying degrees, thus heightening pain perception. It was important for the nurses to provide a supportive environment for Dave and his family.

Nausea

Dave was experiencing nausea on admission which was problematic; a gastroscopy revealed the recurrence of cancer at the pylorus of the immobilised stomach. The lumen from the pylorus had a stricture into the

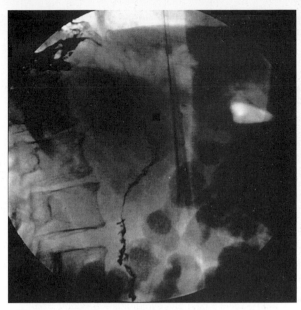

Figure 4.6   Radiograph showing the stricture of pylorus. (By kind permission of South Tyneside District Hospital.)

duodenum caused by the tumour, thus preventing the passage of food or fluids (Fig. 4.6).

A nasogastric tube had been inserted. It was allowed to drain freely and aspirated every 2 hours to keep the stomach empty. Intravenous therapy was started to establish and maintain a fluid intake of 3 litres over 24 hours.

In the hospice, fluids were given subcutaneously (hypodermoclysis). Hypodermoclysis is defined as the infusion of a solution into the subcutaneous tissue to supply the patient with a continuous and sufficient amount of fluid, electrolytes or nutrients (Urdang 1983). This is an easy and effective way to administer fluids.

Dave was kept informed about his treatment and told the findings of the gastroscopy by the surgeon. Surgical treatment to restore the continuity of the lumen could not be considered and other palliative treatments such as radiotherapy and chemotherapy were not an option at this stage. This meant that Dave would continue like this and die soon. Percutaneous gastroscopy (also known as venting gastroscopy) is often a last resort. The stomach drains continuously via a tube placed through the abdomen into the stomach. This allows the patient to drink without vomiting, as the fluids drain into a collecting bag (Ashby et al 1991). For Dave, the option of percutaneous gastroscopy was also impossible as his stomach was in his chest.

To control Dave's nausea, it was decided to give 150 mg cyclizine concurrently with tramadol, via the subcutaneous route. Cyclizine is an antihistamine with added anticholinergic activity. This drug was chosen as symptoms of bowel obstruction may be mediated partly by vagal afferent fibres (Mosby Drug Reference 1994).

Case Study 4.4 – cont'd

Once the nausea and pain were relieved, Dave slept for long periods over night. Sylvia was feeling guilty because he was in hospital and wanted to be at home with his family. Dave reconciled himself that he was in an environment where additional support was available 24 hours a day, should his symptoms return. Sylvia was always in a guilt dilemma and often needed reassurance from nursing staff that Dave was in the best place. Sylvia's own sleep pattern varied and as time moved on she began to look tired and thin.

The next day, after careful consideration and discussion with a radiologist, the team decided that the only option was to try an expansile metal stent implanted in the pyloric stricture to open up the lumen of the bowel. This would alleviate Dave's nausea and he would be able to manage oral medications and a modified liquid diet. He would not need intravenous fluids or nasogastric aspiration. This procedure is not without risks. Incorrect dilatation of the lumen during stent insertion carries the risk of bowel perforation. The recent use of expansile metallic stents had demonstrated an improved survival rate in patients like Dave. He felt at ease with this solution, and agreed to the procedure. The stent arrived within 2 days. During this time Dave's pain and symptoms were controlled. Preliminary radiographs were taken using a contrast opaque solution, instilled via the nasogastric tube. The radiographs enabled the length of the stricture to be measured, and allowed assessment of the extent of the stenosis and a decision on the position of the stent.

Metallic stent insertion

Normally an oesophageal expansile stent is not used in the pylorus and duodenum, because the peristaltic movement in this part of the bowel may dislodge the stent. Dave consented for the procedure, which took place in the radiology department using an image intensifier. When he was positioned (supine) on the table, an electrocardiographic (ECG) monitor was attached and oximetry attached by an ear probe to measure oxygen saturation (normal value greater than 92–94%). Oxygen was given via a nasal cannula throughout the procedure, and his blood pressure was measured before and after sedation with midazolam (increments of 2 mg given every 3 minutes if required). A nurse monitored his airway and vital signs throughout the procedure.

Insertion technique

1. A contrast solution was instilled via the nasogastric tube into the pylorus and stomach; at that time the head end of the table was raised.

2. No contrast solution was seen to enter the duodenum, so a guidewire was passed into the stomach and pushed with some force through the stricture.

3. Dilators were threaded one at a time over the guidewire, to dilate the stricture. At one point, contrast was seen to trickle into the duodenum, indicating a passage could be made.

4. After dilatation to the satisfaction of the radiologist, a special inflatable balloon dilator was threaded over the guidewire. The balloon could be inflated only to a pre-set pressure so as not to rupture the duodenum or pylorus. Only if a final dilatation was successful and satisfactory to the radiologist would the stent be considered.

5. The stent was now threaded over the guidewire encased within its gelatine covering. It proved very difficult to place, taking almost 2 hours, needing removal and re-insertion, and encountering many problems. The procedure was almost abandoned because of the difficulties. Another attempt was made, with extra pressure pushing the stent into the pylorus and duodenum; it was painful for Dave so he was given 50 mg pethidine intravenously with 2 mg midazolam. Finally, the stent was in position; the cover was removed, allowing the holding gel to dissolve and the stent to expand to its maximum size.

6. The stent was expanded internally by the insertion of the balloon dilator, to dilate the internal diameter to 12 mm. This would ensure that the whole stent would remain open.

7. More contrast solution was instilled, via the nasogastric tube. This showed that there was free flow through the stent and demonstrated a complete and successful procedure (Fig. 4.7).

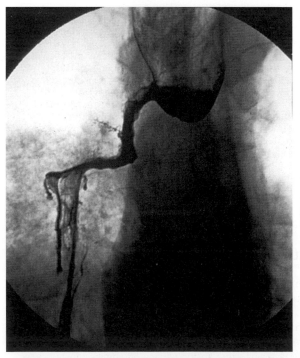

Figure 4.7 Radiograph showing the stent insertion and free-flowing contrast solution through the completely opened stent. (By kind permission of South Tyneside District Hospital.)

Case Study 4.4 — cont'd

Dave returned to the ward for observation; he awoke from sedation to hear the news of a successful positioning of the stent with good function.

The position and function of the stent was rechecked the next day and free clear oral fluids were commenced. It was checked again 5 days later; the extent of expansion was confirmed by radiography (Fig. 4.8).

Nutrition

The stent did not interfere with peristalsis but the pylorus could cope only with fluids. Dave's whole dietary intake was monitored and controlled by the dietician, who provided a high-protein, high-calorie diet. Medication was given in syrup form until his condition deteriorated, after which a syringe driver was used to administer analgesia continuously.

Pain revisited

As Dave's pain increased there was no alternative but to give morphine, as morphine slow-release sachets (MST) in liquid form. The doctor prescribed MST, 30 mg 12 hourly, and 10 mg oral morphine solution for breakthrough pain. Dave was also prescribed a laxative daily, to prevent constipation, and haloperidol subcutaneously at night, to alleviate nausea associated with the morphine. Dave never experienced hallucinations and his pain was well controlled.

The analgesic protocol enabled the registered nurse to respond promptly to Dave's pain without delay or needing to refer to a doctor each time Dave was in pain. Specifically, opioids were given by the clock (Latham 1991).

As Dave weakened, his medications were altered. Diamorphine replaced the MST and methotrimeprazine (30 mg over 24 hours) was given via a syringe-driver to relieve nausea. He responded well as methotrimeprazine (Nozinan) is an antipsychotic drug with anxiolytic and antiemetic properties, and is also a sedative (Joshua & King 1994). The dosage can be increased to 250 mg in 24 hours, and methotrimeprazine can potentiate the action of diamorphine, causing further sedation. Dave continued to weaken and gradually became unconscious. He died later that night surrounded by his family, 4 months after stent placement.

Palliative treatments allowed greater freedom, a relatively pain-free existence and the vomiting never

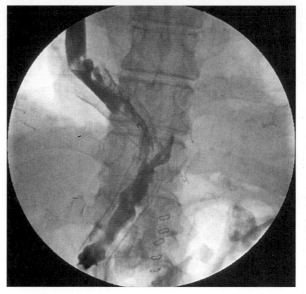

Figure 4.8   Check radiograph 5 days after insertion of the stent. (By kind permission of South Tyneside District Hospital.)

returned. Dave was able to go home occasionally at weekends to be with his family before his condition deteriorated. At Christmas, everyone felt guilty tucking into Christmas dinner, while Dave had a strained soup and Fresubin, a supplementary feed. He did manage some alcohol – he loved Guinness. Open communication with Dave and his family helped throughout the few months that he had left. They were allowed to make informed choices regarding his care. The metallic stent was a great aid to his palliation, allowing Dave to die with dignity, in control and with no vomiting, pain or discomfort.

Without the stent, Dave's life would have been shorter and possibly unbearable. The nursing staff played a valuable role as part of the palliative care team helping to alleviate Dave's anxiety and restlessness and to control his pain and nausea. This allowed him to have quality time to spend with his family.

CONCLUSION

Unfortunately some patients may experience a number of symptomatic problems that could require treatment. Some cancers are becoming more chronic in nature, with patients developing metastatic disease in a number of different sites such as the liver, bone and brain. This presents a great challenge to the patient who has to cope with progressing disease and its impact on their life; it also presents a challenge to the healthcare professionals who support patients through this. As suggested by

Faithfull & Wells (2003), supportive care for patients receiving radiotherapy should not be an optional extra, but something that deserves greater attention.

As Copp (1991) noted, these treatments may prove a stressful and fearful experience for many patients. There are many myths and misconceptions that still surround chemotherapy and radiotherapy. Nurses and healthcare professionals, both in hospital and in the community, are in a unique position to ensure that patients have clear information which they understand.

References

Adams L 1993 Managing chemotherapy-induced nausea and vomiting. Professional Nurse 9(2):91–94

Adamson D 2003 The radiobiological basis of radiotherapy side effects. In: Faithfull S, Wells M (eds) Supportive care in radiotherapy, Churchill Livingstone, Edinburgh, p 71–95

Alison M, Sarraf C 1997 Understanding cancer: from basic science to clinical practice. Cambridge University Press, Cambridge

Archer V R, Billingham L J, Cullen M H 1999 Palliative chemotherapy: no longer a contradiction in terms. The Oncologist 4(6):470–477

Ashby M A, Game P A, Devitt P et al 1991 Percutaneous gastrostomy as venting procedure in palliative care. Palliative Medicine 5:147–150

Aston V 1997 Patient management and docetaxel. International Journal of Palliative Nursing 3(3):175–178

Belcher E A 1992 Cancer nursing. Mosby Year Book, St Louis

Blows W T 2005 The biological basis of nursing: cancer. Routledge, London

Budd K 1995 Tramadol – a step towards the ideal analgesia. European Journal of Palliative Care 2(2):56–60

Burton S 1988 Cytotoxic drugs. Professional Nurse 3(11):447–452

Calvert H, McElwain T 1988 The role of chemotherapy. In: Pritchard P (ed.) Oncology for nurses and health care professionals, 2nd edn, Vol. 1, Pathology, diagnosis and treatment. Harper & Row, Beaconsfield, p 291–303

Campbell I, Illingworth M 1992 Can patients wash during radiotherapy to the breast or chest wall? – a randomised controlled trial. Clinical Oncology 4:78–82

Campbell J, Lane M A 1996 Developing a skin care protocol in radiotherapy. Professional Nurse 12(2):105–108

Coleman R E 1996 Oncological emergencies. In: Hancock B W (ed.) Cancer care in the community. Radcliffe Medical Press, Oxford, p 94

Coleman R E, Hancock B W 1996 Cytotoxic chemotherapy: principles and practice. In: Hancock B W (ed.) Cancer care in the hospital. Radcliffe Medical Press, Oxford, p 49

Colyer H 2003 The context of radiotherapy care. In: Faithfull S, Wells M (ed) Supportive care in radiotherapy. Churchill Livingstone, Edinburgh, p 1–16

Copp K 1991 Nursing patients having radiotherapy. In: Borley D (ed.) Oncology for nurses and health care professionals, Vol. 3. Harper & Row, London, p 38

Davies B, Oberle K 1990 Dimensions of the supportive role of the nurse in palliative care. Oncology Nursing Forum 17:87–94

Day J 1998 Alleviating bone pain using strontium therapy. Professional Nurse 14(4):263–266

Dougherty L 1996 Scalp cooling to prevent hair loss in chemotherapy. Professional Nurse 11(8):507–509

Dougherty L, Bailey C 2001 Chemotherapy. In: Corner J, Bailey C (eds) Cancer nursing care in context. Blackwell Science, Oxford, p 179–221

Downing J 2001 Acute events in cancer care. In: Corner J, Bailey C (eds) Cancer nursing care in context. Blackwell Science, Oxford, p 449–465

Earlam R, Cunha-Melo J R 1980 Oesophageal squamous cell carcinoma. British Journal of Surgery 67:381–390

Faithfull S 2001 Radiotherapy. In: Corner J, Bailey C (eds) Cancer nursing care in context. Blackwell Science, Oxford, p 222–261

Faithfull S 2003 Fatigue and radiotherapy. In: Faithfull S, Wells M (eds) Supportive care in radiotherapy. Churchill Livingstone, Edinburgh, p 118–134

Faithfull S, Wells M 2003 The future of supportive care in radiotherapy. In: Faithfull S, Wells M (eds) Supportive care in radiotherapy, Churchill Livingstone, Edinburgh, p 372–382

Faull C, Barton R 1998 Managing complications of cancer. In: Faull C, Carter Y, Woof R (eds) Handbook of palliative care. Blackwell Science, Oxford, p 177–201

Feber T 1995 Mouth care for patients receiving oral irradiation. Professional Nurse 10(10):666–670

Fenlon D 2001 Endocrine therapies. In: Corner J, Bailey C (eds) Cancer nursing care in context. Blackwell Science, Oxford, p 262–278

Fleisch H 1995 Bisphosphonates in bone disease – from the laboratory to the patient, 2nd edn. Parthenon Publishing, London

Foley K M 1982 Clinical assessment of pain. Acta Anaesthesiologica Scandinavica. Supplement 74:91–96

Green P, Kinghorn S 1995 Radiotherapy. In: David J (ed.) Cancer care prevention, treatment and palliation. Chapman & Hall, London, p 113

Hancock B W, Robinson M H, Rees R C 1996 Other treatments. In: Hancock B W (ed.) Cancer care in the hospital. Radcliffe Medical Press, Oxford, p 67

Hanson E J, Cullihall K 1996 Images of palliative nursing care. Journal of Palliative Care 11(3):35–39

Heals D 1993 A key to well being: oral hygiene in patients with advanced cancer. Professional Nurse 8(6):391–398

Holmes S 1996a Radiotherapy – a guide for practice, 2nd edn. Asset Books, Dorking

Holmes S 1996b Making sense of radiotherapy: curative and palliative. Nursing Times 92(23):32–33

Holmes S 1996c Making sense of cancer chemotherapy. Nursing Times 92(36):42–43

Holmes S 1997 Cancer chemotherapy – a guide for practice, 2nd edn. Asset Books, Dorking

Hoskin P 1994 Changing trends in palliative radiotherapy. In: Tobias J S, Thomas P R M (eds) Current radiation oncology, Vol. 1. Edward Arnold, London, p 342–364

Hoskin P, Makin W 2003a Principles of radiotherapy. In: Oncology for Palliative Medicine. Oxford University Press, Oxford, p 37–49

Hoskin P, Makin W 2003b Metastases involving the brain and meninges. In: Oncology for Palliative Medicine. Oxford University Press, Oxford, p 319–330

Hoskin P, Makin W 2003c Bone metastases. In: Oncology for Palliative Medicine. Oxford University Press, Oxford, p 271–289

Hoskin P, Makin W 2003d Metastatic disease of the thorax. In: Oncology for Palliative Medicine. Oxford University Press, Oxford, p 305–317

Hoskin P, Makin W 2003e Systemic therapy: chemotherapy, hormone therapy, biological therapy. In: Oncology for Palliative Medicine. Oxford University Press, Oxford, p 51–65

Hoskin P, Makin W 2003f Epidemiology and cancer trials. In: Oncology for Palliative Medicine. Oxford University Press, Oxford, p 17–29

Hoskin P, Makin W 2003g Liver metastases. In: Oncology for Palliative Medicine. Oxford University Press, Oxford, p 291–304

Hoskin P, Makin W 2003h Other tumour associated problems. In: Oncology for Palliative Medicine. Oxford University Press, Oxford, p 347–361

Hoy A 1993 Symptom control – other symptom challenges. In: Saunders C, Sykes N (eds) The management of terminal malignant disease. Edward Arnold, London, p 160

Joshua A, King T (eds) 1994 Guy's Hospital nursing drug reference, 2nd edn. Mosby-Year Book Europe, London

Kaye P 2003 A–Z pocketbook of symptom control. EPL Publications, Northampton

Kaye P, Levy D 1997 Palliative chemotherapy. In: Kaye P (ed.) Tutorials in palliative medicine. EPL Publications, Northampton, p 39

Kirkbride P 1995 The role of radiation therapy in palliative care. Journal of Palliative Care 11(1):19–26

Latham J 1991 Pain control, 2nd edn. Austen Cornish, London

Ling J 1997 Clinical trials, palliative care and the research nurse. International Journal of Palliative Nursing 3(4):192–195

Luken J, Middleton J 1995 Chemotherapy and the administration of cytotoxic drugs into established lines. In: David J (ed.) Cancer care prevention, treatment and palliation. Chapman & Hall, London, p 77

Melzack R, Wall P 1965 The challenge of pain. Penguin, Harmondsworth, UK

Moody M, Grocott P 1993 Let us extend our knowledge base: assessment and management of fungating malignant wounds. Professional Nurse 8(9):586–590

Moore J 1995 Biological and hormonal therapy. In: David J (ed.) Cancer care prevention, treatment and palliation. Chapman & Hall, London, p 174

Munro A J 2003 Challenges to radiotherapy today. In: Faithfull S, Wells M (eds) Supportive care in radiotherapy. Churchill Livingstone, Edinburgh, p 17–38

Neal A J, Hoskin P J 1997 Clinical oncology: basic principles and practice, 2nd edn. Arnold, London

Needham P 1997 Palliative radiotherapy. In: Kaye P (ed.) Tutorials in palliative medicine. EPL Publications, Northampton, p 17

O'Brien T 1993 Symptom control – pain. In: Saunders C, Sykes N (eds) The management of terminal malignant disease. Edward Arnold, London, p 33

Oliver G 1988 Radiotherapy. In: Tschudin V (ed.) Nursing the patient with cancer. Prentice Hall, London, p 57–77

Oliver G, McIllmurray M, Ashton V, Harding S, Donovan G 1997 Active palliative anti-cancer therapy. International Journal of Palliative Nursing 3(4):232–237

Powel J M, McConkey C C 1990 Increasing incidence of adenocarcinoma of the gastric cardia and adjacent sites. British Journal of Cancer 62:440–443

Quinton D 1998 Anticipatory nausea and vomiting in chemotherapy. Professional Nurse 13(10):663–666

Regnard C, Hockley J 2004 A guide to symptom relief in palliative care, 5th edn. Radcliffe Medical Press, Oxford

Rice A M 1997 An introduction to radiotherapy. Nursing Standard 12(3):49–56

Richardson A 1995 Fatigue in cancer patients: a review of the literature. European Journal of Cancer Care 4:20–32

Robinson M H, Coleman R E 1996 Treatment of cancer. In: Hancock B (ed.) Cancer care in the community. Radcliffe Medical Press, Oxford, p 38

Roper N, Logan W W, Tierney A J 1980 Learning to use the nursing process. Churchill Livingstone, Edinburgh

Saunders C 1990 Hospice and palliative care – an interdisciplinary approach. Edward Arnold, London

Smith A M 1993 Symptom control – fractures. In: Saunders C, Sykes N (eds) The management of terminal malignant disease. Edward Arnold, London, p 149

Snape D, Robinson A 1996 Radiotherapy. In: Tschudin V (ed.) Nursing the patient with cancer, 2nd edn. Prentice Hall, Hertfordshire, p 61

Souhami R, Tobias J 1995 Cancer and its management, 2nd edn. Blackwell Science, Oxford

Souhami R, Tobias J 2003 Cancer and its management, 4th edn. Blackwell Science, Oxford

Speechley V 1989 Nursing patients having chemotherapy. In: Borley D (ed.) Oncology for nurses and health care professionals, Vol. 3: Cancer nursing. Harper & Row, London, p 74

Stannard D 1989 Pressure prevents nausea. Nursing Times 85(4):33–34

Stein P 1996 Chemotherapy. In: Tschudin V (ed.) Nursing the patient with cancer, 2nd edn. Prentice Hall, Hemel Hempstead, p 78

Stone P, Richards M, Hardy J 1998 Review fatigue in patients with cancer. European Journal of Cancer Care 34(11):1670–1676

Turner G 1996 Oral care. Nursing Standard 10(28):51–56

Twycross R 1997 Symptom management in advanced cancer, 2nd edn. Radcliffe Medical Press, Oxford

Urdang L 1983 Mosby medical and nursing dictionary. Mosby, London

Walding M 1998 Pressure area care and the management of fungating wounds. In: Faull C, Carter Y, Woof R (eds) Handbook of palliative care. Blackwell Science, Oxford, p 284–295

Waller A, Caroline N L 1996 Handbook of palliative care in cancer. Butterworth-Heinemann, Newton

Watkinson A F, Adam A (eds) 1996 Interventional radiology – a practical guide. Radcliffe Medical Press, London

Webb P 1979 Nursing care of patient undergoing treatment by teletherapy. In: Tiffany R (ed.) Cancer nursing – radiotherapy. Faber & Faber, London, p 78

Webb P 1987 Patient education. Nursing 20:748, 750

Wells M 2003 Pain and breathing In: Faithfull S, Wells M (eds) Supportive care in radiotherapy. Churchill Livingstone, Edinburgh, p 160–181

Whale Z 1991 A threat to femininity? Minimising side effects in pelvic irradiation. Professional Nurse 6(6):309–311

Whenery-Tedder M 1997 A positive approach to chemotherapy. Nursing Times 93(23):52–53

Williams C 1994 Causes and management of nausea and vomiting. Nursing Times 90(44):38–41

Further reading

Cancer Research UK. Online. Available: http://www. cancerresearchuk.org

Cancerbackup. Online. Available: http://www. cancerbackup.org.uk

CancerHelp UK. Online. Available: http://www.cancerhelp. org.uk/netscape

Cancernet. Online. Available: http://www.cancernet.co.uk

Institute of Cancer Research. Online. Available: http://www.icr.ac.uk

NHS Direct. Online. Available: http://www.nhsdirect.nhs. uk

Royal College of Radiologists. Online. Available: http://www.goingfora.com/oncology

Chapter 5

Making sense of spiritual care

David Mitchell and Tom Gordon

SPIRITUAL CARE IN CONTEXT

The provision of spiritual care in palliative care has long roots stretching back to the early religious communities. However, the spirituality and spiritual care practised in the 21st century, while capturing the *self-less* caring of these early hospices and the *holistic* care of the modern hospice movement, is a much more structured and accountable area of care.

The struggle for a definition of spirituality and the debate in nursing and medical journals throughout the 1990s have influenced a sea change in thinking, and the *spiritual care* that was once thought impossible to put into words or be audited and measured has come of age for the new millennium.

A key factor in the change has been the clear and focused understanding within palliative care that spiritual care is not an optional extra; rather it is an integral aspect of holistic care that comes into sharp focus for patients, families/carers and health professionals when faced with a life-threatening illness and the processes of dying.

The change has also been influenced by a number of national initiatives that have sought to grapple with the language and concepts of spiritual care, often felt to be woolly and unclear, and to earth it firmly in the modern healthcare framework of standards, guidelines, competence and audit. In particular the following publications have grounded spiritual care and its terminology and practice:

- National Health Service (NHS) guidelines for spiritual and religious care (NHS HDL 76 2002)
- *Clinical Standards for Specialist Palliative Care* (CSBS 2002)
- *WHO Definition of Palliative Care* (World Health Organisation 2003)

- *Standards for Hospice and Palliative Care Chaplaincy* (Association of Hospice and Palliative Care Chaplains [AHPCC] 2006)
- *Spiritual and Religious Care Competencies for Specialist Palliative Care* (Marie Curie Cancer Care [MCCC] 2003)
- *Caring for the Spirit* (South Yorkshire Strategic Health Authority 2003)
- National Institute for Clinical Excellence guidelines (NICE 2004).

This chapter seeks to use the experience of the authors to lead healthcare professionals to a personal understanding of the essence of spirituality in the palliative care setting. By exploring the search for a definition of spirituality, considering how spiritual needs might be assessed and addressed in practice, and encouraging readers to develop an awareness of their personal context of spiritual care, it is hoped that all healthcare professionals will feel enabled and empowered to think 'spiritual' as a natural part of their personal and professional practice.

A DEFINITION OF SPIRITUAL CARE: A USEFUL SEARCH OR A RED HERRING?

The search for a working definition of spirituality is complicated by the common misconception around the relationship between spirituality and religion. Many healthcare professionals, when using the word *spirituality*, are actually thinking of *religion*. Despite the fact that spirituality is a loosely understood term, there is evidence that patients would wish healthcare professionals to address their spiritual needs along with all other aspects of their well-being (Wilkinson 2000). Draper & McSherry (2002) suggest that spirituality needs a definition if it is to be assessed and addressed, but Swinton & Narayanasamy (2002) acknowledge that we readily accept other terms, such as hope and joy, as having an intrinsic recognition without needing a precise understanding and definition. The ever-illusive definition of spiritual care seems no closer. However, this may in fact be a good thing – and the search itself a red herring. Research shows that the essence of spiritual care rests on the need to be open and inclusive rather than clear and precise, and the key element in spiritual care is the focus on 'person-centred care' (Mitchell & Sneddon 1999). This is a view supported by the Scottish Intercollegiate Guideline Network (SIGN) guideline on pain, which acknowledges that there can be no one clear definition of spiritual need, and supports the 'person-centred approach' (SIGN 2000).

One clear distinction that has emerged from the debate and the search for a definition is that spiritual care and religious care are distinctly different. It is now common for guidelines, standards and reports to use both *Spiritual* and *Religious* in their title. NHS Scotland offers a clear description of the two terms:

> **Religious care** is given in the context of the shared religious beliefs, values, liturgies and lifestyle of a faith community.
> **Spiritual care** is usually given in a one-to-one relationship, is completely person-centred, and makes no assumptions about personal conviction or life orientation. Spiritual care is not necessarily religious. Religious care, at its best, should always be spiritual.
>
> (NHS HDL 76 2002)

Such a helpful distinction supports the growing understanding that spiritual care is best described as a journey, and one that does not fit naturally into the familiar religious categories that healthcare professionals have been used to (Cassidy & Davies 2004) – a journey that needs exploring. Consequently, the enabling context of that journey is a person-centred conversation: spiritual care.

REFLECTION POINT

SPIRITUALITY AS MEANING

Spirituality is often equated with meaning and a sense of purpose. Ask yourself the question: What gives you meaning in life? or What is important to you in life? Try to come up with three or four answers.

Draw a line to represent the breadth of your spirituality and place boxes on the line to represent your answers (Fig. 5.1).

The common responses include: family, friends, health, work, faith/religion, happiness, being loved, music, gardening, walking, politics, nature . . .

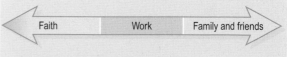

Faith   Work   Family and friends

Figure 5.1   Breadth of spirituality.

What the activity in the Reflection Point box shows is that even a person who might be described as *religious* will have other elements to their spirituality, thus supporting the person-centred approach that engages with the whole person.

It should not be surprising to discover that most healthcare professionals list work as part of their spirituality, and this is certainly true for those working in palliative care. Most people who choose to enter a caring profession have something in them that draws them to caring – their spirituality?

Clearly spirituality is individual to each person. Why then should we expect to be able to create a definition that would suit everyone? Such a definition, which seeks to encompass all aspects of spiritual care and all things that give each of us our sense of meaning, would be so long and diverse that it would be impractical to use, and would, potentially, contain so many omissions and exceptions that it would, more than likely, be unworkable to use.

There is an alternative to the search for a definition that seeks to put into words that which is hard to articulate, yet which healthcare professionals seem to know instinctively. This would be that we should concentrate on the gifts and skills that healthcare professionals have and consider how they can be enhanced and developed.

ASSESSING AND ADDRESSING SPIRITUAL NEED

Accepting, then, that *spirituality* is individual to each person, how should *spiritual care* work in practice?

Many questions arise. Who should provide this care – chaplains, nurses or all staff? How is it to be assessed? How is it measured and audited? What knowledge and skills are required to provide spiritual care?

A validated spiritual assessment tool has been as elusive as a definition of spirituality itself. However, the drive for clinical excellence and accountability in healthcare, combined with a need for measurement and quality of care, naturally leads to the question and importance of assessment in spiritual care (McSherry & Ross 2002). There is no doubt that in the healthcare setting the assessment tool is an essential component in planning care, and has many benefits: it provides a format to work from; it becomes part of a process; and can be a tool to enable measurement and audit. Given that most spiritual assessment is likely to be by nurses, there is a considerable advantage in finding a tool that can be used effectively. As Charters (1999) has suggested, an assessment tool offers an element of structure and security for an area of care that is open to interpretation.

By their nature, assessment tools need to be quick and simple to use. They do, however, lend themselves to a 'tick box' model of care that does not suit a person-centred spiritual assessment. In addition, spiritual needs can change from moment to moment, so we need to consider how often they should be

assessed: on admission, every day, after 3 days, or continuous assessment?

A number of assessment tools have been developed that steer away from the 'tick box' format and are designed to enable staff engage in a spiritual conversation. The HOPE (Anandarajah & Hight 2001) and FICA (Post et al 2000) tools are two examples. Jackson (2004) is a further example which takes the form of guidelines for initiating and sustaining a spiritual assessment. These tools offer sample questions that can be used to guide a spiritual assessment and open up the discussion of spiritual need.

Spiritual care assessment guidelines

"When you were admitted to the hospice you gave us a lot of information. One of the questions you were asked was about your mood at the time. How are you feeling now?"

Depending on the answer the following questions might be explored:

- How easy is it for you to find hope and peace in your life at the moment?
- What makes it difficult for you to find peace at the moment?
- What changes has your illness brought about?
- Do you ever pray or meditate? Does it help you find meaning in life or not?

If the nurse is comfortable, then deal with what comes up. If not – "Would you like to talk to someone further about this?"

(Jackson 2004, p 25)

Instinct and experience

The professional experience of the authors suggests that the healthcare professional's instinct and experience are the essential components for spiritual assessment. Spiritual need must be discerned before it can be assessed. It is the instinctively human skills of healthcare professionals in communication, awareness and a person-centred responsive approach that enable such discernment and assessment to take place (Cobb 2003, Govier 2000). All healthcare professionals should have an awareness of their abilities and limitations, and an understanding of the local procedure for referral to specialist spiritual care.

It is clear in the holistic context of healthcare that assessment of spiritual need does not lend itself to the 'tick and fix' approach. What may be 'ticked' as an appropriate assessment on one occasion or in one set of circumstances may do nothing to define or encapsulate the spiritual need of a patient or carer on another occasion when the prevailing circumstances, mood, influences, and inner turmoil or resolution may be entirely different.

The assessment and delivery of spiritual care requires a real engagement with people and their changing needs and circumstances. It requires the role of the companion rather than repair-person, the fellow-traveller rather than the tick-box analyst. As Harold Kushner and Sheila Cassidy have written:

> When you cannot fix what is broken, you can help very profoundly by sitting down and helping someone cry. A person who is suffering does not want explanation: the person wants consolation. Not reasons, but reassurance.
>
> (Kushner 1981)

> The dying . . . [and here, in respect of those who are searching for meaning and purpose in the face of any life-changing circumstance, we would include all those for whom we care in a healthcare setting] are essentially people on a journey. They are uprooted people, dispossessed, marginalised, travelling fearfully into the unknown . . . Sometimes the movement is barely perceptible, like the moving floors at Heathrow, but sometimes the tracks hurtle through the night, throwing their bewildered occupants from side to side with all the terror of the line to Auschwitz. Above all, the dying are alone and they are afraid. So the spirituality of those who care for the dying must be the spirituality of the companion, of the friend who walks alongside, helping, sharing, and sometimes just sitting, empty-handed, when he would rather run away. It is the spirituality of presence, of being alongside, watchful, available, of being there.
>
> (Cassidy 1988, p 5)

We, as healthcare professionals, are companions on the journey when we offer spiritual care. The essence of spiritual care is not about what we have to say or what wisdom we have to impart, rather it is our presence – that sense of 'being there' and 'being with' – that really matters. How hard this is to put into practice! How often have we felt that we needed to *say* something or *do* something when what was required was simply to be there and let healing take place.

This requires insight from the professional, and self-knowledge.

REFLECTION POINT

EXPLORING YOUR INSIGHT AND EXPERIENCE
Take a few minutes to reflect on a patient or carer in whom you were able to discern spiritual need. What was it that raised your awareness?

- Something in the conversation?
  — Something said or not said?
- A change in the patient?
  — Quieter than usual?
  — A sense of urgency?
  — More withdrawn?
- The patient's reaction to visitors?
  — Were they upset by the visit?
  — Were they different with their visitors than with you?
- A change in the patient's environment?
  — Did the room look or feel different?
  — Was something out of place?
  — Was something added to the room?

You might wish to repeat this exercise for two or three patients/carers and then consider your strengths and weaknesses:

- What aspects of spiritual awareness are you most attuned to?
- Are there other skills you could develop to raise your awareness and instinct?

STANDARDS AND COMPETENCE IN SPIRITUAL CARE

The AHPCC (2006) has published professional *Standards for Hospice and Palliative Care Chaplaincy* which define the context of a spiritual care service. These standards detail the level of service that hospices and palliative care services can expect from chaplaincy services – the profession whose specialist expertise is spiritual and religious care. A key statement in the standards acknowledges that all healthcare professionals can and do provide spiritual care, and it is the role of chaplaincy services to provide advice, education and support to all healthcare professionals in their assessment and delivery of spiritual and religious care. Alongside these professional standards for chaplaincy services sit the MCCC (2003) *Spiritual and Religious Care Competencies for Specialist Palliative Care,* which offers a competency framework for all health professionals in their assessment and delivery of spiritual care. This framework has been recommended by NICE (2004).

A multidisciplinary group from five Marie Curie hospices and the Marie Curie Nursing Service worked on developing a way of capturing the spiritual care that was evident in Marie Curie hospices but could not be audited. Local spiritual care standards had been tried but were considered to be incomplete and ineffective. Spiritual assessment tools were considered, but the findings were that the disadvantages outweighed the advantages in the patient-focused specialist palliative care setting. It was clear from national documents that all staff could and should provide spiritual care, and that chaplaincy, as well as assessing and delivering spiritual care, had an important focus in supporting staff in their provision of care as well as a particular expertise for the more complicated elements of spiritual care.

A four-level competency framework based on knowledge, skills and actions was developed in order to specify levels of spiritual and religious care that could be understood and achieved by all staff and volunteers with patient contact. It was acknowledged that, although the terms used would be familiar to healthcare professionals, the terminology may lack clear definition. However, this was viewed as a strength rather than a weakness for this person-centred area of care.

The approach of this model seeks to *integrate* spiritual care rather than assess it as a specific element of care, thus enabling and supporting healthcare professionals to use and develop their natural instincts and experience in discerning, identifying, assessing and responding to spiritual need. An important part of the process is to encourage individuals to be aware of their own level of competence and to have a clear referral path to the next level of competence.

SPIRITUAL AND RELIGIOUS CARE COMPETENCIES

The competency framework

The competencies have four levels, each level identifying the members of staff and volunteers to whom it applies, followed by a summary statement of the competence expected.

Level 1 – All staff and volunteers who have casual contact with patients and their families

This level seeks to ensure that all staff and volunteers understand that all people have spiritual needs, and distinguishes spiritual and religious needs. It seeks to encourage basic skills of awareness, relationships and communication, and an ability to refer concerns to members of the multidisciplinary team.

Level 2 – Staff and volunteers whose duties require contact with patients and families/carers

This level seeks to enhance the competencies developed at level 1 with an increased awareness of spiritual and religious needs and how they may be identified and responded to. In addition to increased communication skills, identification and referral of difficult needs should be achievable, along with an ability to identify personal training needs.

Level 3 – Staff and volunteers who are members of the multidisciplinary team

This level seeks to enhance further the skills of levels 1 and 2. It moves into the area of assessment of spiritual and religious need, developing a plan for care and recognising complex spiritual, religious and ethical issues. This level also introduces confidentiality and the recording of sensitive and personal patient information.

Level 4 – Staff or volunteers whose primary responsibility is for the spiritual and religious care of patients, visitors and staff

Staff working at level 4 are expected to be able to manage and facilitate complex spiritual and religious needs in patients, families/carers, staff and volunteers, in particular the existential and practical needs arising from the impact on individuals and families from issues in illness, life, dying and death. In addition they should have a clear understanding of their own personal beliefs and spirituality, and be able to journey with others focused on those persons' needs and agendas. They should liaise with external resources as required. They should also act as a resource for support, training and education of healthcare professionals and volunteers, and seek to be involved in professional and national initiatives.

The main body of the framework includes specific definitions of the knowledge, skills and actions of staff operating at each level. The three-column format allows distinctions to be made between theory and practice; for example, a member of the multidisciplinary team may have the knowledge required for level 3 but practise the skills and actions at level 1. This is an important tool in identifying personal and professional training needs as well as affirming levels of competence that may well have gone unnoticed or unaffirmed.

Table 5.1 Progression of skills in spiritual and religious care

Level	Skills
1	An awareness of the nature of spirituality within a palliative care context
	An awareness of the nature of religious needs within a palliative care context
2	An ability to identify individuals with spiritual or religious needs
3	An ability to develop and administer a plan for spiritual care based on spiritual or religious need
4	Demonstrate a wide range of skills to discern, assess and address complex spiritual and religious needs

An example of the progression through the levels of competence is shown in Table 5.1.

It is acknowledged that the vast majority of spiritual care will be assessed and delivered at level 3 – by trained staff who are members of the multidisciplinary team. Therefore, in addition to the communication skills, recognition of confidentiality and awareness of their own spirituality required at levels 1 and 2, level 3 practitioners should demonstrate the following knowledge, skills and actions:

- *Knowledge* – an understanding of spiritual assessment including the ethical dimensions, and an understanding of the skills of other members of the multidisciplinary team
- *Skills* – an ability to elicit patients' concerns, recognise unmet need, respond to emotions and conflict in families, recognise complex spiritual, religious and ethical issues, refer to specialist spiritual resources, and identify their own training needs.
- *Actions* – to document spiritual assessments, interventions and referrals in a way that respects the confidentiality of the individual and the multidisciplinary team.

As with all standards and competencies, to enable audit and assessment of competence there need to be assessment tools. It is envisaged that the competencies will be assessed through appraisal as part of the Personal Performance Review and Development process (PPRD); to support that aim, an assessment tool for levels 1 and 2 and a self-assessment tool for levels 3 and 4 have been published (MCCC 2004).

Integrating the competencies in practice

There is no prescriptive method of introducing the competencies that has been tried and tested, and it is unlikely that one will be developed. It is the nature of palliative care that it is varied in delivery depending on the local setting, needs and culture. However, a number of initiatives have been used by those seeking to implement the competencies into practice. The key is integration, using the existing structures already in place. Examples include: linking the introduction to the local implementation of the NICE (2004) guidance for improving supportive and palliative care for adults with cancer; using existing tutorial, staff-training and reflective-practice opportunities to introduce and discuss the competencies; and including the competencies in PPRD training courses for line managers.

A pilot study using reflective practice sessions supports the anecdotal evidence from those introducing the competencies in the ways described above (Gordon & Mitchell 2004). The study found positive benefits among staff attending the sessions: good practice was affirmed, personal skills and limitations were recognised, and training and development needs identified. What made the process a positive experience for those involved in the study was the recognition that they were already providing spiritual and religious care instinctively as part of their professional role and from that basis of understanding were enabled to explore their individual competencies in more detail, and consider their personal skills and limitations; and that it was expected that there would be a point at which they would refer on to others with a higher level of competence.

The MCCC (2003) document *Spiritual and Religious Care Competencies for Specialist Palliative Care* offers a viable alternative to assessment tools, and enables the healthcare professional to utilise and develop their human and professional instincts and experience to integrate the assessment of the spiritual and religious needs of their patients and their family/carers into their existing practice.

SPIRITUAL CARE IN PRACTICE

Standards and guidelines thus give the framework, and competencies help us look to the knowledge, skills and actions needed to provide spiritual care. In addition, there is the important recognition that our professional experience can lead to enhancing our personal and professional gifts. With this in mind, when it comes to engaging with a patient or family, we rightly ask: How does this work in practice?

There are three key elements that healthcare professionals need to be aware of and consider:

1. You need to have an awareness and understanding of your own spirituality and what you believe about life and death before you can journey with others.
2. If you start on a journey, you need to be prepared to go where the other person leads, or have a strategy to refer on.
3. You need to realise that sometimes you will recognise the issues but remain powerless to help – there are some things that cannot be 'fixed'.

The following section of this chapter will help you to explore the personal context of your spirituality and spiritual care. This section will look at the practicalities of engaging in spiritual care, what to say, when to say nothing, and give guidance in thinking through what you will deal with and what you will refer on.

One of the clearest signs of spiritual distress and one of the most challenging areas for healthcare professionals are the 'Why' questions: Why has this happened to me? Why does God allow suffering? What have I done to deserve this? Rarely are these the real questions on a person's mind, and the clearest and most effective strategy when faced with these questions is an honest answer followed by a question of your own: 'I don't know, but why are you asking that today, what's on your mind?' The answer to your question will determine your ongoing response, and the aim is to engage with the person on that deeper level and to assess what the real issues are and how you are going to respond to and deal with them.

The key here is to be open and responsive to the other person, to identify and understand what the issues are, prioritise them, and work out what is within your competence and where you will refer on what you are unable to deal with.

Sometimes, though, the spiritual encounter does not rely on words – it requires your presence, or simply 'being there'. It is very difficult to assess a patient who is withdrawn and unable to engage or communicate at all. Instinct and experience may tell you that there is some spiritual distress, but what do you do when you don't get an answer to your questions? Do you keep on asking time after time, or adopt a different strategy? There is no right or wrong answer here. However, one strategy is to use your sense of presence. Make time; ask the patient whether it's okay if you sit with them for a few minutes; and thank them for their time before you leave. You can repeat this over a number of days. You may or may not get a response, but what you have done either way is to create the opportunity, and you will have left the patient with a sense that they really matter to you and your caring team.

There will be times, though, when you have been able to discern, assess and identify spiritual needs, and despite your best efforts and those of the team you are unable to resolve the issues.

No matter how experienced we become in discerning, assessing and identifying spiritual and religious needs of patients and their families/carers, the reality is that the solution is not always in our control, and there are therefore occasions when the needs cannot be met in the way we would like. However, good spiritual care is about the willingness to be there and stay with the patient on their journey, which has taken a difficult and unexpected turn.

The essence of spiritual care in practice is to be self-aware; to be prepared to journey with people where they want to go; to know when you are leaving your area of experience and need to refer on to other members of the multidisciplinary team, and to the specialist spiritual care resource available. The flow chart in Figure 5.2 is an example of how spiritual care can work in practice.

Case Study 5.1

Jean has lung cancer, despite the fact that she has never smoked. Her husband died 5 years ago and she has a grown-up son at home. While in the bath, Jean asks Alison (the nurse): 'Why has this happened to me? What have I done to deserve cancer?' Alison could assume that this is a question around the unfairness of a non-smoker getting cancer; however, when asked 'What's put that in your mind today. What are you concerned about?', Jean goes on to explain that she is worried about her son, that they haven't been able to talk about what's happening to her and how ill she is, and that she knows he'll need to arrange her funeral. She's a lapsed church member and does not want a really religious service, and she is worried about whether her son will be able to stay on in their council house once she has died.

Alison now has three issues to deal with and choices to make. She is experienced and comfortable in talking around the issues of families and helping them to talk; she knows the chaplain has particular skills in helping people think through their funeral services; but knows nothing about the local council housing policy. A solution could be to stay with what she is comfortable with and able to deal with and, with the patient's permission, refer to another member of the multidisciplinary team, the social worker, to discuss the housing issue, and the chaplain to discuss the funeral options.

Case Study 5.2

Mary has been admitted for terminal care and is increasingly agitated when her daughter Margaret leaves after visiting. Pauline (the nurse) picks up on Mary's apparent distress and says: 'You seem a bit agitated, Mary. What is it that's troubling you?' After some follow-up questions, Mary discloses that she knows she is dying and would love to see her son Bill, whom she hasn't seen for over 15 years and has lost touch with. Mary has asked Margaret whether she knows where Bill is, but she too has lost touch and has no desire to see her brother again. Mary asks Pauline: 'Will you try to find him for me?'

Pauline agrees to try to contact Bill, but recognises she wouldn't know where to start. She gets permission from the patient to refer to another member of the multidisciplinary team (the chaplain or social worker) to try to trace Bill. The chaplain manages to trace Bill, makes him aware of the seriousness of his mother's condition and of her request to see him. Bill asks for time to think about it and calls the chaplain back later, saying he couldn't in all conscience visit his mother: it would be too painful and he can't forgive her for the past.

This was not the answer anyone wished for or expected. However, it needs to be respected and communicated to Mary. Pauline could have asked the chaplain to see the patient and break the news. However, as she had developed a good relationship with Mary, she decided to break the news to her herself, having discussed with the chaplain how she might word it and respond to other questions that Mary might have.

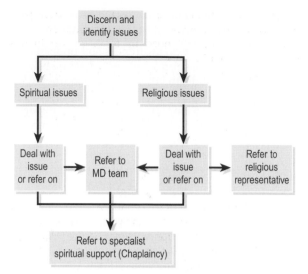

Figure 5.2   Spiritual care in practice.

THE PERSONAL CONTEXT OF SPIRITUAL CARE

The delivery of spiritual care should always be person-centred. As described above, this essentially means journeying with a client or patient on *their* road – and not the road of the healthcare professional. Thus the patient's search for meaning, purpose and fulfilment may take the carer into realms of thought and exploration that are essentially foreign territory, and may reveal issues that are as difficult as they are unexpected. In such circumstances, a number of guidelines must always be utilised by the carer if spiritual care is to be offered in a helpful and healing way.

Listening with focus

If good spiritual care is to be achieved, the carer has to begin and end with the role of being a listener. The drawing out of a story or area of exploration should be facilitated by the use of good reflective listening skills, and a willingness to engage with and take seriously the journey towards meaning. What a person needs most is to be listened to, to be affirmed as a person who matters and whose unfolding story is worth the telling. Such listening should be with focus, and it is often the case that if the right environment is created, through touch, eye contact, helpful body language and the like, a short time of focused attention is worth much more than longer unfocused contact, and an issue shared in a busy ward environment can be more important than a carer and patient finding a more formal and intimate setting of privacy and quietness.

Listening, focus and attentiveness are tools in the creation of an environment where spiritual care works, and where this facet of a person's well-being finds the healing and wholeness that they seek.

A non-judgemental approach

In such moments of supportive intimacy, things will be shared with the carer that may shock and distress. Such is the nature of the spiritual search, for it has to take people into areas of darkness and problems, unfinished business and regrets, which need to be shared and healed. It is often the case, therefore, that in such moments of shock and distress the healthcare professional can be overwhelmed with what is being shared, such that they want to stop the sharing, offer a solution, or even make a judgement or condemnation.

It is natural, sometimes, to be repulsed by what we hear, either because it is shocking or because it is outwith our personal experience to understand. However, the patient needs us to 'hang in there' with their issue. They still need us to listen, for in the telling, and in the trust of sharing an intimacy, a mistake, a darkness or a problem, there is already a healing. To hear themselves tell their story is the beginning of their making sense of it. They have begun to articulate their longings and, as such, they have begun to find their own answers.

The desire to offer our own solutions is also a strong one. 'If I were you I would have done . . .', or 'If that had been me, then I wouldn't . . .', or 'I suggest you do . . .'. Although such things may be the considered opinions of the carer, and, indeed, may be what they would wish to offer to their own circumstances as a way of moving forward, they are heard by the patient as deflection, as rejection of their search, and as an imposition of the value systems of another person.

> Take a walk under my skies, try to see things once the way I do,
> Take a look out through my eyes, take a different point of view.
>
> (James Keelaghan 1993)

What is needed in spiritual care is a willingness to walk under the skies that are above the patient, to see as they see, to understand how they see their world, and to know that they can find wholeness in their own framework and value systems. The patient will always be in a vulnerable position. The establishing of trust with a carer is a risky and costly process. But when trust is established, it can be just the healing environment in which spiritual care can work. To threaten such trust by imposing one's own solutions is to take the caring process backwards and not forwards – and, often, back beyond where the patient started in the first place.

As a consequence, you must beware of making judgements, either out of a desire to condemn or criticise, or because your own value system or set of religious beliefs makes you feel in a position to believe – or even say – that if the patient had only operated in your framework then they would not have found themselves in such a dilemma in the first place. Such judgements serve to push the patient away, and to threaten the trust mentioned above. You might think, and, indeed, you might wonder and be amazed, but you must never say that judgemental thing that is in your mind.

Whatever you share, it has to be supportive to the patient. If spiritual care is to be truly person-centred, the needs of the patient should always have priority. That is not to say that you should not give your opinion when asked, or even reveal how you might have handled a situation if the patient seeks that kind of empathy and insight, for such sharing can be the role of the companion, and can give the patient the much needed support and reassurance that their carer actually understands and appreciates the nature of their spiritual search. But it must never be imposed, or offered as a judgement – for that is not what the patient needs. They have enough negative stuff going on in their own minds without us adding to it. In short, what they need is love and not judgement.

RELIGION – A SUPPORT OR A PROBLEM?

We have already indicated above that religion and spirituality are distinctive from each other, that religion is a shared set of beliefs and values that are common to some, and spirituality is a search for meaning and purpose that is common to all. For some people the spiritual search is worked through in religious terms, using common language, symbols and belief statements. For those who have a clear religious framework in which to operate, and, as a consequence, a set of beliefs and a perspective on life that inform their ability to cope with life's traumas, religion and issues of faith can be major factors in their well-being. If such shared beliefs bring them into contact with a faith community, then the very fact of their sense of belonging to a body of like-minded people can be a vital source of support. There is evidence, anecdotal, experiential and based on research, indicating, for example, that a belief in an 'afterlife', combined with other elements of faith, gives people with a Christian perspective a framework of hope and purpose that assists them with end-of-life issues and the dying process (Gordon 2004). In addition, such a faith perspective helps alleviate a sense of loss and separation from a loved one (Perry & Frankel 1998). Indeed, faith and hope, although fundamental human concepts, are generally associated with religious discourse and language, and are clearly associated with positive attitudes towards life and death (Clarke 2004).

The offices of a person's religion – anointing, prayers, the Eucharist, readings from holy writings – can be of great benefit to them, for they serve as reminders of their continued inclusion in their faith community, and that their journey of faith still matters. It is important to remember, however, that, as with all facets of the care of a patient, such expressions of religion should be individualised and focused on the needs of the patient and not merely made available to serve the needs of the faith community or the person who represents the religious institution. It would not be good patient care to insist that someone is given the Sacraments by the priest just because there is an expectation that this takes place, if the patient expresses no desire to have such religious expressions made available to them.

Faith feeds a person's spirituality when it offers comfort, hope, meaning and fulfilment. But when religion is the only framework in which a person's spirituality is expressed or worked through, and the response of the healthcare professional or religious representative is unhelpful or damaging, then the whole of a person's spirituality is threatened as a result. For some, the faith that they expect to be of help and support, and which they lean on for meaning and purpose when they need it most, actually works in a counterproductive fashion (Gordon 2004). There is evidence, such as the study of the effect of 9/11 on the faith of those affected by the trauma (Dombeck 2002), that people whose cherished beliefs are challenged in the context of traumatic life events are likely to experience 'severe spiritual disequilibrium'.

Some religious people are not spiritual at all, and cannot see beyond their own narrow religious framework to embrace those whose spiritual search is worked out in a different part of the spiritual spectrum. As a consequence, there is the tendency for healthcare professionals who have a strong religious faith or set of beliefs to impose this religion on their patient in the belief that this is good spiritual care. It is not. It is the trap of offering the solutions and judgements that we counselled against above. Of course you can offer your thoughts and perspectives if you are asked – but the patient has to ask. You may find that your religion gives a framework in which you can find meaning and fulfilment. Indeed, you may utilise your religious beliefs to help you understand the struggles of the patient, but religion should never be a 'one size fits all' approach to spiritual care. To see it and use it as such is facile and, ultimately, unhelpful.

There have to be boundaries, therefore, to how much of ourselves, religion included, we share in the pastoral and spiritual encounter. We must wait, often in silence, until the way becomes clearer for our patient, and then allow them to take the first faltering steps on a new way, even though that way may not be of our choosing.

People living with illness or, even more, facing a life-threatening condition find themselves 'dislocated', taken, even wrenched, from familiar places, securities, certainties, beliefs and the like, and dropped into a desert where familiar landmarks and signposts are nowhere to be seen. What they need in this desert place, this environment of loneliness, fear and uncertainty, is for the caring traveller, the healthcare professional that we are, to come out from the secure walls of our city, that which gives us security and safety, and meet them in their fearful place (Gordon 2001). That is true spiritual care. And its value – the ultimate healing – is for the traveller to be confident enough to find a new path on which to travel, while you travel back to your city to find your own security and renewal once more.

BEING GROUNDED

What this essentially means for the carer, therefore, is that you have to be grounded in your own sense of self, your own spirituality. There has, to use the image above, to be a place from which you can go and to which you can return. To stay in your own security and expect the lost traveller to come to you is never to meet the patient in their need and never to offer true spiritual care. To stay outside your own security and expect to have sufficient purpose and strength to meet and travel with many lost travellers in their fearful wanderings is to run the risk of becoming another lost traveller yourself, and of experiencing ultimate burnout in your own fears and loneliness.

Helpful spiritual care is offered by the carer who is grounded in their own spirituality and earthed in their own reality. That does not, and should not, mean that you have all the answers to all of life's difficult questions, and that your own spiritual life is ever and always intact. It simply means that you know what questions to ask, you know how to be comfortable when they are asked by other people, and you are not fearful when you meet them to share these questions in their desert place.

THE COST OF CARING

There is a cost to caring. If spiritual care has to be worth the offering, it has to be worth dealing with the cost to the carer of offering it well.

Involvement with palliative care can help us develop our own sense of spirituality and a sense of what is important (Cornette 1997), as being available, walking alongside, 'tidying mental attics', being supportive of colleagues, and all that is demanded of us, is not easy. It often draws on our spiritual, psychological and physical reserves and can affect our emotional and spiritual well-being (Kinghorn 2005).

Although we connect with the suffering that people share, we need to remain connected with and continue to enhance our own resources (Kinghorn 2005).

Case Study 5.3

William was 54 years old, single, lived alone, and was dying from cancer. He had been referred by his GP to [the hospice specialist community nursing service], but would not allow the specialist nurse into his home when she called, and sent her away with a flea in her ear! So, all [that the hospice] knew about William was his name, address and date of birth, where he lived and what his diagnosis was. And there [they] had to let the matter rest. One day, quite out of the blue, William appeared at the hospice and asked 'to see the boss'. Having identified him as the patient who had been referred [to the hospice] some weeks before, [the] medical director sat down with him to talk, and William expressed his purpose in seeking out the boss. 'I need some help,' he said, 'to clear out my mental attic before I die.'

(Gordon 2001, p 85)

William's spiritual search was, in his terminology, to clear out his attic before he died. Any attic will be an untidy, dust-filled, cobweb-strewn place. There will be many attics that have not been looked at for a long time. To be invited into the attic to assist with and share in the sorting process is the ultimate invitation to offer spiritual care. To stand in the street as an expert in attics and shout instructions to William is to offer solutions, your own solutions, and have no engagement with the sorting process. To invite William to share in your house, and offer him your own security and beliefs, is to deny him the task of tidying his own attic. To respond to his invitation necessitates entering into the messy world of his attic, staying there and, indeed, returning there with him again and again, until it is tidied to his satisfaction.

However, you cannot expect to enter fully into this messy world of a spiritual search and not be affected by it. Some of the dust and cobwebs will stick. It will be disturbing, challenging and threatening. That is the given if we are to be fully engaged with spiritual care. As a consequence, you must be constantly aware of the effect on and the cost to us of such levels of care. You must find your ways of taking 'time out', of withdrawing from the messy attic and dust yourself down, care for yourself, find renewal and regeneration in your own security, if you are to return again to another attic and share in another complicated search for meaning.

And, as you do, you will be challenged to make an attempt to tidy your own attic, to sort your own spirituality. You may have the methodology to do that by yourself, and the confidence to do your own tidying, or you may need to ask for help from someone whom you invite into your attic. Either way, the cost of our caring is the challenge to care for yourself. If the cost is worth paying for the healing and wholeness of the person for whom you are called to care, it is a cost worth paying for your own healing and wholeness, so that good spiritual care can continue to be in your hands to offer others.

Irene began to tell me something of the counselling support she had received when her mother died. The counsellor, she recalled, was terrific – sensitive and warm, focused and professional – and, without her, Irene felt that she would not have been able to see things through. Irene had wondered how the counsellor coped, if she was dealing regularly with other people like her, with all their pain and struggles. It was only looking back on the process, however, that she realised there had been clues along the way. For at the end of each counselling session, with all its tears and anguish, when counsellor and client were taking their leave of each other, the counsellor would always end with something like, 'Well, my husband and I are going out for a meal tonight', or, 'I'm looking forward to my grand-daughter coming at the weekend', or, 'I'm having a girlie shopping trip tomorrow with my friends'. She was, Irene realised, clearly indicating that she had another life, that Irene was not the be-all-and-end-all of her concerns, and that she was taking care of herself. I asked Irene if she felt diminished by that. 'No,' she replied, 'I reckoned that if my counsellor was taking care of herself, she would be all the more able to help me with my stuff the next time we were together.'

(Kinghorn 2005, p 4)

Healthcare professionals have lives other than the lives they give to their patients, carers and colleagues. The ways in which we value and enhance these other, recreational, intimate, relationship parts of our lives keep us whole, and better able to give to our professional roles. Those ways will be varied, but, as they are so often casualties of the demands of our professional life, being kind to ourselves outwith work, and occasionally being self-indulgent, is a must (Kinghorn 2005). Kinghorn quotes this verse from personal communication:

I have a secret garden hidden deep inside,
Where in times of stress I often go and hide,
There I enjoy peace and light,
Shared only with those whom I invite,
I rejoice in their company and happy faces,
With my special people in my most secret places.

CONCLUSION

There can be no doubt that spiritual and religious care is engendering considerable debate at national and professional levels. This chapter has sought to earth the often ethereal vagueness of spirituality into palliative care practice by taking seriously the issues of definition and the assessment and addressing of spiritual needs. Although the practice of developing assessment tools is well established and has many advantages – not least of which is regularising specific assessments in the care of patients – spiritual care does not lend itself to such a set form of assessment. Instead, it requires an individually focused approach that is continual rather than being utilised at set points on our involvement with the patient.

Spiritual and religious care is an area where the language, process and terminology can be loose and vague. However, the publication of spiritual and reli-gious care competencies for specialist palliative care provides an opportunity for all healthcare profes-sionals to consider and develop their personal instinct and experience in their practice, and allow hospices and specialist palliative care units and teams to evidence the level of spiritual and religious care offered in their unit. The competencies are perhaps a first, although important, step forward in developing a measurable and assessable spiritual care.

The personal context in which spiritual care is offered also requires regular review. This ensures that the care offered, and the effect of such care on the carer, continues to enhance the quality of holistic care being delivered and the ongoing attitude and approach of the healthcare professional.

References

Anandarajah G, Hight E 2001 Spirituality and medical practice: using the HOPE questions as a practical tool for spiritual assessment. American Family Physician 63(1):81–88

Association of Hospice and Palliative Care Chaplains 2006 Standards for hospice and palliative care chaplaincy. AHPCC, Help the Hospices, London

Cassidy J P, Davies D J 2004 Cultural and spiritual aspects of palliative medicine. In: Doyle D, Hanks G, Cherny N I, Calman K (eds) Oxford textbook of palliative medicine. Oxford University Press, Oxford, p 955–957

Cassidy S 1988 Sharing the darkness: the spirituality of caring. Darton, Longman & Todd, London

Charters P J 1999 The religious and spiritual needs of mental health clients. Nursing Standard 13(26):34–36

Clarke D 2004 Religion and spirituality: faith and hope. Australasian Psychiatry 11(2):164–168

Cobb M 2003 Spiritual care. In: Lloyd-Williams M (ed.) Psychosocial issues in palliative care. Oxford University Press, Oxford, p 135–148

Cornette K 1997 The imponderable: a search for meaning – whenever I am weak I am strong. International Journal of Palliative Nursing 3(1):6–13

CSBS (formerly the Clinical Standards Board for Scotland) 2002 Clinical standards for specialist palliative care. NHS Quality Improvement Scotland, Edinburgh

Dombeck M 2002 Chaos and self-organisation as a consequence of spiritual disequilibrium. Clinical Nurse Specialist 16(1):42–47

Draper P, McSherry W 2002 A critical view of spirituality and spiritual assessment. Journal of Advanced Nursing 39(1):1–2

Gordon T 2001 A need for living: signposts on the journey of life and beyond. Wild Goose Publications, Glasgow

Gordon T 2004 Recovering our lost saints. Scottish Journal of Healthcare Chaplaincy 7(2):28–33

Gordon T, Mitchell D 2004 A competency model for the assessment and delivery of spiritual care. Palliative Medicine 18(7):646–651

Govier I 2000 Spiritual care in nursing: a systematic approach. Nursing Standard 14(17):32–36

Jackson J 2004 The challenge of providing spiritual care. Professional Nurse 20(3):24–26

Kellaghan J 1993 In: My Skies Album (CD). RedBird/Green Linnet

Kinghorn S 2005 What do you do to look after yourself. International Journal of Palliative Nursing 11(1):4

Kushner H 1981 When bad things happen to good people. Shocken Books, New York

Marie Curie Cancer Care 2003 Spiritual and religious care competencies for specialist palliative care. MCCC, London

Marie Curie Cancer Care 2004 Assessment tools: spiritual and religious care competencies for specialist palliative care. MCCC, London

McSherry W, Ross L 2002 Dilemmas of spiritual assessment: considerations for nursing practice. Journal of Advanced Nursing 38(5):479–488

Mitchell D, Sneddon M 1999 Informing the debate: chaplaincy and spiritual care in Scotland. International Journal of Palliative Nursing 5(6):275–280

National Institute for Clinical Excellence 2004 Improving supportive and palliative care for adults with cancer. The manual. NICE, London

NHS HDL 76 2002 Spiritual care in NHS Scotland: guidelines on chaplaincy and spiritual care in the NHS in Scotland. Scottish Executive, Edinburgh

Perry B, Frankel G 1998 The relationship between faith and well-being. Journal of Religion and Health 37(2):125–136

Post S G, Puchalski C, Larson D 2000 Physicians and patient spirituality: professional boundaries, competency, and ethics. Annals of Internal Medicine 133(9):748–749

Scottish Intercollegiate Guidelines Network 2000 Control of pain in patients with cancer. SIGN, Edinburgh

South Yorkshire Strategic Health Authority 2003 Caring for the spirit: a strategy for chaplaincy and spiritual healthcare workforce. SYSHA, Sheffield

Swinton J, Narayanasamy A 2002 Response to: A critical view of spirituality and spiritual assessment by P. Draper and W. McSherry (2002) Journal of Advanced Nursing 39, 1–2. Journal of Advanced Nursing 40(2):158–160

Wilkinson S 2000 Spiritual recognition within palliative care. International Journal of Palliative Nursing 6(1):4

World Health Organisation 2003 WHO Definition of Palliative Care. Online. Available: http://www.who.int/cancer/palliative/definition/en/ 14 Jan 2007

Chapter 6

Psychosocial dimensions

Robert Becker

INTRODUCTION

There is a character in the popular television series 'Star Trek: The Next Generation' called Deana Troi. She is said to be half human and half Betazoid (a fictional race of people who have the ability to sense others' emotions). In one episode she loses her empathic abilities and finds that she has to rely on her human skills instead to do her job as a counsellor. She truly believes that without her special abilities she cannot function, and becomes frustrated and apologetic to the crew members she sees. One such crew member, who is learning to come to terms with the loss of her husband in a tragic accident, has the foresight and courage to say to her, 'There is more to helping people than the use of some special sense. You have helped me, and continue to do so by your understanding, your openness, your warmth, the relationship we have and by who you are, just as much as by what you do.' It was a sobering lesson for this character, in which she was asked to trust in her natural, intuitive human abilities, and use these in combination with the skills, knowledge and experience that she has to enable her to function well in her job.

I can think of no better example to illustrate the very essence of what is required of the practising nurse to provide psychological help and support to the dying patient and their family in today's complex clinical environments. It is intended that this chapter will explore the issues involved here, make reference to recent government documents and their relevance to psychological care, and be closely linked to everyday nursing practice in the common settings where death most frequently takes place in today's society (Office of National Statistics 2002). The text will concentrate on discussing the psychological issues for the patient and their family, and the nurses' role within these situations. The range of core skills, qualities and knowledge required will be placed in the context of real case studies so that we can learn from the many fine examples of how to foster a compassionate response in this most sensitive area and reflect on its significance for improving clinical practice.

THE NEED FOR BETTER PSYCHOLOGICAL CARE

For a number of years there has been a groundswell of opinion, albeit anecdotal, among patients themselves that their psychological needs are not being met. Running parallel to this has been the development of numerous groups and organisations, most of which exist outside of the National Health Service, catering for the psychological and information needs of patients. Many of these have a high presence on the internet and provide an extremely valuable service to the public and professionals alike. These organisations are mostly of a charitable nature and exist only because of public support. The message from patients is coming across loud and clear and it is important to respond by providing care that will impact upon the quality of life of all those who are dying, regardless of diagnosis.

In an attempt to react to this growing impetus for change the National Council for Hospice and Specialist Palliative Care Services (NCHSPCS 1997) produced a set of guidelines that defined the skills necessary for psychosocial support and assessment at three levels. The UK government has also responded to this impetus by producing extensive guidelines for service development in palliative care including psychological support (National Institute for Clinical Excellence [NICE] 2004). The recommendations are that all patients should undergo systematic psychological assessment at key points in their treatment and have access to appropriate psychological support. Implementation of these guidelines is a slow process and is dependent on adequate resources being available to hospital and primary care trusts. A four-level model of professional psychological assessment and intervention is suggested.

The more formal assessment of psychological morbidity that is required in levels 3 and 4 of the NICE (2004) guidance (Fig. 6.1) requires the use of structured tools. Those in use have been developed from approaches used in psychiatry and consist mostly of structured linear questions asked in an interview style. The reliability and validity of the most common tools for use with advanced illness have been well established (Fitzsimmons & Ahmedzai 2004), and these tools have a useful place in screening for anxiety and depression. They do, however, have their limitations and need to be used in the context of a total quality of life assessment that takes into account the particular psychodynamics of end-of-life care in a culturally sensitive environment.

How realistic and achievable this assessment process proves to be in practice is yet to be seen. Some of the questions that need to be asked are: Do health and social care professionals have the skills, resources and time to undertake repeated formal assessments in their daily practice? Does good quality information exist, and is it suitable and accessible? If

	Level	Group	Assessments	Interventions
Self-help and informal support	1	All health and social care professionals	Recognition of psychological needs	Effective information-giving, compassionate communication and general psychological support
	2	Health and social care professionals with additional expertise	Screen for psychological distress	Psychological interventions (such as anxiety management and problem solving)
	3	Trained and accredited professional	Assessment for psychological distress and diagnosis of some psychopathology	Counselling and specific psychological therapies, such as cognitive behavioural therapy (CBT) and solution-focused therapy, delivered according to an explicit theoretical framework
	4	Mental health specialists – clinical psychologists and psychiatrists	Diagnosis of psychopathology	Specialist psychological and psychiatric interventions

Figure 6.1   Four-component model of psychological support (NICE 2004).

patients' 'needs' and 'preferences' are identified, are suitable options and choices available to them? Essentially, the NICE guidelines dovetail in closely and build on the NCHSPCS (1997) document, but arguably the latter provides a more holistically oriented perspective with a stronger recognition of the role of the family as carers in this area.

There is a need to acknowledge that it will not be possible, at least in the foreseeable future, to find cures for many of the diseases and conditions that afflict our society. Media representations of medical advances often give a false impression of what can be achieved and serve to reinforce the already strongly held beliefs that miracles are just around the corner, and that death can be delayed even further (Aries 1993). The necessity, therefore, to support a more holistic model of patient care that encompasses psychological support and communication skills is paramount. Effective and well thought-out psychological care can be of immense benefit, not only to the minority suffering serious psychological problems, but to all patients. There is also a view that effective communication and psychological support will help to prevent some of the documented psychological morbidity, and in particular help to reduce anxiety (McVey 1998).

Medical opinion is now beginning to follow that of the patients, with the acknowledgement that the palliative approach be integrated into the training of all doctors in the UK (Association for Palliative Medicine 1991). Since that time, the average number of hours devoted to such education has increased significantly (Field & Bee Wee 2002). By contrast, however, the formal teaching of such skills in UK nursing faculties remains *ad hoc* at best (Lloyd Williams & Field 2002) and no such national imperative yet exists (Cooley 2004), despite government recognition of the need (Department of Health 2004a).

THE DISTINGUISHING FEATURES OF THE PSYCHOLOGICAL PERSPECTIVE

It is important to recognise from the outset just what kind of psychological issues the patient and their family find most difficult. This is a very subjective area which will usually be determined by a host of factors such as family dynamics, personality characteristics, access to support systems, previous experience of healthcare and, in some instances, the expectations of the health service itself. There are, however, a number of common denominators that crop up frequently, including (Watson 1994):

- anxiety
- depression
- fears of catching the illness
- pain, which may have a physiological origin, but can seriously impact on mental state
- sexual dysfunction and associated relationship problems
- treatment-related problems, such as psychologically induced nausea and vomiting
- mood swings brought on by treatment with steroids
- social isolation and disruption of job and daily routines
- irritability, tiredness and lethargy
- sleep disturbances
- inability to concentrate.

The nursing profession is perhaps the most well placed of all the healthcare professions to significantly make an impact with many of these difficulties. Payne (1998), in her review of the literature surrounding depression, highlighted widely varying rates of clinical depression of between 3% and 69% depending on the measurement tools and diagnostic criteria used and that females report higher levels of distress than male patients. She argues that nurses should review the psychological state of their patients not only on admission, but at regular periods of continuing care. She considers that healthcare professionals should approach patients directly about how they are feeling and not shy away from this area. Maguire (1999) suggests that problems arise because health professionals make assumptions about what patients need and do not often deliver information in a sensitive way. Cooley (2000), however, reminds us that, although many nurses consider their skills weak in providing psychological support, they possess a core of interpersonal skills learnt through social interaction that can and do provide the basis for good therapeutic relationship building. The long-term benefits to the well-being of patients and families of such support should not be underestimated. The question becomes, therefore, how can nurses understand the problems facing patients and their families and what can be done to support them through the process of coping with these problems?

THE CORE COMPETENCIES REQUIRED TO DELIVER PSYCHOLOGICAL SUPPORT

There are a number of documents that attempt to define the core skills that nurses need in this complex area of palliative nursing practice at both specialist and generic levels (Becker 2004, Royal College of Nursing [RCN] 2002, 2003). All approach the subject from a different perspective and use a range of differing terminology to encapsulate the intended meaning. The underpinning research to support the development of these competencies comes from seminal work by Benner (1984) in the first instance, and has been refined and developed through work by researchers such as Davies & Oberle (1990), Degner et al (1991), Heslin & Bramwell (1989) and Taylor et al (1997). The intention is to provide a coherent framework with which to define the skills of clinical practice at different levels. The outcome has arguably been mixed. At their best, competency statements referring to psychological support offer benchmarks for professional development that practitioners can use to judge their progress in their job, and can form a useful part of a professional development plan linked to the Knowledge and Skills Framework of the Agenda for Change (Department of Health 2004b). At their worst, competencies in this area have created a climate of uncertainty and perceived inadequacy amongst nurses, who find themselves confused and overwhelmed by the proliferation of methodologies which are often written in educational language with which they are unfamiliar (Becker 2000).

Table 6.1 gives examples of the kinds of psychological competency statement that are present in the three documents quoted. Those used relate to registered nurse level in both generic and specialist environments. It is notable that there is no one single category for psychological support mentioned in the more detailed RCN documents. Those competencies referred to come from sections entitled communication, interpersonal, and supportive care, and indicate how such skills have been subsumed into the plethora of terminology used to describe palliative care today. In truth this may not matter as long as the competencies are present and valued; the key issues for most practising nurses are how these skills are to be assessed, at what level, how often, and who is to do it. The reliability and validity of such assessments are fraught with difficulty (Degner et al 1991) and the evidence base to support such judgements must be much broader than academic writing and embrace the more difficult, but essential, area of observable behaviour if the true nature of such skills is to be assessed accurately.

UNDERSTANDING THE EMOTIONAL TRAUMA

The patient's perspective

An interesting paradox crops up whenever clinicians and academics attempt to discuss and analyse the

REFLECTION POINT

Consider a patient you have recently been looking after who has required psychological support, and ask yourself how competent you feel when measuring your performance with the patient against the competencies in Table 6.1. As you progress you may find yourself challenged to be brutally honest and self-critical at times in your self-assessment. This process can be painful and is a strong lesson in self-awareness and professional maturity. You should also be confident enough to give yourself credit where necessary and acknowledge the skills you have. Make no mistake, competency assessment is challenging for all concerned, but if sensitively applied the potential benefits for improved knowledge, skills and attitudes to patient care are self-evident.

If you would like to do a more comprehensive self-assessment of your skills and have access to the internet, log on to http://www.cancernursing.org and follow the links to the Introduction to Palliative Care Nursing Course. It costs nothing to register with the site and undertake the course, and the competency assessment tool used is linked to a challenging case study (Becker 2005).

psychological effects of major illness on the individual. Much of the study in this area has been conducted by health professionals who address themselves in their analysis to the formation of concepts and theories that attempt to explain this phenomenon rationally. This can be seen as a positive thing, in that it contributes to a vast body of serious literature from many eminent authors and helps our overall understanding of what is a complex and intriguing life experience. Yet there remain considerable gaps and limitations in our knowledge, which at present seem to defy contemporary analysis. This, of course, depends on the background to your point of view. Some theologians, for instance, may well argue that their set of beliefs and a particular scripture provide ample understanding and guidance for a follower of a faith. A philosopher, however, will address the issue from a more cognitive viewpoint and ask, 'What is the meaning of this event?', attempting to widen the debate as much as possible. Psychiatrists, psychologists, sociologists and anthropologists will try to analyse from a more humanistic

Table 6.1   Competency for psychological support

The member of staff will:	Who it is aimed at	Reference
• Demonstrate a developing ability to manage emotional issues relating to stages in the patient's journey • Demonstrate knowledge of the support strategies and interventions available to care for patients with complex needs (e.g. patients exhibiting denial/anger following a cancer diagnosis, adverse reactions to alteration in body image) • Have an understanding of the need and be able actively to support patients and their carers to identify and manage their own health and social well-being throughout the cancer journey • Demonstrate knowledge of the impact of advanced disease on family dynamics and the strategies that can be employed • Demonstrate knowledge of support strategies available to manage the complex needs of patient/carers and families during the grieving process and following bereavement • Demonstrate knowledge of differing needs of ethnic, cultural, religious groups and respect for their traditions • Be able to identify own and in some instances colleagues' support needs caring for patients and families with advanced disease • Support patients and their family/carers to explore the issues arising from the transition from curative care to palliative care	Registered practitioner: Nurses working in generic areas, caring for cancer patients and those just entering the specialty, as well as those who routinely use specialist cancer knowledge, skills and experience within their practice	Royal College of Nursing (2003)
• Inspire trust and confidence in the dying patient and family by the use of 'self' in the clinical situation • Recognise and acknowledge the patient's unique personal abilities, giving approval, supporting choices, and providing a realistically hopeful environment within the patient's limitations • Show an awareness and understanding of the beliefs, attitudes and practices of other cultural and ethnic groups within our society • Help patients make sense of their illness and prognosis by offering hope, facilitating reflection of life and values, fulfilling their wishes and attempting to meet spiritual needs • Use sensitive judgement to talk openly about death where appropriate, when patients and families want to do so • Help the patient come to terms with the idea of their own mortality and impending death in a supportive empathic environment • Use knowledge of verbal and non-verbal communication skills to spend time and establish a rapport with the patient and/or significant others to enable trust to develop • Spend time with the patient and family listening to their concerns and worries, respecting their beliefs and opinions in a climate of confidentiality	Registered Nurse working in a generic healthcare environment	Becker R (2000)

Table 6.1   Competency for psychological support – cont'd

The member of staff will:	Who it is aimed at	Reference
• Use the skills of empathy and reflective questioning to enable the patient and family to talk freely if they wish to • Demonstrate a warm, empathic, giving response when appropriate to communicate trust and understanding • Recognise the opportunity, by picking up cues, to hold deeper discussions relating to psychological, emotional or spiritual issues • Confidently facilitate and manage interactions with patients and families • Holistically assess psychological, cultural, social, legal and ethical issues affecting the patient and their carers' well-being, care and treatment • Understand the psychological issues and family dynamics affecting terminally ill people and their carers, and integrate this into practice	Level 2 Registered Nurse: a practitioner with a range of nursing experience who has started training in specialist palliative care, whilst working with responsibility to an experienced practitioner	Royal College of Nursing (2002)

perspective by examining the individual's behaviour and development, to try to come up with a measurable and definable entity. Physicians, however, will refer more to the biophysical model associated with defined pathologies such as anxiety and depression. This latter stance is perhaps the most widely researched and accepted model within current palliative care practice, but does little to address the more existential and holistic element of care. What is abundantly clear is that the whole subject is far more complex in nature than at first appears. From a nursing perspective, demands to acknowledge the whole person and deliver care from this stance underpin palliative nursing practice (Buckley 2002).

The paradox is that very little research has looked in a holistic manner at the experience of major illness as it is lived and perceived by the individual. To do this, of course, one has to acknowledge that subjective reality is central to human experience, instead of looking at humanity from a more biophysical stance, which can be claimed to be reductionist in outlook but more objective overall. It is not unreasonable to conclude, therefore, that in order to gain an evidence base in the study of the lived experience of dying that Western medicine will need to embrace a total paradigm shift in its research thinking and tackle the perennial and difficult ethical issues associated with interviewing the dying. Local and regional ethics committees do not currently look favourably upon such methodology, and some creative thinking is needed within the research community to tackle this major dilemma. Some of the common denominators

that underpin our current understanding of the psychological problems experienced in facing advanced illness are shown in Table 6.2.

As nurses, we would do well to take note of how we can influence the individual's perception of each of these. First, there is a clear nursing duty to develop a high level of skills in active listening and empathy underpinned by knowledge of bereavement theory, so that we may help those people who are suffering loss. Second, the means at our disposal to help influence the prescription of appropriate regimens to control difficult pain and symptoms are vast, and well integrated into nearly every aspect of healthcare. Lastly, if we are getting the first two right then valuing the person as an individual should not become an issue, as it will hopefully be integral to our approach.

The family's perspective

There is an old saying that mental health nurses use to describe the totality of the experience of ill health, which goes something like this: 'It is the patient who experiences the symptoms while it is the family that suffer the illness'. There is a close parallel in this statement to the important role that families play in the psychological support of the dying patient and the way in which they can become consumed by the nature and intensity of what is happening to their loved one, and indeed to themselves.

It is an all too common occurrence for staff to observe that the tiredness and fatigue of visiting rela-

Table 6.2   Common psychological features of advanced illness

Feature	Description
Shock	Often the reaction to a life-limiting diagnosis is one of shock. If no particular symptoms have been experienced, then someone may be completely unprepared for what is said and the shock can be profound.
Anger	There may be anger; people frequently ask: 'Why me?'
Guilt	This is frequently experienced, with people blaming themselves not only for the illness, but also for the indirect suffering it causes to those they love.
Meaning	A person needs to find a sense of meaning or a reason for what has happened. This can involve a search for explanations for why they have developed the disease and a search for spiritual comfort in whatever manner works for them.
Blame	There can be a deep sense of shame where blame is internalised, contributing to a feeling of emotional isolation. Talking about these issues can be particularly difficult, and many of the problems here are associated with gender roles and cultural norms.
Social isolation	There may be a perception that people are repelled by the disease and treat them differently, causing feelings of frustration and of being patronised.
Confusion	There can be a sense of confusion also, and of loss of control over their lives as the healthcare system gears up to deal with the complex issues that arise.
Uncertainty	For the majority of people the knowledge of personal advanced illness means uncertainty about the future, which is a central issue for them. It can manifest itself in a whole range of questions: What will it be like at the end? Will I ever see my children grow up? What about my retirement plans? How will my family cope? These statements and questions can be linked to existential issues about the meaning and relevance of their life so far.
Regrets	These can surface and may cloud the person's ability to maximise and enjoy what life they have left. Indeed, they may feel cheated and angry at missing life's opportunities. For the younger person there is a great poignancy and sense of loss that they will not see their children grow up to adulthood.
Dignity	The compromising of perceived personal dignity is perhaps one of the most significant and complex psychological factors of advanced illness. The gradual physical changes brought about by the illness or its treatments may involve hair loss, weight loss, amputation or some other physical mutilation. There may be loss of mobility and continence, and the necessity to rely on some artificial aid to conduct what were previously normal and private bodily functions. The loss of confidence and the damage to self-esteem can be considerable as the person adjusts to a new way of life.
Culture	The growing diversity of cultures in our society has enriched and deepened our understanding of the wider world, but for many generations in our towns and cities the difficulty of accessing culturally sensitive care at the end of life has been well documented (NCHSPCS 2001). Family support structures may differ; religious beliefs and rituals need to be carefully observed. Ideas surrounding choice, dignity and individuality may differ widely from Western values; norms regarding pain control, expression of grief and truth telling may all be different (Becker 2004).
Chronicity	Advances in treatment regimens mean that many illnesses can continue over long periods of time, and sometimes the effects of treatments can seem worse than the illness itself. Where a person hopes and expects a cure at the outset of an illness, they are often prepared to endure great hardship, but when the focus changes to one of clear time limitation then it is much more difficult to be motivated to continue treatments.
Hope	Maintaining hope in the face of life-threatening illness is immensely challenging, but we know that this multidimensional concept changes focus and moves in other directions. People tell us how they value relationships more, a sense of humour, spiritual issues, happy memories and a stronger self-belief (Herth 1990). We know also that there are a number of realistic and achievable measures that nurses can take to help foster hope in the dying patient (Penson 2000). A more detailed evaluation of the concept of hope and its relevance to health and well-being can be found in Chapter 8.

tives increase as time goes by. They may have to drive long distances, organise their children and work schedules around this crisis, and sacrifice large parts of their normal daily routine in order to be at the bedside. Additional household tasks may be taken on and a spouse or child may now be required to get involved in household management or childcare activities. Along with concerns for the dying person, added work, responsibility and loss of security create an uncomfortable emotional burden. Perhaps the expected help from within the family does not occur, and arguments may ensue. The previous way of life that was so comfortable has been snatched away. Sleep patterns may be disturbed, and eating habits will almost certainly be disrupted owing to the absence of the regular home routines. Snacks on the move will become the order of the day and there may be an increase in minor ailments such as coughs and colds. The consequence of this is increased levels of stress, extra financial burdens and reliance on others for help within the family and social network that may not sit comfortably in our society, which tends to emphasise self-reliance, control and independence. As nurses we can encourage family members to continue with pre-illness activities: illness should not be allowed to totally consume the household, nor should it permanently deprive family members of social activities.

The communication patterns within the family may also become strained in their desire to protect the dying person from outside influences (Hannicq 1995). Clearly, life-threatening illness affects not only the individual but all those around who matter to them. It generates anxiety and alters patterns of behaviour, roles and relationships within that family. Moreover, families play a significant role during a time of illness and their reactions contribute to the patient's response to the illness. Rather than being passive observers, family members are often active and vital participants in the patient's care and treatment (Smith 2004). Issues to do with transport, personal care, household tasks, increased costs on heating and food, alterations in lifestyle and the need for information and emotional support are key issues for the family adapting to caring for a dying relative (Payne et al 1998b).

A comprehensive literature review by Andershed (1999) into the needs of family carers highlighted a predominance of cancer-related articles, but we can extrapolate a number of common denominators from this review that can apply regardless of the patient's diagnosis. Three central themes cropped up that revolved around:

1. Knowing – the need for family members as well as the patient to be informed about diagnosis, treatment options and ultimately prognosis
2. Being – spending time together and being close to one another, sharing and supporting each other through difficult times
3. Doing – involvement in the practical tasks and activities of daily life and caring.

Although this pattern has a useful framework that can offer us a clearer understanding, the complex dynamics of family life often dictate otherwise. The strong, almost instinctive, desire to protect extends not just from the relatives towards the patient, but vice versa. The dying patient can be extremely perceptive of the moods, behaviours and reactions of those around them and may assist their loved ones in a mutual pretence of normality to help them cope with the daily visits. This active and conscious denial is a normal coping mechanism and must be seen in the context of the complete family unit and the state of knowledge of the patient of their condition. It is all too easy for a nurse to make a judgement of such a situation and to challenge individuals in the belief that no-one is facing reality, only to find a hostile retort. This denial strategy is far more subtle and effective than at first appears, and demands of the staff a close communication network to keep abreast of the changing daily scenes and dynamics.

Indeed, patients themselves may well introduce cues and clues into conversations about their illness and its progression, waiting for someone to react in the context of the real facts in order to help them come to terms with things. Each person shares some responsibility for either maintaining or breaking the unwritten code of avoidance, and the transition to an open awareness may be sudden or gradual.

As 24-hour carers, nurses are in a unique situation to be party to this change in perception and can help facilitate its smooth transition where possible. The nursing role here is dependent on the trust and rapport that has been built with the respective family members. It places the nurse potentially at the centre of this major life crisis and all the consequent cathartic emotional release that may go with it. The opportunity to shape and influence the coping strategies of the patient and family at this crucial and vulnerable time is immense, and is surely at the very core of palliative nursing practice. There are no guarantees, of course, and it is just as possible to hinder the situation rather than help it. The key word here is opportunity.

The psychological reaction of the nurse

When nurses care for the dying they know that they are expected to provide not only physical care but also understanding, comfort and emotional support for the patient and their family. Indeed, this holistic emphasis on care is clearly emphasised in a number of reports and definitions of palliative care (European Association of Palliative Care 1989, NCHSPCS 2001a, NICE 2004, World Health Organisation [WHO] 2002). However, our culture tends to emphasise youth, life and avoidance of the taboo subject of death (Aries 1993). Nurse education itself has a high emphasis on all aspects of individual health maintenance, as one would expect, and new nurses learn very quickly about the complexities of defining and promoting health from both an academic and an individual perspective, until, that is, they are introduced in the classroom to the care of someone who is dying and caring for their family. The looks of astonishment and anxiety are almost universal, regardless of age and life experience. Nurses care for the dying more than any other health-care professional, but it is very clear that they are ill prepared for this part of their role (Payne et al 1998a). Death anxiety is a frequent experience and arises from a number of factors (Boyle & Carter 1998):

- society's attitudes
- personal death experience
- relevant clinical experience.

There is evidence that qualified nurses also have high anxiety levels and may distance themselves from the dying (Mills 1990).

There can be a sense that being a professional carer confers some passive immunity from confronting issues to do with personal death. Educational and life experience tells us that death is something that happens to others and on the television, and yet we are expected to face this fundamental issue directly in order to deliver quality nursing care. There is a need, therefore, for nurses to develop close personal relationships with their patients and to be conscious of the increased risk of emotional damage that may result from such closeness. Farley (2004) recognises such situations of cognitive dissonance as both a challenge and an opportunity for development. It is possible, however, to deal with such intensity in caring at different levels, and work by Rittman et al (1997) demonstrates that experienced nurses make conscious decisions to do just that, depending on the demands they are presented with. What is not clear is whether such strategies are a means of emotional survival or avoidance of patient contact which contributes to one of the patient's major problems, that of loneliness and isolation (Benner & Wrubel 1989).

EXPLORING THE PRACTICE-BASED REALITY

Patients in hospital

See Case Study 6.1.

Research-based analysis

A number of valuable learning points arise from Case Study 6.1 that can shape and influence our nursing practice when providing psychological support:

Case Study 6.1   A patient in hospital

Anne was first diagnosed with cancer 3 years ago and underwent a mastectomy. After the operation she received a course of adjuvant chemotherapy on an outpatient basis. Despite the loss of her hair, which concerned her greatly, her recovery was steady. On a routine 6-monthly visit to her consultant, she complained of lower back pain and a swollen left eye. Soon afterwards she was admitted for investigations that revealed a large metastasis in her lower spine and one in her left orbit. Radiotherapy was given and after a full assessment for her pain an extensive analgesic regimen was prescribed.

Anne's son, Alan, and daughter, Rachel, and her husband had travelled some 200 miles from their homes in Scotland to be by her side. Anne was well informed of the situation and presented as a stoical, smiling and uncomplaining woman, with great strength of character. Her determination to adopt a positive approach throughout her illness had clearly helped her and, to some extent, her children, who now had to deal with the very real prospect of their mother's death.

Alan, in particular, was finding it very distressing and was often angry about his impotence to change the situation his mother was in. He would change the subject whenever his mother wished to discuss her illness and would excuse himself from the room whenever he could. He clearly did not know what to do or say, and this made him feel uneasy when he was sitting by her bed. The key nurse involved quietly suggested that he try holding her hand, and reassured him that he need not always have to say anything.

Rachel used her husband for support and appeared to be coping better with the reality of her mother's impending death. It was Anne's now pale and sallow complexion that caused them much distress. Anne realised this herself and would weep quietly after her family had left. It was important, therefore, for staff to be available to be with her at this sensitive time. Anne was an articulate and intelligent woman, whose need for accurate information was clearly expressed on many occasions.

In small ways, both children became involved in their mother's care, by providing her with her favourite music to listen to, a regular supply of magazines and her own nightclothes and make-up. They would often read to her, selecting brief items of news.

After several days Anne began to slip in and out of consciousness with occasional moments of lucidity; she died peacefully one lunchtime with her family at her side. Alan broke down in tears almost immediately and was comforted by his sister. Rachel and Alan stayed at their mother's side for some 20 minutes saying their goodbyes, and thanked the staff before they left. Alan commented that he felt satisfied that he had been able to communicate with his mother and appreciated being able to be there and help a little.

Anne's body image and perception of self is clearly a major nursing concern. Not only has she lost her breast and hair, but also her face is becoming disfigured due to the swelling in her left eye. Studies of the factors affecting body image have shown that issues such as self-confidence, self-criticism, media influence and relationships with partners are critical (Paquette & Raine 2004). There are two main factors here (Cronan 1993):

1. Body perception – how individuals visualise their body
2. Body attitude – how individuals value their body and their feelings towards it.

A change of body image may also be defined as a loss of psychological self, including loss of self-concept, self-esteem and self-identity. From a cultural perspective there can be a loss of social role and identity (Paquette & Raine 2004). In Anne's case this was significant.

The psychological reaction of the son, Alan, and daughter, Rachel, to their mother's fate can be understood better by reference to research into grief and loss. Current thinking in this area reinforces the multidimensional, subjective and normalistic nature of the grief experience (Walter 1999) and, while the process-centred staging theories can give us a useful framework with which to aid our understanding, the shock, despair, denial, anger and sense of impotence that Alan felt, coupled with his eventual reconciling to the situation as he adapted, are all indicative patterns of normal behaviour that the nurse can place into context for Alan.

Anne's stoical reaction to her illness is very culturally contextual to Western society. The focus within a family tends to be on organisation of the practicalities and coping with day-to-day life rather than dealing with feelings, anxieties and thoughts (Payne et al 1998b). Clearly, all members of this family had a need to support one another in whatever way they could, and it is up to the nurse to facilitate this.

The need for the nurse to foster better communication both verbally and non-verbally was of paramount importance to this family if they were to attempt to come to terms with the impact of Anne's impending death. Any serious illness or condition where recovery is unlikely or impossible serves to remind people of their own mortality and increases their sense of fear and vulnerability (Maguire 1999). There has been a vast multitude of appropriate research into the way that nurses communicate with the dying and their relatives, with conflicting results dependent on the methodologies used. Much of this work highlights the limitations of busy clinical environments and the impediments that mitigate against successful communication (Field 1989).

The use of touch – that most basic form of communication – was evident in this case study. Touch has the ability to convey a huge amount of reassurance and empathy (Le May 2004). Anne was very concerned about Alan, who was younger than his sister and had been living at home until very recently. Encouraging him to hold on to his mother's hand may have also helped to reduce Anne's anxieties. We should never underestimate the potency of this form of non-verbal communication with another person (Hallett 2004).

Alan's tears can be difficult to deal with, as there is an expectation in most Western societies that men will remain in charge of their emotions in most situations (Staudacher 1993). We also know quite clearly that encouraging and allowing the expression of such grief is a healthy thing (Worden 2003). There is a need, therefore, to allow Alan time and space to express himself as he sees fit, and to understand the psychological contradictions that confront men in these sensitive situations. In her book *Men and Grief*, Staudacher (1993) considers that Western men are under considerable cultural pressure to behave in a certain way when dealing with grief; she cites a range of the most common behaviours that are not expected (Box 6.1).

While these somewhat unrealistic expectations may make life bearable in the short term, they can make the successful resolution of loss a difficult issue. Allowing the family to stay at the bedside to say their goodbyes is a very positive and supportive part of the nurse's role. It can, nevertheless, be difficult to achieve in a busy acute clinical environment, because of the incessant pressure on bed occupancy. Gone are the days when a body would be left on a ward for 6 hours or more to allow relatives to visit. There is anecdotal evidence to suggest that 1 hour is more common today – and even that is in jeopardy at times.

Box 6.1   Unexpected behaviours (Staudacher 1993)

- Lose control over a situation
- Cry openly
- Be afraid or dependent
- Be insecure, anxious or passive
- Express loneliness, sadness or depression
- Express the need for love and affection
- Be playful and touch other men
- Exhibit what are considered typically 'feminine' characteristics

Patients at home

See Case Study 6.2.

Case Study 6.2   A patient at home

Maureen was a 58-year-old woman who lived in a small rural village with her husband, Tom, and several dogs. She had been diagnosed with multiple sclerosis some 3 years previously and took early retirement from her job as a result. Up until 3 months ago her mobility and control over her life had been good, but following their return from a short holiday abroad she had begun to deteriorate rapidly, and was now housebound and very weak. The district nurses visited twice a week to help her shower and provide some psychosocial support. Maureen was a woman who valued her independence and privacy. During the visits it was thus important for the nurse to maximise the opportunity to talk to Maureen about her situation, her fears and coping strategies. Inevitably, therefore, the time spent in the bathroom was sometimes more than an hour. Maureen's husband was very supportive and grateful for the help. As the main carer, he was frequently exhausted, and very protective towards his wife.

Often he could hear laughter coming from the bathroom. For example, one day the zip on Maureen's dress burst and she commented: 'I've come this far without a diet and I'm not starting now for anyone'. At most visits after the shower the nurse would sit and take coffee with them both. The conversation revolved around grandchildren, parenting, social activities and, when appropriate, Maureen's illness. There was a comfortable and respectful honesty between all concerned.

As she deteriorated, Maureen's bed was brought downstairs to a lounge room that overlooked their large and well tended garden. This gave her the opportunity to be near her dogs, which she adored, and to be close to natural light and her much cherished garden. They had a wide circle of friends who used to call round, but these visits began to diminish as Maureen got progressively worse.

The visits from the nurse were therefore much more than merely attending to practical tasks; they became a 'lifeline to normality', as Tom put it, and a chance also to speak honestly to someone independent about the attitudes of their friends and their sense of abandonment.

As Maureen's death became imminent the visits increased, and on one occasion she was particularly low. She spoke not about herself, but of the effect that her condition was having on Tom's mental health. Although they were open with each other about her condition, she noticed that he was becoming very joking and yet distant at the same time, which she felt was out of character. His attitude and demeanour towards the nurse changed, and he kept conversations very brief and dismissive of the situation approaching.

Maureen died a peaceful death about 10 days later, with her husband and dogs by her side. The district nurse visited soon after and encountered a tirade of verbal hostility from Tom which was mixed with many regrets. The nurse tried to calm the situation down, but without success, and left soon after. She visited again 2 days later and found a tearful, remorseful and rather drunk Tom, who apologised for his previous behaviour. The nurse made some strong coffee, sat down with Tom and listened carefully over the next hour to his story. At times he sank into tearful despair, alternating with an appropriate light-hearted comment about Maureen's life and her habits. As she left that day, Tom squeezed her hand gently, smiled and nodded his head.

Research-based analysis

The district nursing team recognised that unhurried visits early in the terminal illness would help to make caring later on more effective. Lugton (2001) suggests that a supportive relationship will not develop where contacts are hurried.

Clearly the time spent in building a trusting and empathic relationship with Maureen paid off in the conversations in the bathroom. The very personal nature of assisting with someone's hygiene involves the nurse in an intimacy of touch, which is implicit within the job itself (Le May 2004).

Maureen's right to as much independence and control over her choices in care as possible was respected, and the need for self-determination and autonomy as a vital aspect of her psychological well-being is discussed in detail in the NICE (2004) document 'Improving Supportive and Palliative Care for People with Cancer'.

The laughter was used by Maureen as a way of coping with her situation; when initiated by the patient, this is both appropriate and desirable as a healthy way of dealing with difficult situations. Although widely recognised for its therapeutic value in well people, humour is only just becoming more socially and professionally accepted in an illness situation. Kanninen (1998) has conducted a comprehensive review of the literature in this area and argues that all healthcare professionals should start to pay much more attention to the value of humour in care settings. Its use in a palliative context is a potentially sensitive issue, but there is a growing body of evidence to back up its clinical efficacy in terms of patient well-being and also as a useful strategy for staff to use to build and maintain a good rapport (Morris & Page 2004).

The practical task of moving Maureen's bed to the lounge had the more crucial effect of supporting her needs in a more spiritual sense. In order to maintain a sense of hope and quality to life, it is important to maximise these aesthetic experiences as a strategy and skill. Spiritual care includes such simple things as observing a sunrise or sunset, taking a walk at some favoured beauty spot, enjoying a glass of wine, coffee or special food, seeing a film, reading a book or having a new hairstyle (Becker & Gamlin 2004).

The interpersonal skills used throughout these encounters are fundamental to good communication. The district nurse is a guest on private property, unlike the patient in hospital or a nursing home, who is on the nurse's territory. This changes the dynamics of the interaction and places an onus of responsibility on the nurse to be extra sensitive to the changing felt meanings of what is encountered in a person's home (Thomas 2003).

Tom's rather jocular and uncharacteristic reaction to Maureen's impending death is cognisant of his inner fears and worries about losing her, and manifests itself in a daily superficiality and denial in order to cope. It is a simple thesis: 'Why expose myself to the extreme pain I know is there, if I can put it to one side in order to cope?' The important thing to remember is to place this behaviour in context as a normal reaction to the situation. Worden (2003) talks of the necessity to experience the pain of grief, but also recognises along with the majority of authors who have written in this area that this denial, although worrying for Maureen, should be handled carefully.

To be exposed to verbal aggression in someone's home as a caring professional can be both frightening and challenging. There is a need to be acutely aware of the verbal and non-verbal signals that you are sending out in such a situation, so that you can avoid escalating the aggression (Bentley 2004). The district nurse here made the decision to go, because she clearly felt that to stay would cause that escalation. After an event such as this, it is vital that the nurse herself makes an opportunity to discuss this with a colleague, manager or supervisor, to reflect and learn from the experience (Stephenson 1995). Equally, the district nurse was able, from her knowledge of loss and grief reactions, to see this in context. It is not uncommon for relatives to vent their anger on the people who represent the health services, as they feel let down. It goes back to our cultural expectation of a long life, and is part of a search for meaning to the death itself.

It took courage to go back to the house 2 days later, but the district nurse clearly felt that sufficient time had elapsed for Tom to calm down, and a familiar face may be more welcome than someone unknown.

Her decision proved correct and she used her skills to help Tom talk through his feelings and anxieties. The seemingly simple, yet therapeutic, activity of allowing someone to tell their story is well recognised in bereavement counselling theory (Worden 2003) and enabled Tom to gain a better sense of perspective on things.

As the nurse left that day she received a thanks and acknowledgement from Tom for her help. No words were spoken and it could be argued that none was necessary. This spontaneous gesture of warmth in many ways represents to the nurse that intangible and often indefinable element we call 'job satisfaction', and is bound up in the complexities of the human condition. It is also about the often undervalued and yet acknowledged skill of 'presencing'. The power of true presence is when the patient and/or family acknowledge that they feel heard, understood and supported, as in this case (Mullard 2005).

KEY NURSING STRATEGIES

When dealing with an impending death and the situation soon after, there are a number of simple strategies and core skills that the practising nurse can employ to help give psychological support to the patient and family; these are now considered.

Spend time with dying patients

It is all too easy to avoid the dying patient and their relatives. Sometimes they need to be left alone, but there are many times when the need for human contact, comfort and reassurance is vital (Mullard 2005).

The caring concept of 'being available' and 'presencing' is acknowledged by a number of authors. It is synonymous with Parse's (1992) concept of 'true presence' and is one of the carative factors used by Watson (1994). Benner & Wrubel (1989) note that the ability to presence oneself and to be with a patient in a way that acknowledges a shared humanity is the basis of nursing as a caring practice.

There will always be a sense of powerlessness when confronted with death. This is something that no-one can change. The real skill is in learning to be comfortable with that powerlessness and using it to help the patient and family. We do this by the sensitive use of what is intuitive and felt, as much as by what is learnt (Benner 1984). Sheila Cassidy (1988, p 64) summed it up very well when she said:

> Slowly I learn about the importance of power-lessness. I experience it in my life, and I live with

it in my work. The secret is not to be afraid of it – not to run away. The dying know we are not God . . . All they ask is that we do not desert them.

Answer questions

A patient may ask a nurse, doctor or any member of the caring team at any time questions about their prognosis and diagnosis. They may also wish to discuss their thoughts and feelings surrounding this. All members of the direct caring team should have up-to-date knowledge about a patient's condition and should be prepared to share this if requested. There is much anxiety expressed by practising nurses about this area, but there is no code, rule or law that forbids a nurse to give this information if in their judgement it is the right thing to do at the time. Indeed, this responsibility and accountability is enshrined in the Code of Professional Conduct (Nursing and Midwifery Council 2004). We need to be sensitive, however, to the working relationships we have with our colleagues and to our responsibility to the patient to handle the questions with the utmost care. Equally, as nurses, there is a clear responsibility to advise non-professional and junior staff on how to deal with questions, and when to seek help. (Chapter 7 of this book explores this in more depth.)

Allow the patient to die

This may sound rather obvious, but one of the major challenges of palliative nursing in non-specialist environments is empowering staff to reach a considered decision regarding the care orientation of the patient. Ideally, this should be done in conjunction with the patient, if possible the relatives and all members of the team. Much distress can be caused if efforts to initiate resuscitation or other procedures are fruitless, when the quality of the remaining life is poor (Resuscitation Council 2001). It is the simple ethical principle of 'non-maleficence' or, in other words, that we should do the patient no harm. The Nursing and Midwifery Council (2004) Code of Professional Conduct makes this quite explicit. It requires an assertive and knowledgeable nurse who has a good understanding of accountability and confidence to challenge the status quo where necessary if the patient's best interest is to be served.

Understand the family's needs

It is good practice to assign a member of staff to discover what family there is, how they wish to be involved in care and what, if any, special needs they may have. This is not only part of the admission procedure but a continuing responsibility thereafter as relationships change and staff come and go. Although difficult to achieve, in some clinical environments, the sense of continuity achieved by this approach is highly valued by both patient and relatives.

Consider the patient's choice about where they wish to be

Although many patients, when asked, express a wish to die at home, the reality of care today is that only about 25% will actually achieve that desire (Office of National Statistics 2002). Thus, with the bulk of the population dying in some form of institution, careful attention to the environment can provide good psychological support by creating a milieu that the patient is comfortable with. Some patients may prefer peace and quiet, and wish to be in a side room. Others, however, like to be part of life on a ward. Some may like to be moved closer to the office or staff desk. Such choice may not be available within the nursing and residential home, but the opportunity to personalise care within that environment is usually better as a result of greater continuity in staff and often more long-term relationships. Those who die at home can have a wide variety of services to support them (depending on diagnosis, unfortunately), but the psychological comfort of being in familiar surroundings is a powerful element. The key word to consider is choice.

Respect patients' interpretation of their dignity

Don't build yourself a set of beliefs and values that unconsciously communicate to the patient and family that their loved one's death should represent an ideal. There is no right or wrong way to die, and many people die with unfinished business in relationships and personal difficulties that are impossible to influence or change; this does not negate or devalue the care that has been given. Let the patient decide what their priorities are and work towards these. There is a need to recognise and accept that, despite the best efforts of the multiprofessional team, there will be a nucleus of people who choose to reject the help offered to them. We must therefore learn to evaluate care based on what we know of the patient's values and beliefs, and not our own.

SUMMARY

This chapter has concerned itself with attempting to explore the knowledge and skills necessary to practise what is essentially one aspect of the art of nursing care. The professional nursing skills and attributes necessary to support the terminally ill and those close to them are now becoming much clearer. Equally the organisational and resource reasons that limit our practice in this area are well known. If we are to rise to the challenge of dealing with the complex psychodynamic issues that surround the provision of psychological support, the question we really have to ask ourselves is: 'Do we have the will and the confidence to change?' Current government initiatives have laid the groundwork for a more logical and systematic strategy for psychological support for the first time ever, so the imperative is very much in the hands of the clinicians to make it work.

I am convinced in my own mind that nurses consistently underestimate and undervalue the skills they have. Like many of you, I have seen some outstanding examples of care, compassion and support given in sometimes tortuous circumstances, yet the value we ascribe to this area of nursing practice is consistently less than that afforded to the skills involved in the science of practice. In the continuing debate surrounding how palliative care is defined and resourced, nurses should not lose sight of these vital elements. There is a disturbing paradox beginning to emerge here. Anecdotal evidence is growing that in specialist units nurses are abdicating the more psychosocial and psychological aspects of their role to other health professionals at the first opportunity, and the same is happening in acute hospitals where the presence of a growing number of Clinical Nurse Specialists in palliative care is beginning to have the same effect.

When we attempt to deliver psychological support, this begins as soon as the patient and family become active participants in care. Considerable responsibility lies therefore on all professionals to shape this intense and disturbing life experience by their strategies and interventions. Patients and families require an interested person who can establish a trusting relationship, help them sort out their life and assist them in determining future directions. It is an opportunity to use a diverse range of interpersonal skills, utilising the techniques of active listening, attending, questioning, understanding, facilitating, supporting and assessing problems and being involved in an ongoing therapeutic relationship.

There is no simple answer to the question of how to give good-quality psychological support to the dying; it will always remain a sensitive subjective area simply because it deals with the human condition in perhaps its greatest life crisis and as such, it could be argued, defies complete analysis. With this in mind, therefore, when we make an active decision to respond to our patients with an open, non-judgemental and empathic response, remember the quote from 'Star Trek' made at the beginning of this chapter:

> You have helped me, and continue to do so by your understanding, your openness, your warmth, the relationship we have and by who you are, just as much as by what you do.

REFLECTION POINTS

- To what extent does the apparent 'business' of a nurse's daily clinical work impact on the potential for quality psychological care?
- What are the obstacles and opportunities created by a more systematic assessment-based approach to psychological care?
- How can we influence the difficult adaptation to change that takes place within family structures, and provide the kind of psychological support that is valued and useful?
- Why is it that difficulties with communication are perhaps the single most difficult barrier to overcome when dealing with the emotional support of the dying person and their family?
- How can nurses influence and promote the psychological component of care into the undergraduate curriculum?
- People's reactions to death and dying have their basis in the psychological maturity and the personality characteristics of the individual. In what way do a person's own beliefs, values and experiences significantly influence their attitudes in this area?
- What priority do we currently give to the conscious use of self in a palliative care situation to effect a change in the ill person?
- Should we be looking towards what we mean by 'therapeutic nursing' from a psychological perspective and how it is characterised?
- What are the challenges that researchers in palliative care have to face if we are to get a true picture of the needs of dying people and their families?
- There will come a time in all our lives when we are faced with the necessity to give active psychological support. Consider carefully the value that the culture of nursing and healthcare currently places on our responses to this issue, despite the well meaning aspirations of government guidelines, and ask yourself whether providing high-quality psychological support will continue to be seen as a luxury, affordable only in well-staffed specialist units, and not the basic human right it should be in all caring environments.

References

Andershed B 1999 The role of the family carer at the end of life: an evidence based literature review. Swedish Board of Health and Welfare, Stockholm

Aries P 1993 Death denied. Cited in: Dickenson D, Johnson M (eds) Death, dying and bereavement, Ch. 2. Sage, London

Association of Palliative Medicine of Great Britain and Ireland 1991 Palliative medicine curriculum. Cited in: National Council for Hospice and Specialist Palliative Care Services 1995 Specialist palliative care: a statement of definitions. Occasional Paper 8, p 23. NCHSPCS, London

Association for Palliative Medicine 1992 Palliative medicine curriculum for medical students, general professional training and specialist training. Cited in: National Council for Hospice and Specialist Palliative Care Services 1996 Education in palliative care. Occasional Paper 9. NCHSPCS, London

Becker R 2000 Competency assessment in palliative nursing. European Journal of Palliative Care 7(3):88–91

Becker R 2004 Education in cancer and palliative care: an international perspective. In: Foyle L, Hostad J (eds) Delivering cancer and palliative care education. Radcliffe Press, Oxford, p 189–202

Becker R 2005 An introduction to palliative care nursing. Online. Available: http://www.cancernursing.org/informationarea/courses/futurecourses/furtherdetails.asp?Area=InformationArea&Section=Courses&SubSection=FutureCourses&CourseID=34 15 Jan 2007

Becker R, Gamlin R 2004 Fundamental aspects of palliative care nursing. Quay Books, Salisbury

Benner P 1984 From novice to expert. American Journal of Nursing March:402–407

Benner P, Wrubel J 1989 The primacy of care. Addison-Wesley, Menlo Park, CA

Bentley J 2004 Taking steps to ensure personal safety. British Journal of Community Nursing 9(12):518

Boyle M, Carter D E 1998 Death anxiety amongst nurses. International Journal of Palliative Nursing 4(1):37–43

Buckley J 2002 Holism and a health promoting approach to palliative care. International Journal of Palliative Nursing 8(10):505–508

Cassidy S 1988 Sharing the darkness: the spirituality of caring, p 64 Darton, Longman & Todd, London

Cooley C 2000 Communication skills in palliative care. Professional Nurse 15(9):603–605

Cooley C 2004 Core skills nursing cancer patients. International Cancer Nursing News 16(2):45

Cronan L 1993 Management of the patient with altered body image. British Journal of Nursing 2(5):257–261

Davies B, Oberle K 1990 Dimensions of the supportive role of the nurse in palliative care. Oncology Nursing Forum 17(1):87–94

Degner L F, Gow C M, Thompson L A 1991 Critical nursing behaviours in care for the dying. Cancer Nursing 14(5):246–253

Department of Health 2004a Government response to House of Commons Health Committee Report on Palliative Care. Fourth Report of Session 2003–04. Department of Health, London

Department of Health 2004b Agenda for Change: final agreement. Department of Health, London

European Association of Palliative Care 1989 European Association of Palliative Care by-laws. EAPC & National Cancer Institute, Milan

Farley G 2004 Death anxiety and death education. In: Foyle L, Hostad J (eds) Delivering cancer and palliative care education. Radcliffe Press, Oxford, p 73–84

Field D 1989 Nursing the dying. Routledge, London

Field D, Bee Wee 2002 Preparation for palliative care: teaching about death, dying and bereavement in UK medical schools 2000–2001. Medical Education 36:561–567

Fitzsimmons D, Ahmedzai S 2004 Approaches to assessment in palliative care. In: Payne S, Seymour J, Ingleton C (eds) Palliative care nursing: principles and evidence for practice. Open University Press, Maidenhead, p 163–185

Hallett A 2004 Narratives of therapeutic touch. Nursing Standard 19(1):33–37

Hannicq M 1995 Family care: new principles. European Journal of Palliative Care 2(1):21–24

Harper B C 1977 Death: the coping mechanism of the health professional. Southeastern University Press, Greenville, SC

Herth K 1990 Fostering hope in terminally ill people. Journal of Advanced Nursing 15:1250–1259

Heslin K, Bramwell L 1989 The supportive role of the staff nurse in the hospital palliative care situation. Journal of Palliative Care 5:20–26

Kanninen M 1998 Humour in palliative care: a review of the literature. International Journal of Palliative Nursing 4(3):110–114

Le May A 2004 Building rapport through non verbal communication. Nursing and Residential Care 6(10):488–491

Lloyd Williams M, Field D 2002 Are undergraduate nurses taught palliative care during their training? Nurse Education Today 22(7):589–592

Lugton J 2001 Communicating with dying people and their relatives. Radcliffe Medical Press, London

Maguire P 1999 Improving communication with cancer patients. European Journal of Cancer Care 35(10):1415–1422

McVey P 1998 Depression among the palliative care oncology population. International Journal of Palliative Nursing 4(2):86–93

Mills J 1990 A study of the relationships between hospice nurses and college students in the area of death anxiety. University Microfilms International, USA

Morris S, Page W 2004 Humour in cancer and palliative care: an educational perspective. In: Foyle L, Hostad J (eds) Delivering cancer and palliative care education. Radcliffe Publishing, Oxford, p 173–187

Mullard E 2005 Presencing: the unseen therapeutic relationship. In: Nyatanga B, Astley Pepper M (eds) Hidden aspects of palliative care. Quay Books, Salisbury, p 45–57

National Council for Hospice and Specialist Palliative Care Services 1997 Feeling better: psychosocial care in specialist palliative care. Occasional Paper 13. NCHSPCS, London

National Council for Hospice and Specialist Palliative Care Services 2001a What do we mean by palliative care? A discussion paper. Briefing No. 9. NCHSPCS, London

National Council for Hospice and Specialist Palliative Care Services 2001b Palliative care services for different ethnic groups. Seminar Proceedings. NCHSPCS, London

National Institute for Clinical Excellence 2004 Improving supportive and palliative care for people with cancer. NICE, London

Nursing and Midwifery Council 2004 Code of Professional Conduct: standards for conduct performance and ethics. HMSO, London

Office of National Statistics 2002 Mortality statistics: review of Registrar General on deaths in England and Wales 2002. HMSO, London

Paquette M, Raine K 2004 Socio-cultural context of women's body image. Social Science and Medicine 59(5):1047–1058

Parse R 1992 Human becoming: Parse's theory of nursing. Nursing Science Quarterly 5:35–42

Payne S 1998 Depression in palliative care: a literature review. International Journal of Palliative Nursing 4(4):184–191

Payne S A, Dean S J, Kalus C 1998a A comparative study of death anxiety in hospice and emergency nurses. Journal of Advanced Nursing 28(4):700–706

Payne S, Smith P, Dean S 1998b Identifying the concerns of informal carers in palliative care. Palliative Medicine 13:37–44

Penson J 2000 A hope is not a promise: fostering hope within palliative care. International Journal of Palliative Nursing 6(2):95–98

Resuscitation Council 2001 Decisions relating to cardiopulmonary resuscitation. A joint statement from the British Medical Association, the Resuscitation Council (UK) and the Royal College of Nursing. Resuscitation Council, London

Rittman M, Paige P, Rivera J, Godown I 1997 Phenomenological study of nurses caring for dying patients. Cancer Nursing 20:115–119

Royal College of Nursing 2002 A framework for nurses working in specialist palliative care: competencies project. RCN Publications, London

Royal College of Nursing 2003 Core competency framework for cancer nursing: delivering effective patient care. RCN Publications, London

Smith P 2004 Working with family care givers in a palliative care setting. In: Payne S, Seymour J, Ingleton C (eds) Palliative care nursing: principles and evidence for practice. Open University Press, Maidenhead, p 312–328

Staudacher C 1993 Men and grief. New Harbinger Publications, Oakland, CA

Stephenson S, Holm D 1995 Reflection: a student's perspective. In: Palmer A, Burns S, Bulman C (eds) Reflective practice in nursing: the growth of the professional practitioner. Blackwell Science, Oxford, p 53–62

Taylor B, Glass N, McFarlane J, Stirling C 1997 Palliative nurses' perceptions of the nature and effects of their work. International Journal of Palliative Nursing 3(5):253–258

Thomas K 2003 Caring for the dying at home: companions on the journey. Radcliffe Medical Press, Oxford

Walter T 1999 On bereavement. Open University Press, Buckinghamshire

Watson M 1994 Psychological care for cancer patients and their families. Journal of Mental Health 3:457–465

Worden W J 2003 Grief counselling and grief therapy: a handbook for the mental health practitioner, 3rd edn. Brunner Routledge, Hove

World Health Organisation 2002 Palliative care. Online. Available: http://www.who.int/cancer/palliative/en/ available 20 Mar 2006

Chapter 7

Communication in advanced illness: challenges and opportunities

Shaun Kinghorn, Sandra Gaines and Gill Satterley

INTRODUCTION

Effective communication is central to promoting high-quality palliative care. Inadequate communication may be the source of much distress for patients and their families, and mitigates against adjustment to cancer and other life-threatening illnesses (Kruijver et al 2000). Effective and sensitive communication is the heart of comforting, assessment of need, expression of psychological/social/spiritual distress, as well as planning for what may be perceived to be an undesirable and premature end to life. The compelling search for ways of improving communication is ongoing and there is evidence to suggest that little has improved despite a plethora of initiatives to improve the situation (Maguire 1999, Wilkinson 1991).

This chapter seeks to explore the nature of effective communication as it relates to palliative nursing, and discusses the principles that underpin the handling of awkward questions, breaking bad news and handling collusion. The focus on principles that might guide practice is supplemented by consideration of selective frameworks that may be directly relevant to the work of practitioners within a palliative care context. The chapter also considers factors that influence the development of nurses' communication skills, including training, attitudes of staff, clinical supervision and evaluation of communication practice. It is acknowledged that it is not possible to cover all communication challenges and it is recommended that reference is made to associated chapters on psychological issues, loss and grief, looking after yourself, hope and spirituality to develop a broader understanding of communication issues in advanced illness.

COMMUNICATION IN ADVANCED ILLNESS: THE CONTEXT

The National Institute for Clinical Excellence (NICE 2004) comments that good face-to-face communication between health and social work professionals and patients and their carers is fundamental to the provision of high-quality care. Good communication ensures that patients' and carers' concerns and choices are elicited, and yet patients and carers frequently report communication skills of practitioners to be lacking (NICE 2004). Such conclusions may be linked to the rapidly expanding expectations that patients and their families have, and to our ability to keep pace with these expectations. The expression of these expectations is receiving political and social affirmation in order that the patient can feel in control, and justified in articulating their need. Field & Copp (1999) mention that over the past 40 years there has been a progression from a closed awareness to a more open awareness with regard to communicating with the dying. Such an assertion cannot be applied universally. Not all patients are able to articulate their needs clearly. Illness, sex, social class, fatigue and other distressing symptoms impact on the individual's capacity to express need and the emotional pain that may accompany advanced illness. It is argued that palliative care needs to be attuned to the needs of the disadvantaged dying who cannot always express their needs and fears, because of coexisting learning disabilities or mental health issues.

Advanced illness is a quagmire of painful emotions, difficult decisions and loss. Patients and their families requiring palliative care may have made contact with these services within a timeframe of weeks, or months, following an initial diagnosis. Alternatively, some require palliative care after enduring a constellation of emotionally and physically taxing therapies over a period of years. In such situations, uncertainty becomes a constant companion. The pathway, timeframes and reasons that accompany the palliative care journey are both complex and unique. An acknowledgement by the nurse that the individual has specific and unique communication needs is essential to high-quality palliative care. Lugton et al (2005) suggest that the individual confronted by a life-threatening illness is faced by a number of threats, which include the threats to identity and future plans, to social roles, to physical and psychosocial independence, to body image, to relationships, of stigma and isolation, and to faith and hope. A lot of these challenges

are highly dependent on the use of communication skills for assessment and resolution of concerns.

Enhancing our capacity to support patients with advanced illnesses is dependent on the development of appropriate skills and the possession of specific attitudes. This simplistic proposition fails to acknowledge the complex social context in which communicating with those with a life-threatening illness occurs. Helping patients to make sense of the past and come to terms with the present and future has to acknowledge the factors that might influence our capacity constructively to support patients and their families (Box 7.1).

> Communicating significant news should normally be undertaken by a skilled clinician who has received advanced level training and is assessed as being an effective communicator.
> (Key Recommendation 5, NICE 2004, p 56–64)

However, this is not always practical and all staff should be trained to respond appropriately to patients' and carers' concerns before referring to a more senior professional. Several issues, in particular, form a common theme in that practitioners find them challenging in everyday practice. These are breaking bad news, dealing with difficult questions and the situation of collusion.

Breaking bad news

Developments in nursing have led to nurses having an active role in some of the more challenging aspects of supporting the patient through a life-threatening illness. Although the responsibility of sharing bad news at diagnosis at present is generally in the hands of our medical colleagues, nurses are increasingly being involved in sharing bad news. The development of nurse-led initiatives and a more active role in diagnostic and treatment stages of incurable illnesses will inevitably lead to nurses needing to enhance their skills in breaking bad news.

Penson (2000) commented that the sharing of the whole truth is often associated with taking away hope. If we get it right, the patient will never forget us; if we get it wrong, they will never forgive us (Buckman 1996). The degree of trauma associated with the news is determined by the gap between the patient's expectations and the presented truths associated with the progress of the disease. The handling of the emotions associated with 'giving bad news' can equally be distressing for the deliverer (Franks 1997). Bad news is not linked just to sharing the

Box 7.1 Factors that might create communication difficulties

- *Age of the patient* – The elderly may have hearing, sight or speech difficulties that impact on the expression and reception of communication needs. The age of the practitioner may also influence their attitude on how much the patient should be told regarding their illness (Gillhooly et al 1988). Communicating with the young who are dying is often considered to be a source of professional distress.

- *Factors linked to the disease or associated treatments* – These may inhibit constructive dialogue, for instance radiotherapy or surgery to the head or neck, confusional states resulting from pharmacological interventions or the disease process.

- *The patient and family members' previous experiences of a life-threatening illness* – These experiences may come in the form of memories of a relative or friend having had . . . or died from . . . These experiences may form a route map for the patient to the point where they resist healthcare professionals' efforts to portray things as they really are.

- *Presence of distressing symptoms* – The unremitting experiences associated with breathlessness, pain, vomiting and other symptoms not only lead to emotional distress but themselves create communication difficulties. Good symptom management is therefore a key to sustaining meaningful communication channels.

- *Blocking behaviours* (Wilkinson 1991) – These behaviours can be initiated by nurses, patients and family members as a coping mechanism. The desire to maintain control over the present and the future may manifest itself in the patient and family blocking attempts from professionals initiating additional support. Blocking may be a reasonable coping strategy when the patient is being supported by a large number of professionals who all have a vested interest in obtaining the patient's story.

- *Cultural issues* – The various ethnic groups that now reside in the UK have different philosophical orientations towards life and death that are likely to impact on the style and methods of communication adopted by the practitioner.

initial life-threatening diagnosis; it may accompany any of the following scenarios: the patient is invited to consider being admitted to a hospice; the patient is starting an opioid for pain control; the patient is informed that the side-effects of drugs will promote certain disturbances in physical appearance as well as ease symptoms.

It is the patient who determines what news is bad news. The professionals involved in delivering palliative care may have their own concept of what constitutes bad news; these perceptions may not be totally congruent with those of the patient.

The principles behind the practice

Breaking bad news is viewed as one of those tasks that were traditionally associated with medical staff. This responsibility may have been assumed without assessment of competence, further questioning of performance or ongoing supervision.

A number of authors have proposed frameworks for breaking bad news (Baile et al 2000, Buckman 1992, Faulkener 1998, Kaye 1996) that can guide the practitioner in sharing the news of a life-threatening illness or the advent of a crisis. The sharing of bad news cannot be dependent on intuition, but requires careful assessment, interpersonal competence, sensitivity and a capacity for handling a wide range of distressing emotions. These skills need to dovetail with a framework of principles that systematically and sensitively broach news and is paced to meet the needs of the individual. It is essential that these principles are applied consistently to each 'bad news' event in order that the person can come to terms with the life change. Box 7.2 outlines the orientation of each of the above authors to the breaking of bad news. Baile et al (2000), in their six-step protocol for delivering bad news, go further and provide a detailed guide, stressing the need for adequate preparation of self, environment and the patient. Management of the interview and how to provide adequate support to the patient and carers is discussed, highlighting the need to end with a clear plan that the patient and family are in agreement with, followed by the importance of clear documentation and records of the event.

Each of these frameworks has a high degree of consensus. The emphasis on preparation, follow-through and allowing the patient to determine the pace and volume of the news seems to represent reconciling features of these models. These models are underpinned by a concern that individual anxieties and emotional responses are acknowledged and allowed to surface.

Box 7.2   Frameworks for breaking bad news

BUCKMAN (1992)
1. Getting started
2. Finding out how much the patient knows
3. Find out how much the patient wants to know
4. Sharing the information (aligning and educating)
5. Responding to the patient's feelings
6. Planning and follow-through

KAYE (1996)
1. Preparation
2. What does the patient know?
3. Is more information wanted?
4. Give a warning shot
5. Allow denial
6. Explain if requested
7. Listen to concerns
8. Encourage ventilation of feelings
9. Summary and plan
10. Offer availability

FAULKENER (1997)
1. Identify current knowledge or suspicions
2. Warn of impending news (warning shot)
3. News at patient's pace and in manageable chunks
4. Allow the patient to choose when they have heard enough
5. Give space
6. Handle reactions

SPIKES FRAMEWORK – BAILE ET AL (2000)
1. Setting up the interview
2. Assessing the patient's *Perception*
3. Obtaining the patient's *Invitation*
4. Giving *Knowledge* and information to the patient
5. Addressing the patient's *Emotions*
6. Strategy and *Summary*

Such pacing can reduce the risk of denial being an inevitable consequence of breaking the news. Faulkener (1998) sees a systematic approach as being fundamental to ensuring that psychological damage is not an inevitable consequence of breaking bad news.

The sharing of a diagnosis of a life-threatening illness may evoke strong emotional responses, including grief, isolation, depression, despair and shock (Morley 1997). Some responses are designed to help the individual and/or family cope with the devastating news. One such coping mechanism is denial: this permits the person to avoid the harsh realities that often accompany a cancer diagnosis and subsequent alterations in prognosis. The difficulty with this coping mechanism is that it often creates tension amongst staff and family members. The gap between truth and reality may hinder planning towards a peaceful death, and lead to non-acceptance of services that could ease the burden of the patient and family members.

As bad news may be a frequent experience, supporting colleagues who often break bad news is essential. The current emphasis on weeding out bad practice needs to be countermanded by an equal determination to support and praise good practice when it is witnessed.

Collusion: 'You won't tell him, will you?'

Irrespective of your sphere of practice, whether it be hospice, nursing home, community or hospital, the challenge of collusion remains a major communication issue. Its prevention, persistence and resolution can be influenced significantly by the skills, knowledge and attitudes of staff. Even though the mentally competent patient has a legal right to information concerning their diagnosis, prognosis and treatment, it is still practice in some areas that relatives are briefed on the situation before the patient.

Collusion is defined as protecting another from bad news (Faulkener 1998). There are various types of collusion. The first type is initiated by relatives, who may confront the nurses by strongly asserting that patients must not be told their diagnosis, or they 'will just go to pieces'. Correspondingly, the patient may be insistent that the relatives are not to know.

Collusion may be also initiated by professionals, who may establish a set of unwritten rules that are aimed at concealing the full implications of a life-threatening illness. Often the act of collusion is initiated by the desire to maintain short-term goals rather than examining the long-term consequences of such actions.

Withholding information creates a number of ethical and practical problems. There is little evidence to suggest that sharing a diagnosis will be psychologically damaging to a patient (Buckman 1992, Franks 1997).

The rationale for colluding may be founded on a desire not to harm another party, fearing that the individual will 'go to pieces'. The strength of feeling associated with the desire to withhold information on the surface is not consistent with an act of kindness. There are a number of options open to the professional: to collude with relatives and honour this assertion, or alternatively to try gently to break the collusion. Each pathway merits careful consideration, with its own unique set of consequences which must be explored.

Anxiety is a common emotion following the sharing of bad news, but is not an emotion that is permanent or beyond the realms of successful management. If the patient is described by the relative as not being able to cope with bad news, careful consideration must be given to previous life experiences and psychological resilience which may dampen the impact of the bad news. By doing nothing, the patient will become aware of a gradual functional deterioration, body image disturbances and the emergence of potentially distressing symptoms. The web of deceit, if sustained to this point, could be significant in determining whether access to specialist cancer/palliative care services is to be sought. Often patients are requested to attend cancer centres or palliative care units that are clearly signposted, or appointments are made on headed paper that clearly states the nature of the service provided. Of more long-standing impact is the effect of missed opportunities (Box 7.3), should collusion be allowed to persist to the time of death. Although little research has been done in this area it is possible to speculate that allowing collusion to continue will impact on the depth of pain experienced by those who are bereaved.

Dilemmas also exist for the nurse who confronts the situation directly. In a hospital or hospice situation it is all too easy to pass the task on to another professional. This is not the case for the community practitioner, who often faces collusion alone in the patient's home where the carer and the patient hold the strongest power base.

Close relationships with family members are fundamental to ensuring that the patient receives the

support of nurses and other professionals. Untimely confrontation of this issue may create a volatile situation. Nevertheless, in the short term it may be appropriate for the nurse to emphasise in a supportive manner that if he or she is asked by the patient or questioned regarding his/her condition then these issues will need to be tackled.

In a similar manner to breaking bad news, it is important that handling collusion is broached in a systematic and sensitive manner. From experience in delivering workshops on communication, practitioners have found it useful to follow principles that guide practice when an individual insists that the truth must be withheld:

- Identify to whom you are speaking – Are they the next of kin? Are the views of this relative consistent with those of other family members?
- Explore the reasons why the relative believes the bad news should be withheld.
- Explore with the individual(s) the difficulties they are experiencing in visiting or caring for their relative.
- Explore what will be the medium- and long-term consequences of withholding the bad news for themselves and the patient.
- Decide on the response.

You will note from these guidelines that the response follows a number of perceptual explorations that will govern the final response. Often the issue of long-term consequences is not explored. The nurse can facilitate a new perspective on the situation that may ultimately lead to a free flow of information.

Situations in which relatives are insisting that bad news is not shared with a patient and other variations on this theme are preventable. Nurses at the diagnostic end of life-threatening illness ought to reflect on the consequences of supporting a protocol that encourages withholding the sharing of information from the patient. Initiating and sustaining collusion leaves unfinished business (Faulkener 1998), and the opportunity to express many things that matter is important to the patient. Vivian (2006) is of the opinion that the nurse's role in truth-telling is an important element and therefore significant in avoiding collusion. She further comments that the law indicates the importance of providing sufficient information to patients in order for them to make informed choices; this may involve divulging prognosis. However, as Vivian states: 'It is unwise . . . to state that all dying patients should be told the truth because each case is different and may be complex'. Case Study 7.1 demonstrates the complexity of some scenarios.

Box 7.3 Leaving collusion alone: missed opportunities

- The chance to say . . .
  Goodbye
  Thank you
  I am sorry
  If only
  I will miss you
  I am going to miss
- To go on a last holiday together
- To invest time and energy in developing a life history that may be written, videotaped or audiotaped, or a combination of all three
- To put financial affairs in order
- To write that last will and testament

Case Study 7.1   Collusion

A frail 69-year-old man was undergoing the diagnostic procedures for bowel cancer. His daughter, a specialist nurse and his only close family member, felt strongly that she alone should be the first point of contact regarding information on her father's progress.

The ward staff struggled with this situation as the patient tried unsuccessfully to get information from them. The surgeon, when confronted by the daughter, discussed the results with her before telling the patient herself. When it was discovered that the patient had spread of his disease with liver metastasis, the daughter insisted that her father not be told.

This created a situation in which the patient was informed that surgery would no longer be performed, leading to a great deal of anxiety and worry for the patient as no explanation could be offered. The ward team felt helpless and deceitful in not being able to address the patient's concerns. Eventually, after much heated and emotional discussion with the ward team, the daughter reluctantly agreed that her father could be told. The daughter later required much support from the Macmillan team as she was angry and upset that her father had been told.

On reflection, the ward team felt that, although the daughter was 'difficult', they could have handled this situation better.

- What do you feel the main issues are here?
- What were the consequences for staff involved in the care of the patient in this situation?
- What are the consequences of withholding of information from the patient?
- Using the guiding principles above, consider how the situation may have been more effectively dealt with.
- What is the role of the nurse in preventing such situations from arising?

You may find it useful to discuss this case study within your own team.

Acknowledgement
Case study provided by Audrey Rowe, Nursing Team Manager, Marie Curie Nursing Service, Marie Curie Hospice Newcastle.

Handling awkward questions

One of the key features of palliative care is the infinite number of difficult questions that may be posed by patients and relatives. Breaking bad news is almost an elective situation, in which communication needs can be anticipated and prepared for. With awkward questions this is not always the case: the question or statement may be spontaneous and seemingly unprovoked, and for the nurse is anxiety-provoking. You may be able to identify some of the following questions and statements that you have heard from patients and their families:

- How long have I got?
- Am I going to get better?
- How will she cope when I am gone?
- What will it be like when I die?
- Will you help me on my way? I can't cope with this any longer.
- It's just not fair!
- There must be other treatment they could use.
- What would you do in my situation?
- The doctor could be wrong!
- Why?

There are probably many more questions that could be added to this list. The delivery of these questions is often well thought out and may have been preceded by a lot of personal reflection. The above questions may be awkward for one or more of the following reasons:

- The answer may not be known.
- The practitioner may not have the authority to answer the question.
- The timing of the question may not be congruent with the practitioner's time allocation.
- The individual may not have the skills to handle the question and the subsequent issues.
- The question may be accompanied by intense emotion, such as anxiety, anger and other forms of distress.
- For the nurse, the question may rekindle powerful personal memories of past difficult situations, both personal and professional.

There are, of course, no stock phrases or answers that can adequately respond to such questions. The answer lies in the sensitive application of the following principles which are designed to elicit the most pressing concerns beneath the question. First, it is important to:

1. Acknowledge that the question is important to the individual and merits your undivided attention.
2. Use skilful questioning, preferably with open questions, to help facilitate the ventilation of feelings and elicit what the real issues are.
3. Listen intently throughout.
4. Summarise what has been said to clarify the nature of the problem.
5. Decide on the appropriate response.

Once again, exploration precedes response. The application of these principles is manifest in the situation given in Case Study 7.2.

Case Study 7.2   Handling awkward questions

John is a 55-year-old man with a carcinoma of the colon who is being cared for in your surgical unit. He has secondary deposits in his liver and has recently undergone palliative chemotherapy. He is married with two daughters aged 24 and 21 years who no longer live at home with their mother, Grace. Melinda, the eldest daughter, is expecting a baby in 3 months' time. John is fatigued, anxious, and complains of back pain and upper abdominal pain. You are helping him to get ready one morning when he starts to mutter: 'I am not getting any better'. This quiet statement is followed by: 'How long have I got?' How will you respond?

Perhaps the application of the following principles to Case Study 7.2 may help. It is not suggested this should be a template for every similar situation, but nevertheless it is there to illustrate how awkward questions require systematic exploration to ensure the response is helpful to the patient:

1. Acknowledge that the question is important to the individual and merits your time

You could allow a little silence to pass by if nothing further comes; then make sure John is in a quiet, comfortable position where there is some privacy. It may be appropriate to repeat the question back to John and ask him to offer some background to the question.

2. Use skilful questioning, preferably with open questions, to help facilitate the ventilation of feelings and elicit what the real issues are

Questions that may help promote further discussion could include:

- What is your impression of what the future holds?
- What would you want to do with the time you now have?
- How can we help?
- You look . . . ?

3. Listen intently throughout

There is a possibility that John may expand on his awareness of lost future opportunities and the total pain of being confronted with a time-limiting illness. During this period the carers develop greater insight into the real issues and perhaps witness John coming to terms with the realities of the future. This may include not seeing the arrival of his first grandchild.

Aspirations, when verbalised by the patient, can then be confirmed or highlighted as being difficult.

4. Summarise what has been said to clarify the nature of the problem

In the outpouring of concerns and emotion that may accompany the handling of awkward questions, a mini-summary helps to ensure that what is being presented by the patient has been interpreted correctly. In this instance, the following example may be appropriate:

> John, we started by you asking me a fairly direct question in which you asked, 'How long have I got?' You have mentioned that there is much you wish to do and have expressed concerns over the fact that you may never see your first grandchild. It appears that this may be your biggest concern as well as concerns over how Grace, your wife, will cope.

5. Decide on the appropriate response

In this situation, in view of John's continual deterioration, it is probable that he may not see the arrival of his grandchild. This uncertainty cannot be replaced with false reassurances. Further assistance and support can be offered to help him and his wife to plan for the future, whatever shape or form that might take.

Situations like the above place high demands on the communication skills of the practitioner, and support mechanisms such as clinical supervision are essential when this type of situation is encountered frequently.

REFLECTION POINT

- List the questions and queries from patients and their families that you have found difficult to handle, and consider what made them difficult.

WHICH FRAMEWORKS CAN GUIDE YOUR COMMUNICATION PRACTICE?

Developments in palliative care for cancer patients and those with other life-threatening illnesses have led to the requirement that practitioners continually review and develop their repertoire of communication skills. Good communication is not just about possessing the verbal and non-verbal skills and the background knowledge to deal with awkward questions. More and more practitioners have to explore difficult issues such as preferred place of care (Lugton et al 2005). As has been already illustrated in the 'Breaking bad news' section above, high-quality communication is also about having the frameworks and principles to work through such difficult communication issues.

NICE (2004) offers the following key recommendations relating to face-to-face communication (p 56–64):

- People affected by cancer should be involved in developing cancer services
- There should be good communication, and people affected by cancer should be involved in decision making
- Information should be available free of charge
- People affected by cancer should be offered a range of physical, emotional, spiritual and social support
- There should be services to help people living with the after-effects of cancer manage these for themselves
- People with advanced cancer should have access to a range of services to improve their quality of life
- There should be support for people dying from cancer
- The needs of family and other carers of people with cancer should be met
- There should be a trained workforce to provide services

These guidelines place emphasis on the fact that some professionals may feel inadequately trained in some aspects of communication. Part of developing your practice is having frameworks to guide how you respond to difficult communication areas, especially those involving psychosocial support.

Consistency in delivering advanced practice may require the nurse to base the helping relationship on counselling/communication frameworks. A significant portion of the chapter has considered practice, which is guided by principles. These principles have to a greater extent emerged in order to guide the practitioner and cope with the emotional chaos that may accompany breaking bad news, handling awkward questions, or preparing the patient and family for death. Using these principles is appropriate in handling short-duration communication issues. In some instances it is necessary to base practice on counselling frameworks that may help patients to resolve past, current and anticipated problems related to the threat of a limited lifespan. Counselling frameworks do not only provide frameworks for practice, but can also offer preferred attributes that may facili-

tate a genuine helping relationship which can be the basis of helping patients adjust to the challenges associated with a limited lifespan.

Burton & Watson (2000) noted that healthcare professionals have a number of frameworks to choose from to guide their practice, including psychodynamic models, client-centred models and the cognitive behavioural model. It is beyond the scope of this chapter to provide an in-depth review of all frameworks, but examples will be provided of Heron's client-centred model and the cognitive behavioural model. Irrespective of which model you use, it is important that the practitioner emphasises and explores the resource and competencies of the patient and their family in working through their difficulties (Davy & Ellis 2000).

Heron's client–centred model

John Heron (1993) promoted the notion of the helper as someone who can support, enable and promote well-being in the individual. It is further suggested that the helper may have five key attributes:

1. Warm concern and acceptance for another
2. Openness and attunement to the other's experiential reality
3. A grasp of what the other needs for his or her essential flourishing
4. An ability to facilitate the flourishing of such needs in the right manner at the right time
5. An authentic presence.

Heron's assertion that the helper has to possess desirable attributes is supported by Bailey & Wilkinson (1998), who conducted a study involving 36 patients with advanced cancer designed to elicit patients' views on nurses' communication skills. Twenty-seven patients suggested that good verbal and non-verbal skills, demonstration of approachable personal attributes and having knowledge of their subject were highly desirable. The attributes mentioned in essence form the core values that underpin some of the six categories of counselling intervention. The creative communicator is one who can successfully reconcile desirable personal attributes with established counselling/communication frameworks. The application of Heron's theory of human nature has been explored more fully in a paper by Liossi & Mystakidou (1997). Heron describes the six categories as having the following dimensions:

Authoritative

1. *Prescriptive* – A prescriptive intervention seeks to direct the behaviour of the client, usually

behaviour that is outside the practitioner–client relationship.

2. *Informative* – An informative intervention seeks to impart knowledge and information to the client.
3. *Confronting* – A confronting intervention seeks to raise the client's consciousness about some limiting attitude or behaviour of which they are relatively unaware.

Facilitative

4. *Cathartic* – A cathartic intervention seeks to enable the client to discharge, to abreact a painful emotion, primarily grief, fear and anger.
5. *Catalytic* – A catalytic intervention seeks to elicit self-discovery, self-directed living, learning and problem-solving in the client.
6. *Supportive* – A supportive intervention seeks to affirm the worth and value of the client's person, qualities, attitudes or actions.

The authoritative interventions are very much lodged in a hierarchical domain, whereas the facilitative interventions are more dependent on the client leading the agenda, discharging feelings, and discerning the nature of the problem and potential solutions. Case Study 7.3 illustrates the scope of using this model in a palliative care situation. It is acknowledged that the timing and appropriate sequencing of these interventions needs to be mediated by Jenny's family.

Applying the six-category intervention model to Case Study 7.3, it is clear that the facilitative interventions will need to be applied consistently by all staff to create a climate of trust and reassuring presence. Unconditional positive regard and calm communication will help nurture a rapport with family members.

Case Study 7.3   Intervention model

Jenny is a 51-year-old woman who has advanced carcinoma of the lung. She has been recently admitted to the hospice for pain and symptom control. Jenny has been married to her husband, Brian, for 26 years. Brian is self-employed, running his own electrical contracting business. Jenny and Brian have two sons, Grant aged 17 years and David aged 25. David lives 4 hours' drive away and is married to Sheila; they are expecting their second child in 3 months' time. While at home Jenny was becoming increasingly dependent on her family to meet her daily needs. Prior to admission, Brian and her younger son, Grant, were looking after Jenny with assistance from the district nurse and the general practitioner. Jenny is anxious, and nocturnal panic attacks have been an emerging problem.

Supportive

Staff should affirm the worth of Jenny and her family, and elicit the depth of suffering she and her family are experiencing. As Brian visits his wife regularly, this will affect his capacity to maintain a regular income, which will be a source of concern for Jenny. Her fear of dying during a panic attack and the role shift accompanying dependence 'on her family' for care may be concerns that could be expressed.

Cathartic

Both Jenny and her family may have concealed a wide range of fears relating to the present and the future. It is likely that each member will have their own emotional profile, which may include anger, uncertainty and anxiety: no-one may want to unburden to another member of the family. As a result, the hurt and distress may be carefully contained. The therapeutic value of simply listening to patients ventilating their feelings, which may be manifest in tears, shouting or anger, cannot be underestimated. Heron acknowledges the centrality of unconditional positive regard as a key to the door in sometimes unleashing painful emotions. It is often the case that during these outbursts the real fears emerge. Statements such as, 'You look close to tears . . .', 'You look angry . . .' and 'How are you coping with what is happening to you?' may offer an opportunity for the practitioner to unlock the door. Jenny may be upset at the possibility that she may not be remembered as a grandmother. In a similar vein, David and Sheila may have reflected on the possibility that their children may never see their grandmother.

Informative

The emergence of panic attacks may have been precipitated in Jenny by a fear of dying in her sleep. It may be helpful for the practitioner to take time to explain the antecedents to panic attacks and that they can be controlled. There is also the possibility that Jenny may want to know how exactly she will die and seek the advice of a practitioner on how appropriate it would be to have family members present 'when that time' arrives. Information regarding the availability of services that could support Jenny and her family at home in the future could be offered.

Catalytic

A catalytic intervention aims to seek solutions in what may appear to be seemingly impossible situations. Utilising this approach, the team could help

Jenny and her husband look towards the future and 'get things in order', such as finances, funeral, etc. With this intervention, the pace at which issues are explored requires delicate treatment in order that Jenny is empowered with a sense of control. Catalytic interventions can be helpful in ensuring that Jenny might be able to explore ways in which she would want to be remembered in the future.

Confronting

Palliative care is often perceived to be a 'gentle' discipline that does not embrace confrontation as a core value. Nevertheless, it may be appropriate in a sensitive manner for the practitioner to reflect back to Jenny or her family the consequences of actions that may not be conducive to a peaceful death.

Not all of the six interventions may be indicated in every given situation; neither is it the responsibility of one practitioner to utilise all the strategies. The social worker may find themself 'on the receiving end' of Brian's and other family members' distress, whereas the nurse and medical team may be principally involved in informative/supportive interventions.

The cognitive behavioural option

The use of cognitive behavioural therapy (CBT) has received increasing attention concerning its application to palliative care. Although research into its application in a cancer/palliative care situation is in its infancy, the evidence for its use in handling depression and anxiety is compelling (Blackburn & Davidson 1990, Bottomley 1998, Enright 1997, Moorey et al 1998, Payne 1998). Anxiety and depression are common adjustment reactions to living under the cloud of a life-threatening illness. CBT is a problem-oriented approach that helps people to identify and deal with unhelpful, dysfunctional thinking patterns, assumptions and patterns of behaviour.

In mental health settings CBT is well established, with compelling evidence to suggest its efficacy, especially in anxiety and depression (Blackburn & Davidson 1990, Moorey et al 1998). The application of this framework in a palliative care situation is becoming more recognised, and there is a need for more research in this field. Adjuvant psychological therapy (APT), developed by Moorey and Greer, is based on a CBT framework especially for cancer patients, and may be applied across a broad spectrum of patients from early diagnosis to end-stage disease. Moorey et al (1998) conducted a study comparing APT with supportive counselling for cancer patients. The study concluded that APT produced greater changes in anxiety and adjustments to cancer.

CBT is a brief, patient-focused therapy based on the premise that it is not the illness itself that produces the emotional response, but the meaning of the illness for the person involved (Moorey & Greer 2002). For example, one patient may view his cancer only as a death sentence and consequently feel hopeless and depressed, whereas another may perceive it as a challenge and feel hopeful. For the hopeless depressed patient, CBT may enable them to recognise negative and unhelpful thoughts or behaviours that will reinforce emotional distress.

This basic CBT model (Fig. 7.1) illustrates the interaction between thoughts, moods/emotions, physical manifestations of emotions and associated behaviours. The key features of this approach are illustrated in Box 7.4.

Case Study 7.4 illustrates how a CBT may be applied to a palliative care patient.

Box 7.4   Some characteristics of cognitive behavioural therapy (adapted from Moorey & Greer 2002)

- Short term – usually 6 to 12 sessions are offered, initially lasting for 1 hour, but patients with more advanced illness may receive much shorter, more frequent, sessions.
- Structured – Each session is structured with an agenda agreed by patient and therapist.
- Problem-focused and collaborative – Patient and therapist work together to define and solve current problems.
- Exploratory and experimental – A variety of treatment techniques are employed: non-directive methods, behavioural, cognitive and interpersonal techniques.
- Educational – Patient is taught coping strategies.
- Socratic questioning style – Patient is invited to challenge their understanding of thought or events by asking questions that clarify their thinking.
- Homework – Patient is often given homework between sessions. This may entail identifying negative cognitive or behavioural patterns, or conducting experiments to test negative beliefs and predictions.

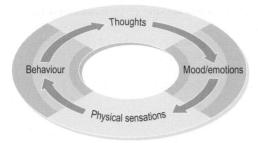

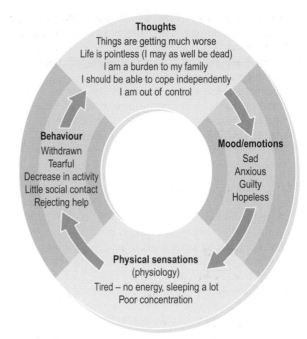

Figure 7.1 Cognitive model: basic CBT model showing the interaction between aspects of human experience. (Based on Greenberger & Padesky 1996 Mind over mood. Change the way you feel by changing the way you think. The Guildford Press, New York.)

Case Study 7.4

Liz is a 46-year-old divorced woman who lives alone. She has a son aged 23 years and daughter aged 20, both living nearby. Liz was diagnosed with motor neurone disease 1 year ago. She is now wheelchair-bound and experiencing difficulties caring for herself, but is reluctant to accept help from carers. She has suffered persistent low mood since diagnosis and, despite antidepressant medication, there has been no significant improvement in her mood. She also presented with symptoms of anxiety relating to her ability to cope with her rapidly progressing illness. She is withdrawn, has little social contact and has abandoned many activities she once enjoyed. She spends most of the day in bed.

Liz was referred for CBT in an attempt to improve her mood and help her with coping strategies. She cried throughout her initial assessment session. Overwhelming feelings of helplessness and hopelessness were prevalent. One of the first things she said to her therapist was: 'It makes no difference what you try to do or say to me, I'm going to die anyway.'

The vicious cycle depicted in Figure 7.2 served to reinforce Liz's low mood and associated behaviours that maintained the cycle. For patients such as Liz, CBT techniques aim to break this cycle and improve mental adjustment to advancing disease.

Techniques used may be cognitive or behaviourally focused. Although an extensive review of techniques is not within the scope of this text, a brief summary of some techniques used with Liz may help illustrate the approach.

Behavioural techniques

- Encouraging increasing levels of activity that may initially help low mood. This may include asking

Figure 7.2 Liz's cognitive model – a vicious cycle.

the patient to complete activity schedules or timetables. This does not mean filling every minute of each day, but introducing some structure to the day with particular emphasis on pleasurable activities, however small, that patients may have abandoned.

- Encouraging the patient to carry out simple 'experiments' to test negative thoughts or beliefs. For example, a patient who believes: 'What's the point in doing anything anymore – it's not worth the bother' may be challenged to list any small activities they can still manage and guess how much pleasure they get from each, predicting pleasure as a score out of ten. Their task is then to try one or two activities from the list and immediately score the actual pleasure derived. Usually, this demonstrates that predictions of pleasure are lower and the pleasure actually experienced is greater, resulting in reappraisal of the negative thought or belief and perhaps beginning to initiate change.

Cognitive techniques

- Helping patients to identify negative thoughts about their situation – in Liz's case: 'Things are getting much worse' and 'I am out of control'.
- Enabling patients to recognise the connection between their thoughts, mood and behaviour. Often thought/mood diaries are used.

- Teaching patients how to challenge these negative thoughts, as they often contain thinking distortions.
- Encouraging patients to consider evidence for and against negative thoughts.
- Enabling patients to think of alternatives and develop more balanced thoughts, often by the use of Socratic questions such as: 'Could there be any other way of looking at this?' or 'Have you had to deal with anything like this in the past? How did you manage then?'

Box 7.5 illustrates a cognitive technique used with Liz.

After collecting the evidence together, Liz was encouraged to review it closely, particularly as she had produced more evidence against the negative thought. Consequently Liz concluded that this thought may not be accurate after all, and was able to generate her perception towards a more positive bias.

There are many challenges when applying CBT techniques to patients with advanced disease. One of the most obvious is that, for many patients who experience negative thoughts about their cancer, some of these thoughts may not be distorted but an accurate reflection of the problems they are facing, for example: 'My cancer is getting worse'. Although this may be a realistic negative thought, such thoughts are unhelpful and the patient will be taught techniques to help modify them and generate more balanced thoughts. Exploring these realistic negative thoughts by means of cognitive techniques may enable patients to see the effect of these ruminations on the ability to enjoy their remaining life to the full.

The aim of CBT is not to attempt to change the patient's view into one of unrealistic optimism, but to empower them by teaching effective coping strategies, thus enhancing feelings of control and self-reliance. Application of a CBT approach may also be of value when communicating with both patients and carers in the following situations:

- Facilitating adjustment to advancing disease
- Promoting adaptive coping strategies
- Understanding and coping with anxiety/panic attacks
- Increasing activity
- Increasing self-esteem
- Elevating mood
- Improving communication with family members (e.g. handling collusion).

When working with very ill patients, time is often limited. Several weeks of therapy may not be possible owing to rapidly progressing disease or the patient being too weak or exhausted for 'full-blown' CBT sessions. Interventions when patients are so ill should be brief and focused on immediate problems causing distress. 'Cognitive first aid' (i.e. the immediate application of CBT techniques) may also be applied to patients suffering overwhelming distress who may require a one-off short intervention to deal with a situation such as panic attacks, mood disturbance close to death, euthanasia or suicidal ideation.

The NICE (2004) document states that there are: 'insufficient numbers of professionals equipped to support patients and carers in psychological distress' and further advocates the use of specific psychological therapies delivered according to an explicit theoretical framework. Communication within a CBT framework will enable the palliative care nurse to elicit concerns, identify distress, and ensure that patients and carers access appropriate support (p 56–64).

DEVELOPING COMMUNICATION PRACTICE: THE OPTIONS

The issue of enhancing communication practice via training with seriously ill patients has received considerable attention (Booth et al 1999, Heaven & Maguire 1996, Wilkinson 1991, Wilkinson et al 1998, 1999). Teaching that raises awareness of issues surrounding death and dying may facilitate an increased willingness to approach the dying but not positively impact on eliciting patient/family concerns or improve competence in handling awkward questions.

Box 7.5 Evidence for and against the negative thought 'I am out of control'

EVIDENCE SUPPORTING THE THOUGHT
- I can't control my legs.
- I'm wheelchair-bound.
- The doctors and nurses try to push equipment on to me that I don't want.

EVIDENCE AGAINST THE THOUGHT
- I live alone.
- I organise and run my home and finances.
- I look after my pets well (including a diabetic dog).
- I plan my day – do what I want.
- I direct my carers.
- I am able to choose whether and when I need help.

Heaven & Maguire (1996) mention that simple skills training is insufficient to alter clinical behaviour. This conclusion emerged from a study involving 44 hospice nurses who participated in an evaluation of a 10-week communication course that had a particular focus on the nurse's ability to elicit patients' concerns. The programme was very much based on the skills of assessment. These skills were evaluated by analysis of audiotaped conversations with patients. It was concluded that there was a lack of improvement in the outcome of communication, demonstrated by the fact that before and after training nurses identified fewer than 40% of the concerns that patients raised. As hospice care encompasses a multiprofessional ethos, it is possible that the socialisation of hospice nurses mitigates against them taking sole responsibility for eliciting total concerns. It is possible, despite the impact of trying, that they may be cognitively attuned to specific concerns and conscious that it is the combined efforts of the whole team that produce a comprehensive picture of the patient/family concerns.

Wilkinson et al (1998) evaluated the value of nurse–patient communication in a palliative care programme that involved 110 nurses completing a 26-hour training programme over a 6-month interval. The training programme had a broader base than the study previously cited, and included knowledge and attitudes as well as assessment skills. The content of the programme included coverage of topics such as counselling skills; loss, grief and bereavement; body image; and anxiety and depression. A pre- and post-course audiotape was used to elicit competence in patient assessment skills. In addition, students had the option of formal assessment by conducting a written critique of their skills. It was concluded that there was a statistically significant improvement in assessment skills from pre- to post-test scores, with 90% of participants having increased their scores. Audiotape recordings, self-critique and feedback sessions were described as being the most valuable elements of the programme.

It would appear if there is to be a significant development in nurses' skills, training programmes will need to include feedback and review of audiotape/videotape situations, and the opportunity for practitioners to examine their own skills and attitudes in relation to patients requiring palliative care. These difficulties are clearly compounded by uncertainty regarding the type of competencies that need to be established in guiding the novice and the expert practitioner alike. Husband et al (2000) highlight the need for cancer training and education using a competency-based approach. One of the nine competencies specified in the paper was that of communication. Using the competency-based approach, the novice practitioner could evolve from merely being able to identify a patient and family in distress to a higher-level skill of delivering a range of systematic therapeutic interventions that may have a demonstrable effect on reducing anxiety and depression.

The randomised controlled trial conducted by Fallowfield et al (2002), involving an intensive 3-day training course on communication skills for oncologists, concluded that training courses significantly improve doctors' skills. Furthermore, Fellowes et al (2004), in a systematic review, concluded that the training programmes assessed in the trials they included appeared to be effective in improving the communication skills of cancer care professionals.

The need to improve communication is further emphasised within the recently developed NHS Knowledge and Skills Framework (2006). The identification of competencies and the designation of programmes to meet these competencies (Box 7.6) may contribute to resolving the problems highlighted by previous research in nurses failing to elicit patients' and family members' primary concerns.

Although research has indicated the positive influence some training packages can have, sustainable change and communication skills are likely to be enhanced by a programme of clinical supervision. Clinical supervision has an established history in social work, counselling and mental health nursing (Haynes et al 2002).

In view of the likelihood that the nurse in palliative care is confronted by difficult communication scenarios, the practice of clinical supervision would seem commensurate with the development of high-quality clinical practice. The emotional labour of palliative nursing has been represented graphically in a study by Jones (1999), who cited the case of a Macmillan nurse who mentioned that: 'The patient will look at me without a single word and convey the message I know that you know'. Jones (1999) further mentions that supervision can help the nurse make sense of the complex feelings that may accompany difficult communication issues, and provides an opportunity to process and refine feelings, thoughts and actions that emerge from professional practice. In essence, palliative care nurses may be participating in momentous experiences in the lives of patients and their families (Jones 1997). Involvement in such experiences is not without its problems. Concerning the hazards of helping, Hawkins & Shohet (1997) mention that we may find ourselves in a position where we consider ourselves to be helpers rather than a channel for help. Such self-awareness is essential if the professional is

---

Box 7.6   Developing communication practice for the multidisciplinary team

Title of workshop: Communicating with patients and their families with advanced illness

Facilitators: Sandra Gaines and Shaun Kinghorn
Duration: 1 day
Audience: In total, 280 multiprofessional staff represented by specific multidisciplinary teams (MDTs). Staff attending included palliative care consultants, oncologists and oncology surgeons, nurses, specialist nurses, dieticians, therapy radiographers, occupational therapists, physiotherapists, lead nurses, nurse consultants, pathologists, healthcare assistants, social workers, cancer genetics staff (8 to 16 staff attended each workshop).

Content/approach: The workshops utilised a participant-centred agenda to identify and explore the individual team issues in communicating with cancer patients and their families. Use of strategies included role play by facilitators, case study and video analysis, sculpting, reflection and discussion.

WHAT DID THE PARTICIPANTS SAY? – A SELECTION OF COMMENTS

'I feel that I will be more self-aware and conscious of the need for good communication skills.'

'To look at patients as individuals with a history and not just their cancer.'

'Change might not be the word, but an evaluation of what I do already might add something to my practice.'

'I enjoyed the team approach to discussing the evaluation of our communication skills.'

'As a busy surgeon I felt I couldn't afford the time to attend today and doubted the benefit for me. Now, having completed the workshop, I feel it is one of the most relevant training days ever, both for myself and the team, and feel all my colleagues should attend.'

'This was the first time our whole team has been together in one room, and that in itself has been beneficial.'

FACILITATORS' COMMENTS – LESSONS LEARNED

'The aims of the workshops were to raise awareness of the issues and not to primarily develop skills. The workshops provided a forum for the MDTs to reflect on their individual and team approaches to communicating with cancer patients and their families. This was often the first time the MDT had actually reflected on this important area of practice. As such it was a revealing experience, allowing them the time and space to challenge aspects of their practice that had been formerly taken for granted, such as how and where bad news was broken. Action planning for future practice resulted in the MDTs identifying several immediate improvements that could be made, as well as the need for more advanced communication skills training for various professionals within the MDTs. The feedback from cancer network patients' forums was that they had noticed a reduction in complaints about unsatisfactory patient/professional communication within the cancer team.'

---

to be consistent in maintaining his or her effectiveness as a communicator with the seriously ill. Such awareness can be facilitated in a variety of ways, including clinical supervision.

A significant portion of the palliative care nurse's role is conducted in one-to-one situations, and the process of the developing nurse–patient relationship may take place beyond the gaze of other colleagues. Physical care for the highly dependent may be given in twos, whereas handling sensitive communication may be handled alone. This lone practice is commensurate with privacy and the promotion of a climate where the patient may freely express fears and major concerns. It is this scenario that creates a situation where the nurse may feel: 'How do I know if I got it right?', 'Did I say the right thing?' or 'Perhaps I could have listened more'. It is argued that clinical supervi-

sion is essential if communication practice is to be enhanced.

Developments in communicating with the seriously ill could be facilitated by palliative care staff having a more active role in auditing practice. The King's Fund (Walker et al 1996) has published guidelines for delivering a cancer diagnosis. The guidelines focus primarily on the primary–secondary interface, the communication of bad news and organisational issues. Such a document is welcome in view of the ever-mounting concerns that patients and families express regarding lack of communication. Even though we might provide training programmes and have started to instigate clinical supervision, the development of a communication audit will help palliative care nurses ascertain the quality of communication they offer to patients and their families.

CONCLUSION

Practitioners are increasingly entrusted with the responsibility of playing an active role in handling some of the more difficult communication issues that have until now been the domain of medical staff. The development of nurse-led clinics will place new demands on the communication skills of nurses. Such responsibilities need to be accompanied by adequate preparation, based on clearly defined competencies, evaluation and ongoing supervision. These prerequisites are essential in facilitating excellence in communicating with the seriously ill. The current drive to network with other specialties and disciplines is encouraging palliative care nursing to consider other models of supportive communication, such as cognitive behavioural therapy. Being equipped with the skills to evaluate the application of such frameworks within a palliative care context will help enhance the evidence base of palliative care.

References

Baile W, Buckman R, Lenzi R et al 2000 SPIKES – a six step protocol for delivering bad news: application to the patient with cancer. The Oncologist 5:302–311

Bailey K, Wilkinson S 1998 Patients' views on nurses' communication skills: a pilot study. International Journal of Palliative Nursing 4(6):300–305

Blackburn I, Davidson K 1990 Cognitive therapy for depression and anxiety. Blackwell Scientific, Oxford

Booth K, Maguire P, Hillier V F 1999 Measurement of communication skills in cancer care: myth or reality? Journal of Advanced Nursing 30(5):1073–1079

Bottomley A 1998 Group cognitive behavioural therapy with cancer patients: the views of women participants on a short-term intervention. European Journal of Cancer Care 7:23–30

Buckman R 1992 How to break bad news: a guide for health care professionals. Papermac, Basingstoke

Buckman R 1996 Talking to patients about cancer: no excuse for not doing it now. British Medical Journal 313:699–700

Burton M, Watson M 2000 Counselling people with cancer. Wiley, Chichester

Davy J Ellis S 2000 Counselling skills in palliative care. Open University Press, Buckingham

Enright S 1997 Cognitive behavioral therapy. British Medical Journal 314:1811–1822

Fallowfield L, Jenkins V, Farewell V, Saul J, Duffy A, Eves R 2002 Efficacy of a Cancer Research UK communication skills training model for oncologists: a randomized controlled trial. Lancet 359:650–656

Faulkener A 1998 When the news is bad: a guide for health professionals. Stanley Thornes, Cheltenham

Fellowes D, Wilkinson S, Moore P 2004 Communication skills training for health care professionals working with cancer patients, their families and/or carers. Cochrane Database Systematic Review (2):CD003751

Field D, Copp G 1999 Communication and awareness about dying in the 1990s. Palliative Medicine 13:459–468

Franks A 1997 Breaking bad news and the challenge of communication. European Journal of Palliative Care 4(2):61–66

Gillhooly M, Berkeley J, McCann K, Gibling F, Murray K 1988 Truth telling with dying cancer patients. Palliative Medicine 2:64–71

Hawkins P, Shohet R 1997 Supervision in the helping professions. Open University Press, Milton Keynes

Haynes R, Corey G, Moulton P 2002 Clinical supervision in the helping professions: a practical guide. Wadsworth Publishing, London

Heaven K, Maguire P 1996 Training hospice nurses to elicit patient concerns. Journal of Advanced Nursing 23:280–286

Heaven C M, Maguire P 1997 Disclosure of concerns by hospice patients and their identification by nurses. Palliative Medicine 11:283–290

Heron J 1993 Helping the client: a creative practical approach. Sage Publications, London

Husband G, Banks-Howe J, Boal L, Hodgson D 2000 A competency-based tool for education. European Journal of Cancer Care 9:36–40

Jones A 1997 A 'bonding between strangers': a palliative model of clinical supervision. Journal of Advanced Nursing 26:1028–1035

Jones A 1999 'A heavy and blessed experience': a psychoanalytic study of community Macmillan nurses and their roles in serious illness and palliative care. Journal of Advanced Nursing 30(6):1297–1303

Kaye P 1996 Breaking bad news: a ten step approach. EPL Publications, Northampton

Kruijver I, Kerkstra A, Bensing J, Van der Wiel H 2000 Nurse/patient communication in cancer care: a review of the literature. Cancer Nursing 23(1):20–31

Liossi C, Mystakidou K 1997 Heron's theory of human needs in palliative care. European Journal of Palliative Care 4(1):32–35

Maguire P 1999 Improving communication with cancer patients. European Journal of Cancer 35(10):1415–1422

Moorey S, Greer S, Bliss J, Law M 1998 A comparison of adjuvant psychological therapy and supportive counselling in patients with cancer. Psycho-oncology 7:218–228

Moorey S, Greer S 2002 Cognitive behavioural therapy for people with cancer. Oxford University Press, Oxford

Morley C 1997 The use of denial by patients with cancer. Professional Nurse 12(5):380–381

National Health Service Knowledge and Skills
Framework 2006 NHS KSF. Online. Available:
http://www.nhsu.nhs.uk/ksf/index.html Aug 2006

National Institute for Clinical Excellence 2004 Improving
supportive and palliative care for adults with cancer.
NICE, London

Payne S 1998 Depression in palliative care patients.
International Journal of Palliative Nursing 14(4):184–192

Penson J 2000 A hope is not a promise: fostering hope
within palliative care. International Journal of Palliative
Nursing 6(2):94–97

Vivian R 2006 Truth telling in palliative care nursing: the
dilemmas of collusion. International Journal of Palliative
Nursing 12(7):341–349

Walker G, Bradburn J, Maher J 1996 Breaking bad news:
establishing an auditable procedure for giving the cancer
diagnosis. King's Fund, London

Wilkinson S 1991 Factors which influence how nurses
communicate with cancer patients. Journal of Advanced
Nursing 16:677–688

Wilkinson S, Roberts A, Aldridge J 1998 Nurse–patient
communication in palliative care: an evaluation of a
communication skills programme. Palliative Medicine
12:13–22

Wilkinson S, Bailey K, Aldridge J, Roberts A 1999
A longitudinal evaluation of a communication
skills programme. Palliative Medicine
13:341–348

Chapter 8

Facilitating hope in palliative care

Rosemary McIntyre and Jackie Chaplin

INTRODUCTION

The concept of hope has long been of interest to philosophers, psychologists, theologians and health-care professionals. Furthermore, the nebulous and dynamic nature of hope has generated significant professional debate and research within the field of palliative care as practitioners grapple with its practical application to patient- and family-focused care.

Although this chapter will, in part, draw on the authors' original research with relatives of cancer patients (McIntyre 2002), and with research and palliative care practice with cancer patients (Chaplin 1996), we believe that the insights gained can be applied to practice that extends beyond cancer to encompass the wider spectrum of illness requiring palliative care.

This chapter aims to:

- Explore the concept of hope within the context of palliative care
- Propose a framework to support professionals in fostering hope within palliative care
- Using selected case studies, apply the framework to the care of patients and families
- Debate the wider implications for palliative care practice of facilitating hope in patients with cancer and other illnesses.

Fostering hope is an important aspect of palliative nursing practice, but it should be noted that this is not exclusively a nursing responsibility, as it requires a multiprofessional approach. As such, this chapter should be of interest not only to nurses but also to other members of the multiprofessional palliative care team.

BRIEF REVIEW OF SELECTED LITERATURE

In palliative care the increased levels of professional discussion and research activity over the past two decades have focused on a number of key areas. First, the focus has been in defining hope and determining its meaning for patients, families and professionals (Benzein & Saveman 1998, Benzein et al 2001, Dufault & Martocchio 1985, Farran et al 1995, Herth & Cutliffe 2002a, Hinds 1984, Nekolaichuk & Bruera 1998). Second, there have been attempts to measure hope and its relationship to a range of psychosocial variables (Chapman & Pepler 1998, Felder 2004, Nekolaichuk & Bruera 2004). Third, there is a growing body of literature that identifies strategies that foster or sustain hope (Appelin & Bertero 2004, Buckley & Herth 2004, Duggleby 2001, Herth 1990).

Initial research into the concept of hope originated in the USA, but there is now a growing body of international research focusing on hope (Benzein et al 2001, Farran et al 1995, Herth & Cutliffe 2002a, 2002b, Klyma & Vehvilainen-Julkunen 1997, Nekolaichuk & Bruera 2004). Early research into hope in patients with cancer identified hope as a dynamic energising life force that is essential for survival (Dufault & Martocchio 1985). Hope is diametrically opposed to hopelessness; it is inextricably linked to coping and is therefore particularly important within the context of life-threatening illness (Farran et al 1995, Hegarty 2001).

In one of the first qualitative studies of hope in palliative care, Herth (1990) found it to be an enduring feature in the experiences of terminally ill hospice patients. Herth also confirmed that hope in terminally ill people can be influenced both positively and negatively by a range of different factors, and especially by the nature of the patients' relationships with others.

Herth's findings are supported by more recent research into the meaning of hope for palliative care patients. A growing body of literature reveals a consensus that hope operates as an inner resource that not only acts as a source of psychological and physical energy, but is associated with finding meaning in living (Benzein et al 2001, Buckley & Herth 2004, Duggleby 2001, Duggleby & Wright 2004, Flemming 1997, Post-White et al 1996). It is also increasingly clear from the literature that having positive personal relationships with family members and with health professionals is essential to fostering hope in patients who are receiving palliative care (Buckley & Herth 2004, Duggleby & Wright 2004). There is now a consensus that hope is of relevance to palliative care practice and that healthcare professionals working in palliative care can play an important role in fostering hope in the patients and families for whom they provide care. In the next section a model for facilitating hope in palliative care will be presented and discussed (McIntyre & Chaplin 2001).

A CONCEPTUAL MODEL OF HOPE WITHIN PALLIATIVE CARE

When considering ways in which healthcare professionals might facilitate hope in patients and families receiving palliative care, whether for cancer or other illnesses, we thought that it might be helpful to offer a simple conceptual model that captures the main elements of care that might facilitate hope. The model has been developed around the key themes of Comfort, Attachment and Worth. These themes are not separate or discrete entities. Each in its own right is essential to sustain hope, but together the themes represent an interrelated, dynamic and synergistic framework for planning care.

The first theme, that of 'comfort', provides a focus for activities that might foster and sustain hope in those caught up in palliative care. Fundamental to this is effective symptom management, as uncontrolled pain and other distressing symptoms increase the patient's and the family's vulnerability and distress, and thereby reduce their capacity for hope. A range of actions aimed at enhancing the patient's physical comfort and well-being, and not only direct symptom management activities, can have the potential to enhance the patient's sense of hope and can confirm for them that life is still worth living.

The second theme of 'attachment' highlights the importance of caring relationships, especially in advanced illness where uncertainty and fear diminish feelings of hopefulness for the present and the future. Many people nearing the end of life fear being abandoned and isolated, and having access to supportive family and professional relationships can help sustain feelings of hope. Many palliative care practitioners can attest to the importance of establishing a relationship at a personal level and of 'being there' for patients and families as they confront the profound emotional and spiritual challenges of facing death.

'Worth' is the third theme in our conceptual model. This theme is concerned with those activities that acknowledge the intrinsic value of the patient or relative as a unique and valued person. Worth is also linked to having a sense of meaning and purpose in life and has a number of perspectives: the present, the future and the past. Sensitive communication skills and individually focused care can support the patient's sense that they are being valued for themselves as a person, and are not merely being seen as someone with an illness.

The interrelated and synergistic nature of the themes within the conceptual model of hope must be stressed. Effective relationships are fundamental to promoting physical comfort and to making the person feel that their worries, concerns and wishes are important. If needs relating to any one of these three themes are unmet, the individual's capacity for hopefulness about their current situation and future prospects will be compromised.

The butterfly model we provide offers a visual summary of the themes that we believe are associated with fostering hope in end-of-life care. This image was adopted as the butterfly reflects very aptly the fragility and vulnerability of hope within palliative care.

In the section that follows the butterfly model will be applied as a visual framework to help readers conceptualise and integrate the various elements of hope-facilitating care. We will draw on research data from patients and families who have faced the challenges of advanced illness (Chaplin 1996, McIntyre 2002). Hearing the voices of the patients and the relatives should help to illuminate their feelings and needs, and illustrate the ways in which palliative care professionals may facilitate hope within their practice.

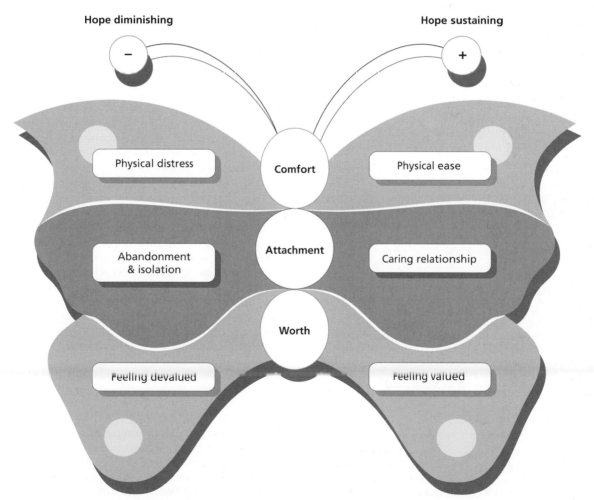

Figure 8.1 The butterfly model of hope: a conceptual model for exploring experiences and interventions.

FACILITATING HOPE IN PALLIATIVE CARE PATIENTS

A person who is required to confront the reality of their own dying will experience many challenges to their capacity to sustain hope (Hegarty 2001). Advancing disease, diminishing physical functioning, and the social and emotional impact of terminal illness can all contribute to an experience in which hope may appear to be lost or given up (Hockley 1993).

It is intended that the conceptual framework used in this chapter will facilitate an inclusive and holistic approach to the exploration of some of the complex issues that surround hope in palliative care.

THEME 1: COMFORT

Physical distress .... **Physical ease**

Pain and other symptoms are commonly experienced in the last years and months of life in patients with advanced cancer and other illnesses. Pain has long been recognised as having psychological, spiritual and social as well as physical dimensions, and as a result pain and other symptoms have a multidimensional impact on the individual who experiences them (Twycross 1997).

Case Study 8.1 illustrates the complexities of providing high-quality palliative care that is truly holistic in approach, and that recognises and addresses the challenges to hope that such situations present.

Case Study 8.1   Sadie's story

Sadie is a 43-year-old married mother of two children with advanced apical lung cancer. She experienced severe pain, which was poorly controlled initially while she was nursed at home. This was a very difficult time for Sadie, who became very withdrawn yet at the same time acutely anxious. Eventually the pain was identified as being neuropathic in nature and was controlled by antidepressants. Later in her illness Sadie experienced a spinal cord compression due to spinal metastases which responded partially to steroids and radiotherapy. Sadie's backache resolved, but she continued to experience urinary and faecal incontinence. In the last few weeks of her life she was cared for at home by her family with support from the primary healthcare team.

Comment on Case Study 8.1

Sadie's symptoms threaten her capacity for hope in a number of ways. Pain, and suffering due to her many symptoms, challenged her ability to cope with her illness experience. Sadie's experience, which was multidimensional in its nature, generated fears and concerns for the future. These fears included uncertainties regarding the future severity of the pain and other symptoms, and concerns about her capacity to cope in the future. In addition, difficulties in controlling Sadie's neuropathic pain because of the pain's resistance to opioids made Sadie fearful for the future and thus diminished her levels of hope. Sadie had coped with this by focusing on her children's needs until the pain had such an impact on her daily life that this was no longer effective. This was manifested by her withdrawal and introspection. Sadie's hope was to stay at home with her children for as long as possible, yet the uncontrolled pain threatened this hope.

Research confirms that the impact of pain on an individual's capacity to hope is a complex phenomenon that is not associated purely with the intensity of the pain experienced (Coyle 2004). The meaning of the pain, the perceived lack of effectiveness of treatment, and the impact that the pain has on the individual's daily life have all been identified as factors that diminish hope in those near the end of life (Chen 2003, Lin et al 2003). Many of these factors can be seen in Sadie's experience, where Sadie's confidence in healthcare professionals' abilities to control her symptoms was shaken. Sadie's fear was born out of her experiences that greater pain was ahead, and concern that it would not be effectively managed by her general practitioner, in whom she had lost trust.

Furthermore, the final stages of progressive non-curative illnesses often include diminishing control over body functions. Increased fatigue and muscle weakness associated with many illnesses – cancer, motor neurone disease, end-stage cardiac failure, etc. – result in individuals affected by these illnesses having to come to terms with the fact that, rather than themselves, it is the disease process that controls their ability to carry out normal activities, such as walking, eating, micturition and defaecation. This lack of physical control can diminish levels of hope as it threatens autonomy and can affect the social roles that individuals normally fulfil.

If we explore the impact of this lack of control in Sadie's situation, the incontinence diminished hope because, in effect, the disease has robbed her of control. The enforced physical dependence challenged her integrity as an autonomous adult and also detracted from her ability to fulfil her role as a mother, forcing her physical dependence on her husband and children. Again, this raised Sadie's fears about the future: uncertainties and concerns about what symptoms she might experience in the last weeks and days of life detracted from her ability to enjoy life now and reduced her hopes that she could enjoy life in the future. In addition, both the fears for the future and physical dependence detracted from Sadie's abilities to live a normal life with her husband and children.

Sadie's circumstances clearly highlight that having a sense of control and maintaining dignity through physical independent living can be adversely affected by advanced disease. Furthermore, although the relationship between a sense of control, dignity and hope is not well understood, maintaining a sense of dignity in terminal illness has been identified as being of significant importance to patients and also supportive of feelings of hope (Chochinov et al 2002). This also highlights the interconnectedness between different aspects of the hope experience in palliative care.

THEME 2: ATTACHMENT

Abandonment and isolation ... Caring relationships
An important element of palliative care is the emphasis on the provision of care in a holistic manner, and therefore the provision of emotional and social support is essential to high-quality palliative care. The existence of satisfying relationships and connectedness with others is an important factor in the maintenance of psychosocial well-being in patients with advanced cancer (Lin & Bauer-Wu 2003). The nurse is thus in a unique and privileged position to establish a relationship that fosters the individual's capacity to cope with their current life situation and reduces their fear of being abandoned. In Case Study 8.2, a patient describes, in his own words, the positive contribution to hope that nurses can make.

Case Study 8.2   John's story

To me I was special . . . I felt as if I was special . . . you never seemed to be left out of anything. You were part of their . . . part of the ward, everything put you at ease really, you never seemed to get left out of anything that was going on. You know when the doctors came up. You knew what was happening, the nurses and that . . . were absolutely fabulous, the staff and the nurses and even the auxiliaries . . . nothing was a bother, which was really good . . . You know nothing was a bother, I thought they were really brilliant . . . I just got the feeling that you were part of a family, it was just something that they gave me . . . you know. I wasn't just a number I was a person . . . You were treated like a person . . . which is like a hope. Just something they gave me and that . . . that helped me.

Comment on Case Study 8.2

The nurse–patient relationship, therefore, can be a powerful way by which the nurse communicates respect for the individual's intrinsic value as a person, a willingness to share this difficult experience, and a caring attachment that is non-judgemental. John clearly experienced these aspects of such a relationship, and this contributed to his feelings of hopefulness. The interwoven nature of attachment and worth will be evident in the discussion that follows.

Caring can be demonstrated in a number of different ways. First, by being there for the individual, active listening can demonstrate a willingness to try to understand the person as an individual as well as trying to understand their current life situation. Second, listening to the patient provides the patient with the opportunity to discuss their concerns, fears and worries with someone whom they do not feel a need to protect. Such a discussion requires a warm and emotionally safe environment, which fosters a sense of belonging. John's narrative indicates that such an environment was provided.

The person nearing the end of his or her life is coping with loss of self as a healthy adult whose death is an imminent reality rather than a future event. The experience of this loss has a profound effect on an individual's level and nature of hope. Not only may the focus of living change, but also the focus of the individual's hope. During the dying process the patient may, through reflection and discussion, redefine their goals and priorities in life.

Self-exploration and reflection offers the potential for self-knowledge and personal growth (Byock 1996). In turn, this process may have a profound effect upon the relationships that the patient has with other family members. The nurse can play a key role in fostering relationships within the family at this difficult time by reassuring relatives that they can make a positive contribution to the patient's care by being there.

Finally, personal introspection is energy demanding and cannot be sustained 24 hours a day. Just as individuals need the opportunity to discuss issues that are deeply important, they also require the freedom not to do so. It should be recognised that many people cope with the stresses of living by using humour. Throughout life, humour can and often does play an important role in maintaining a sense of normality, and has been identified as being an important element of the nurse–patient relationship (Christie & Moore 2004). The palliative care nurse has a responsibility also to foster light-heartedness and normality, as a sense of normality can in turn support the individual's sense of control.

THEME 3: WORTH

Feeling devalued .... Feeling valued

For some individuals the process of dying raises fundamental fears about their integrity and value as a person. Lair (1996) suggests that a diagnosis of a terminal illness constitutes a life crisis that calls for a re-evaluation of values and goals, and that this life crisis may also challenge the identity of self.

Feelings of reduced self-worth may arise not only from the image of advancing illness eroding the person but also from previous experience. Case Study 8.3 describes one man's view of the dehumanising effects of cancer and the fears this triggered when he himself was diagnosed with lung cancer.

Case Study 8.3   Jimmy's story

Well, when I was told I had cancer, I accepted the fact, before I spoke to the doctors, I accepted it might be incurable . . . The first thing I've got to think about, I've got to face that, but I've got to think of them (his family) . . . I've got to think of my wife because I saw my father going from a man of the build of myself to someone the size of a . . . monkey . . . about four stone, five stone, in a bed . . . just shrinking away because anybody who gets cancer that's incurable, anybody, everybody goes the same way, they just lie there and waste away and I didn't want that for them (his family) . . . Well, I had my mind made up if I thought I had incurable cancer . . . It's not fair to your family . . . I genuinely think you could top yourself . . . rather than see them suffering . . . I don't see why you should make other people you are attached to go through 6, 9 months, a year, to see whoever it was they lived with turning into something . . . they didn't get married to . . . turning into something that's unrecognisable . . . My father worked all his life, he worked all his days and retired, and then he took the cancer and he just went away. I had to go up to the bedroom every day and sit and watch this man I admired as a man . . . gone from a man into just a thing lying between the sheets.

Comment on Case Study 8.3

Jimmy's narrative demonstrates how his previous experiences of cancer with his father were brought sharply to the fore on the discovery of his diagnosis of cancer. His perceptions of the dehumanising effects of cancer are graphically illustrated in his image of his father that he has carried for over 40 years. The wasting effects of this disease and the possibility of turning into something 'unrecognisable' was something he feared not only for himself but also because of the impact this might have on his family. Note the words 'a monkey' . . . 'just shrinking away' . . . and 'something that's unrecognisable' . . . 'gone from a man into just a thing lying between the sheets'. This raises important issues regarding both self-worth and attachment.

Another aspect of worth is the need for individuals to feel autonomous and to have a sense of meaning and purpose in life. It is essential, therefore, that nurses support the patient in making large and small decisions, as a lack of autonomous decision-making can have a profoundly devaluing effect on the person with advanced disease whose sense of personal control may already be threatened by the disease process itself (Chochinov et al 2002). It has also been recognised that hope is enhanced if the individual feels able to die at peace with their inner self. Some elderly people die at peace because they feel they have lived their life fully, have put their affairs in order and are ready to say goodbye. This acceptance of death is a positive action which surprisingly sustains hope, whereas having 'unfinished business' may detract from the individual's ability to move on. Kubler-Ross (1969) described the acceptance of death in an attempt to understand the psychological stages involved in the process of dying. The concept of this adaptive process being in stages is often criticized, and thus the professional carer's acceptance of the individuality of each person's response to the loss of self that they are experiencing as part of the dying process is crucial in fostering self-worth. To support the person's feelings of personal worth, health professionals must recognise that responses to loss in terminal illness, denial, anger, bargaining, depression and acceptance can be experienced in unique and individualistic ways rather than in sequential stages.

Another factor influencing hope is the individual's sense of a personal future. In haematology/oncology patients the sense of a personal future which is a factor in the sustenance of hope is firmly linked to hope for survival (Perakyla 1991, Post-White et al 1996). In a palliative care context, the sense of a personal future is not necessarily focused on a physical future. It is related to three aspects: the affirmation of what one has been; the knowledge that opportunities still exist to live life meaningfully; and a belief that one will 'live on' after physical death.

Confirmation of self-worth can often be achieved by review of what has been (Lair 1996). Nurses who care for people who are dying will recognise that, commonly, patients feel the need to talk about their life. This life review can be very beneficial to the patient, reaffirming their self-value and allowing them the opportunity to put death into the perspective of living.

The concept of providing support to ensure the opportunity to live life fully until death occurs is fundamental to palliative care (DeRaeve 1996). The belief that good days, happy times or meaningful moments can be enjoyed can be supported only through the provision of holistic palliative care, symptom management, emotional support, financial and physical care, and family care.

Furthermore, the belief that one is able to 'live on' in the memories of others or that a bit of 'self' lives on in children and grandchildren can be a positive supporter of hope. Family members can be encouraged to contribute positively to the patient's hope by reminiscing and remembering family memories. Individuals may also find support for hope in religious beliefs which may encompass faith in spiritual life after death. Again, the nurse can play a key role in supporting the individual religious beliefs of both the patients and family.

FACILITATING HOPE IN PATIENTS – A SUMMARY

A range of interventions has been identified that nurture hope in patients receiving palliative care (Table 8.1). These interventions are intended as a guide and are not considered to be all-inclusive. A key aspect of nurturing hope is that interventions are

Table 8.1   Interventions to facilitate hope in people with palliative care needs

Theme	Aim	Interventions to nurture hope in relatives
Comfort	To promote physical ease in patients	• Comprehensively assess the individual's comfort needs • Implement appropriate pharmacological and non-pharmacological interventions to ensure effective pain and symptom control • Utilise appropriate support surfaces to prevent further tissue damage, taking account of patient's comfort preferences • Sensitively meet personal hygiene needs by utilising an individual and caring approach • When in bed, nurse in an appropriate position to minimise discomfort and distress • When in the last days or hours of life, review goals and need for nursing and other interventions, for example by initiating the Liverpool Care Pathway for the Dying • Minimise avoidable distress by preventing constipation and/or incontinence
Attachment	To establish an effective relationship with the patient and promote caring relationships between patient and family	• Provide a caring environment that is welcoming and recognises the patient's ongoing needs for information and support • Establish an effective relationship with the patient that recognises the need for honesty, sensitivity and trust • 'Be there' when added support is required, such as when redefining goals and expectations • Facilitate communication and expressions of caring between patients and relatives by offering support and privacy as needed • Engage in informal dialogue about 'normal' topics with patient and relatives, and utilise humour as appropriate
Worth	To ensure the patient feels valued as a unique human being	• Show genuine concern for the patient as an unique person with individual needs, concerns and preferences • Support the patient to set and achieve realistic goals within limits of condition • Facilitate life review so that patient is able to share personal memories and life stories • Sensitively explore spiritual/religious beliefs and provide access to support as appropriate • Explore wishes (e.g. desired place of care and death) and promote and support decision-making • As appropriate, support patient in formulating plans for after death (e.g. funeral arrangements)

potentially synergistic in nature and, while discussed individually, the holistic nature of palliative care requires that an integrated approach be adopted. The interrelatedness of all these themes cannot be overstressed. The following interventions are offered as ways in which palliative care nurses can nurture hope in their patients.

FACILITATING HOPE IN RELATIVES

When a family faces the profound challenge of a terminal illness in one of its members, there are many and significant demands on the family members' coping resources and on their capacity to sustain hope. There is the anticipated loss of the dying loved one and of the existing relationship, and the pain of seeing a loved one's health deteriorating and suffering from the effects of their illness. There is also the sense of helplessness at being unable to do anything to make the sick person better and the stress of assuming additional and new roles within the family. Some of these burdens can be addressed more readily than others. For example, some distressing symptoms can hopefully be alleviated by providing high-quality palliative care. However, the distress of impending loss and the wider impact of serious illness on the family as a unit is less amenable to amelioration. The quote below offers a powerful image of the lasting effects that serious illness can have on a family and its members. It also highlights the challenge of professionals in supporting the family as they struggle through the illness experience.

> Visualise a mobile with four or five pieces suspended from the ceiling, gently moving in the air. The whole is in balance, steady yet moving, some pieces are moving rapidly; others are almost stationary. Some are heavier and appear to carry more weight in the ultimate direction of the mobile's movement; others seem to go along for the ride. A breeze catching only one segment of the mobile immediately influences the movement of every piece, some more than others, and the pace picks up with some pieces unbalancing themselves and moving about chaotically for a time. Gradually the whole exerts its influence on the errant parts until stability is restored but not before a decided change in direction of the whole may have taken place.
>
> (Allmond et al 1979)

The following section focuses on ways in which nurses can support the coping efforts of families whose loved ones are receiving palliative care. For more detailed coverage of coping theory, family theory and family nursing practice in palliative care, readers should consult McIntyre & Lugton (2005), Whyte (1997) and Wright & Leahey (2000).

APPLYING THE CONCEPTUAL MODEL TO THE CARE OF THE RELATIVES

Examples of relatives' experiences of hope-diminishing and hope-sustaining care will be considered, drawing on data from McIntyre's (2002) study. This action research study focused on working with nurses in the acute hospital setting to develop research-based interventions to support relatives of dying cancer patients. Later in this section consideration is given to the needs of those families whose dying relative's care is provided in the home and where there are children in the family. The key themes of Comfort, Attachment and Worth are used as a framework for considering the support needs of families in each care setting.

Theme – comfort

Physical distress .... Physical ease

Being in the role of the close relative of a dying patient is exhausting, both physically and emotionally. McIntyre's research findings revealed that in the final weeks of the patient's life, where the patient is being cared for in hospital, relatives greatly appreciate having access to a comfortable private area where they can rest and muster their emotional resources. In the brief exemplar below, a relative (Mary) is expressing her appreciation of the recently improved facilities provided in the ward where her father was dying. Being able to retire to a private space for brief periods of rest and reflection was sustaining her coping resources so that she could continue to remain with her father in the hospital during his final days:

Mary: Well, this relatives' room is a real Godsend. I actually prefer coming along here rather than going downstairs to the canteen. Because at this stage sometimes other people just annoy you and coming along here . . . well, really it feels like a sanctuary. Just to come in here to the quietness and just sit. It's just fantastic. If you are sitting *all* the time at the bedside you get to feel like a zombie, but if you can get away for a break it is a really soothing, calming thing. It even makes dad seem less demanding.

Relatives who stay overnight in the ward can present challenges for the nursing staff. However, when the family is made to feel welcome in the ward, and when simple steps are taken to optimise their comfort, this can yield far-reaching benefits. In the dialogue below an elderly woman (Edna) confirms that the efforts made by the ward staff for her comfort were not only supporting her but had significant benefits for her dying husband (Jim):

Edna: I have been staying overnight in the ward since last Wednesday (four nights). My friend has twice stayed overnight with me. The nurses gave me a bed. A nice wee fold-up bed right in beside him. And they brought in a recliner chair for my friend so she could get some rest too.

Researcher: Has you being there overnight helped Jim?

Edna: Yes. Oh yes. He gets agitated if I'm away from him.

Edna went on to explain that she and her husband had never before been apart and they were both 'more contented' when she could stay beside him. However, Edna also knew that if Jim had seen her weary and in need of sleep he would have insisted that she leave. In this situation the provision of a simple folding bed set up beside the patient offered a significant coping resource for both patient and relative. They wanted to remain together at this crucial time, and by this measure the nurses had supported them in their hopes and had reduced the potential for future regret.

A less positive experience is reported below by Shona, who had recently returned from the USA to be with her dying father. At the time of interview Shona and her brothers were keeping a round-the-clock vigil at their father's bedside in the open ward with screens around the bed. Shona describes the discomfort and the lack of privacy that they are experiencing.

Shona: No, you're not comfortable in the ward. I put two seats together with a stool in between them and tried to lie down because my legs were swelling from sitting upright all night. You can't rest or relax. Also, I know it's difficult with lack of resources but I do feel that in a case like ours, where time is so very short, a single room would have been much more ideal.

The distress of these relatives was intensified by lack of basic privacy as they sat at the bedside of their dying relative. The family were unable to communicate in an intimate way with their father, or with each other. At this stage of intense emotion and stress, and when family communications are so crucial, access to a single room for the patient, and to a rest area to provide a break away from the bedside for the family, was the ideal that was frequently expressed by relatives. During this emotionally demanding period a sense of intrusion may be experienced when the dying patient and family are constantly exposed to the noise and activity of a busy ward; this is illustrated in the quotes below:

Cathy: No. When he was in a four-bedded room I wasn't comfortable. I felt he (father) was agitated with all the noise that was going on all around him. In fact we got to the stage that we couldn't even talk to each other.

George: When he (father) was eventually moved to a room of his own it really was the best thing. He was a lot happier and we were much more comfortable. We couldn't sit in the big ward with any real privacy and the way we were feeling we just wanted to be alone with him.

This suggests that a point is reached in the illness trajectory when the patient and the family's primary needs are to be in an environment that offers them some quiet and privacy, where they can communicate with and support one another. During this emotionally intense period nurses should be acutely sensitive to the subtle shifts in the illness progression, and to changes in the family's interactions, so that they can respond by offering access to a private area where the family can be together. Nurses should also maintain regular contact with the family in order to ensure their ongoing comfort both at the bedside and in a rest area in the ward. This includes offering access to facilities for toilet and rest and light refreshments within the ward.

Relatives can also suffer by proxy if they see their loved one in physical or emotional distress that is not being managed adequately. The provision of high-quality symptom management is crucial to the comfort of both the patient and the close family. Taking simple steps to provide for the physical comfort and emotional support of both patient and family can have powerful and reciprocal benefits, thus facilitating hope in circumstances where hope is fragile but crucial.

Theme – attachment

Abandonment and isolation .... Caring relationships

Although the relatives in McIntyre's study all firmly stated their needs for regular contact with nurses who were caring for their dying relative, most said that they felt hesitant about approaching the nurses whom they perceived to be too busy to be interrupted. Quotes below from Sarah and James illustrate relatives' anxiety about disturbing busy staff and their concerns about being a 'nuisance' by approaching the nurses too often:

Sarah: I don't like approaching the nurses in case they're too busy with something else. So I really appreciate it when they say to me, 'Excuse me, could I have a word with you?' Yes, I really do appreciate that.

James: It would really help if families were told at the outset that the nurses could be approached with any questions or worries we might have. If relatives knew that at the start and were reminded from time to time it would help a lot.

The research data also confirmed that relatives observe nurses closely to pick up cues to which nurses might be most approachable. Nurses with an open and friendly manner conveyed accessibility, but relatives said they would hesitate to approach those nurses who rarely smiled or made eye contact with them. Graham sums this up below:

Graham: There are some nurses that you would approach more readily than others. It really depends on their attitude. If you feel that their attitude is good and that they're quite happy to talk to you, then that's the ones you'll seek out. The attitude of the nursing staff is really important.

In addition, when the ward climate was informal and where relaxed staff–relative contact mechanisms were in place, relatives could relax and not feel they were 'in the way'. The following comments are typical of the positive experiences that some relatives had in the wards:

'Most definitely the nurses have approached me. I haven't had to seek out a nurse at all. They obviously sense your need.'

'When we came in this time, Nurse S immediately came up to us and said who she was and that she would be looking after Mary.'

The climate of friendship and warmth that relatives experienced in some of the study wards was highly praised by the participants in this study. The quote below from Janice confirms the very positive effect that such a climate can have on the relatives:

Janice: The nurses are talking to me a lot. They're asking how my mum is and they're also asking me how I am. I would say over the past few days that the nurses are concentrating just as much on me and my well-being, as they are in caring for my mother.

Relatives also gained significant comfort from seeing a bond of attachment develop between the nurses and their sick relative. It seemed that they felt much comforted and reassured when they saw their dying relative being treated by the staff as 'someone special'. Seeing this gave the relatives confidence that the staff actually cared *about* their dying loved one. Kim and Janice both illustrate the value that families place on this:

Kim: Some nurses put in that wee bit extra. They treat my mum like she's a little friend. They come right up to her and chat to her, and they always come to say 'cheerio' to her before they go home.

Janice: It's very comforting to me just knowing that they are there. Not just for their medical expertise but for their *comfort* as well. They are so nice and friendly to my mum,

and to the whole family. It is really excellent. It has made such a big, *big* difference to us.

When the emotional climate was warm, and relationships between staff, patients and relatives were relaxed and friendly, this was hope sustained and supported the family. Jennifer (quoted below) was interviewed in the early stages of the study before the improvements in family care had been implemented. At the time of the interview she had just spent four consecutive days and nights at her dying mother's bedside:

Jennifer: When I was in that room with my mother I was alone. It was just her and me. I was alone. Very, very much alone.

In a few short words, Jennifer conveys a profound sense of abandonment. Physical and emotional isolation had exhausted her resources and diminished her capacity for hope.

Another woman (Sue) also conveys her desolation when she was unable to establish any real connection with the nursing staff:

Sue: I'm not just talking about the ward facilities (weeping) but just to have a nurse greet you . . . Not necessarily as a long lost friend . . . but just so that if you have any questions then you know you can go to her. If they could just come over and say a wee word to us . . . To let you know if he's had a bad night or whatever. I mean I know it's a job to them but he's family to me. That way you would see there's a bit of care in there.

Jennifer and Sue's experiences confirm that, when caught up in the emotionally charged situation of impending loss, it can be alienating and hope crushing to encounter staff who are aloof and distant in their manner. In a climate where relationships are cool and where reassurance is lacking, relatives can also experience escalating concerns for the safety and well-being of their ill relative (McIntyre 2002).

Theme – worth

Feeling devalued .... Feeling valued

When a much loved family member is dying, relatives need to have the intrinsic value and the worth of their dying loved one acknowledged and respected. Relatives also need to know that some members of staff know and care *about* their loved one. In the quote below, Catherine is appealing for the worth of her dad to be recognised by the nurses:

Catherine: I would ask the nurses to try to look beyond the difficulties that they are experiencing with him and see that, if there are relatives who care *so* much for him, there must be more to him than they're seeing at this point of time . . . Some of them do know that. I'm talking of my particular old man now. He is my Dad and, though he has not always been an easy man to deal with, we love him very dearly. He is a very loveable old man.

When relatives could see evidence of liking and respect being conveyed to the patient, this seemed to support their own feelings of security and hopefulness. However, any perceived lack of respect generated significant distress. Adam (below) illustrates the hurt that resulted when he believed that his Dad's worth as a person had been undermined:

Adam: The doctors did their rounds and they never even came near him. I just felt that they were treating him like a lost cause. I'm not being critical but it was just like he's a lost cause. That really stuck in my throat. They didn't even come over to let him feel he was still worth having a look at.

Insensitive communications with the family can undermine the relatives' own sense of worth and crush their capacity for hopefulness. In the quote below, an elderly woman (Edith) reports on a conversation she had with the doctor who was looking after her dying husband. The bad news about her husband's prognosis was conveyed to Edith as she stood in the corridor. The distressing impact of the message was increased and her needs for support went unmet during this communication. As a result Edith was bleak and hopeless.

Edith: There was nowhere where we could go to be alone for a minute or two. I mean, what would that doctor have done if I had fallen at his feet or burst into floods of tears? I mean, I just flew for my daughter and we had a cup of tea in the staff canteen. But even there you had no privacy. She was crying and I was crying and we'd nowhere we could go to be alone.

In this study relatives placed the very highest value on seeing their ill loved one physically comfortable and free from distressing symptoms. Their next priority was to receive regular information about their loved one's condition and to get regular access to the medical staff. Relatives also valued receiving regular contact and support from nursing staff. Most relatives also appreciated being offered facilities for their comfort and privacy, and a friendly, informal and supportive ward climate.

Relatives also appreciated dealing with nurses whom the family knew and who also seemed to know and like their sick relative as a person. Nurses who took the time to talk to the relatives, and to listen to them, were found to be a crucial source of support. When nurses reduced the emotional distance and connected with the family on a person-to-person level, this conveyed genuine empathy from which relatives derived great comfort and support. Supported in these ways, they were better able to cope with their situation and to retain some capacity for hope within the family.

The final quote from Patricia offers a particularly clear example of the potential that nurses have to facilitate hope in the dying patient's relatives:

Patricia: The nurses have to realise that in dealing with relatives in my situation it's just different from a normal patient's visitors. You have got to have that little bit extra. Possibly some of the nurses won't have that little bit extra to give, but I've discovered these nurses do have it.

Researcher: How does that 'little bit extra' help?

Patricia: It reassures me that Peter is going to be all right, that they have his interest at heart, and mine too. It makes me feel better when I can feel and see that contact between him and them, and I think, 'She's a lovely girl. She knows. She feels'.

FACILITATING HOPE IN RELATIVES OF DYING PATIENTS IN HOSPITAL

As the needs of every family and family member vary, and as different care settings present different challenges and needs, the interventions set out in Table 8.2 should not be seen as either prescriptive or comprehensive. In addition, as hope-facilitating interventions are potentially synergistic in their effects, it is emphasised that an integrated and holistic approach is needed when acting to support hope in families of dying patients.

HOPE IN RELATIVES IN THE HOME CARE SETTING

There is an increasing trend, supported by UK policy, towards supporting choice in the place of death. This has implications for palliative care provision within the community setting. Wherever the patient may ultimately die, they are likely to spend most of their last year of life in their own home being cared for by close family members. When the patient and the family's hopes are focused on allowing the patient to die in his or her own home, the general practitioner (GP) and district nurses need to be acutely sensitive to the shifting needs of the caring family. Support from palliative care clinical nurse specialists such as Macmillan nurses and/or accessing the Marie Curie Nursing Service to provide extended periods of care in the home, often overnight, can provide crucial support to the family, perhaps avoiding late crisis admission to hospital due to caregiver strain (Brazil et al 2005).

The challenges to hope in the close relatives of patients being cared for at home will now be considered with reference to Case Study 8.4. Readers will be asked to analyse this case study and to consider the shifting focus of hope for the couple, the child and the extended family.

Table 8.2   Interventions aimed at supporting families in the hospital setting

Theme	Aim	Interventions to nurture hope in relatives
Comfort	To promote physical ease for relatives who are spending long periods of time in the ward area	Ensure the patient's personal and environmental comfort is optimised and symptoms are well managed Provide access to a private area away from the bedside for relatives to rest and receive information and support Provide a recliner chair, pillows, blankets and/or camp bed for relatives staying overnight by the bedside Reduce intrusive noise (e.g. TVs) around the bed area Ensure relatives can access toilet and washing facilities Provide hot/cold refreshments at ward level and direct to hospital canteen for meals
Attachment	To promote caring relationships between relatives and the patient, and between relatives and staff	Provide a caring environment that is welcoming and recognises the relatives' needs for regular contact, support and information Be available when added support is required, such as when redefining goals and expectations Show genuine concern and caring for the patient as a person Facilitate expressions of caring between patients and relatives by offering support and privacy as needed Engage in informal dialogue about 'normal' topics with relatives when appropriate
Worth	To enable the relative to be valued as a vital part of the care team	Show genuine concern for the relative's own well-being Allow relatives to see the patient being treated with dignity and respect, and with all main needs met Explore wishes (e.g. desired place of death) and promote and support decision-making Facilitate life review so that relatives are able to share personal memories with the patient (and with staff) Sensitively explore spiritual/religious beliefs and provide access to support as appropriate

Palliative care in the home setting

Case Study 8.4   The Watson family

James Watson is a 37-year-old career soldier whose work has allowed him to travel widely. He has always been proud of his job and enjoyed the close camaraderie of fellow servicemen. James currently lives on an army base in the Midlands with his wife of 6 years (Anna) and their son Jake aged 3. Two years after they married James had a seizure. A brain tumour was diagnosed. This was treated by surgery and radiotherapy followed by chemotherapy. Although this was traumatic for the couple, within a year James was deemed fit to return to his army job, albeit on restricted duties. All seemed to be back on an even keel and so the couple decided to try for a baby; the arrival of their son Jake was much celebrated. Anna left her job as a care assistant to look after Jake and all was going well for the family.

Eight months ago James started to experience further symptoms. His balance and coordination were gradually deteriorating, and to his distress he dropped little Jake whilst carrying him. Investigations confirmed that the brain tumour had returned and had grown.

Palliative management now offered the only option. Despite radiotherapy and ongoing palliative chemotherapy, James' difficulties are increasing. Although lucid and alert, he can now say only a few words. He has right-sided weakness, is unsteady on his feet, and is experiencing nausea and vomiting. James has recently been retired, on medical grounds, from his military post and the family are moving from army accommodation into their own home. James' care has been transferred to the local GP and community palliative care services. Fiona, a clinical nurse specialist in palliative care, is now involved in looking after the family.

Anna's parents live 40 miles away. They are the family's main source of support. Jake often stays over with his grandparents for days at a time so that Anna can look after James. James' parents live a lot closer but there are tensions between them and Anna. Whilst Anna and James are fairly realistic, James's mother is angry and unable to accept the situation. She is convinced that with prayer her son will recover.

Facilitating hope in the Watson family

It has already been stated that hope has reciprocal and transactional qualities in that hopefulness in one person within a close relationship has the potential to 'rub off' on others, so helping them to sustain hope. Conversely hopelessness in one person can diminish hope in others within a close relationship. This characteristic of hope underscores the need to facilitate hope in the family as they will have a crucial role in supporting the dying patient.

Readers are now asked to use the themes of Comfort, Attachment and Worth as a framework for assessing the impact of this illness on different members of the family. In particular, we should consider the threats to hope that different family members face, and the potential that healthcare professionals might have for facilitating hope in this family, albeit in a constantly shifting form. Some questions about the family's capacity for hope are suggested below. Readers should consider these and any other questions that their own analysis of the case study might raise.

James

- In what ways is his illness currently threatening James's comfort and well-being?
- What interventions might optimise his physical comfort and safety?
- What impact has the illness had on James's relationships within the nuclear and extended family and with his wider circle of contacts?
- What interventions or resources might help James sustain his close attachments?
- In what ways has James's illness impacted upon his family, social and gender roles?
- What support might be put in to help James optimise his sense of self-worth?

Anna

- What might the physical and emotional impact be on Anna of being James's main carer?
- How might the illness have affected Anna's relationships with James, Jake, her parents and parents-in-law, and her friends?
- Anna has watched her husband go from being a 'fighting fit' soldier to a mute, disabled person. In the face of this, how might James and Anna be supported to sustain their relationship?
- The relationship difficulties with her in-laws is happening just when Anna, James and his parents all need considerable support. How might they all

be helped and the potential for future regret reduced?

Jake

Jake is being well cared for by his grandparents but he is very young and his routine and key attachments have all been disrupted. In addition, Jake's dad has changed over recent months and he can no longer talk to him, hold him or play with him.

- What resources and services might be mobilised to support Jake during this time and also after his dad has died?
- How might the risk of longer-term negative consequences for Jake be minimised?

IMPLICATIONS FOR PRACTICE

Having now considered the concept of hope, and having discussed how a simple conceptual model may be used as a framework for facilitating hope in patients and families receiving palliative care, discussion will now focus on the wider implications for palliative care.

It has already been clearly stated that hope is an essential feature of life that persists even in those with an incurable life-threatening illness. Yet, for healthcare professionals, the level awareness of the concept of hope, and its practical application in the care of palliative care patients and families, is variable. Greater professional debate is needed within the literature and in practice. This would help to increase professional understanding of the importance of hope to palliative care practice where the focus must be on quality of life.

This chapter offers a simple conceptual model that may be used to help healthcare professionals turn what is a nebulous concept into practical activities that have the potential to foster and sustain hope in people who are receiving palliative care. Furthermore, activities to support hope in patients and families are pertinent regardless of diagnosis. The key themes of Comfort, Attachment and Worth are drawn from human experiences of advanced illness, not the illness itself, and as such this framework can be applied to the care of people who are dying from a range of conditions, including cancer, heart failure, motor neurone disease or dementia. The challenge for professionals is to see past the diagnostic label and respond to the person, whether the patient or the relative.

A further challenge for healthcare professionals is that the facilitation of hope in those nearing the end of life requires a range of advanced communication skills that are adaptable and thus able to respond to the ever-changing needs of individuals. As with communication skills, skills in facilitating hope require not a universal approach but an individually focused approach that responds to the needs of the individual at each point of the illness progression. Considerable emphasis has been placed on the development of advanced communication skills for healthcare professionals caring for people with cancer, but this is less evident for those caring for people with end-stage heart disease, lung disease or dementia. Indeed, it could be argued that the challenges of facilitating hope in a person dying with advanced dementia are even greater than for someone with cancer, as the professional is faced with the added difficulty of caring for a person with cognitive impairment. Facilitating hope in people with palliative care needs in non-malignant illness undoubtedly warrants further investigation and research.

It is apparent that, although research in relation to hope in palliative care has grown over the past decade, a number of areas merit greater investigation. Of primary interest is whether, and in what ways, hope at the end of life differs for people with non-malignant disease compared with that in those with cancer. To what extent, if any, is the experience of hope different for someone with chronic pulmonary disease or motor neurone disease, compared with someone with cancer? Second, what is the exact relationship between hope and depression in palliative care? A diagnostic feature of depression is a sense of hopelessness, so could the implementation of hope-fostering activities early during people's illness experiences reduce the prevalence of depression in palliative care patients? Third, in the context of palliative care, how does hope or hopelessness in the patient affect the level of hope experienced by the relatives, and what is the role of the healthcare professional in facilitating hope within families?

The reciprocal nature of hope is known, yet in practice many nurses have witnessed differences within families as to the focus of hope at different times. These, and many other areas, are worthy of further research in palliative care. Finally there is the ever-present challenge as to how research findings can be translated into improved care for patients and families. We hope that this chapter will make some contribution to illustrating how research can lead to developments in palliative care practice.

CONCLUSION

Hope represents an essential feature of the experience of being human that endures even when individuals are experiencing incurable illnesses and are at the end of life. Hope is a dynamic energising force that is linked to coping and is sustained in part by positive relationships with others. There has been a growing interest in the concept of hope and its relevance to cancer and palliative care practice over the past two decades, and more recently there has been some expansion to include a focus on hope in palliative care for those with non-malignant diseases.

Nurses and other healthcare professionals have the potential to influence hope significantly in patients and families receiving palliative care. Our conceptual model of hope has concentrated on the three key themes of Comfort, Attachment and Worth. This model has been applied to patients and relatives, presented in the form of case studies and research exemplars, thus highlighting the synergistic nature of the three themes and the profound impact that significant relationships have on hope in palliative care.

The chapter concluded by highlighting some wider implications for palliative care practice, not least the challenge of increasing healthcare professionals' awareness and understanding of hope and its relevance to palliative care across the diagnostic spectrum.

References

Allmond B, Buckman W, Gofman H 1979 The family is the patient. C V Mosby, St Louis. Cited in: Wright L, Leahey M 2000 Nurses and families. F A Davis, Philadelphia, p 37

Appelin G, Bertero C 2004 Patients' experiences of palliative care in the home: a phenomenological study of a Swedish sample. Cancer Nursing 27:65–70

Benzein E, Saveman B 1998 Nurses' perception of hope in patients with cancer: a palliative care perspective. Cancer Nursing 21:10–16

Benzein E, Norberg A, Saveman B 2001 The meaning of the lived experience of hope in patients with cancer in palliative home care. Palliative Medicine 15:117–126

Brazil K, Bedard H, Krueger P et al 2005 Service Preferences Among Family Caregivers of the Terminally Ill. Journal of Palliative Medicine, Feb 2005, Vol. 8, No. 1: 69–78

Buckley J, Herth K 2004 Fostering hope in terminally ill patients. Nursing Standard 19:33–41

Byock I 1996 Beyond symptom management. European Journal of Palliative Care 3:125–130

Chaplin J 1996 An exploration of the quality of care received by individuals having lung cancer surgery:

perceptions of patients, relatives and nurses. University of Glasgow, Glasgow

Chapman K J, Pepler C 1998 Coping, hope and anticipatory grief in family members in palliative home care. Cancer Nursing 21:226–234

Chen M L 2003 Pain and hope in patients with cancer: a role for cognition. Cancer Nursing 26:61–67

Chochinov H, Hack T, McClement S, Kristjanson L, Harlos M 2002 Dignity in the terminally ill: a developing empirical model. Social Science and Medicine 54:433–443

Christie W, Moore C 2004 The impact of humour on patients with cancer. Clinical Journal of Oncology Nursing 9:211–218

Coyle N 2004 In their own words: seven advanced cancer patients describe their experience of pain and the use of opioid drugs. Journal of Pain and Symptom Management 27:300–309

DeRaeve L 1996 Dignity and integrity at the end of life. International Journal of Palliative Nursing 2:71–76

Dufault K, Martocchio B C 1985 Hope: its spheres and dimensions. Nursing Clinics of North America 20:379–391

Duggleby W 2001 Hope at the end of life. Journal of Hospice and Palliative Nursing 3:51–64

Duggleby W, Wright K 2004 Elderly palliative care cancer patients' descriptions of hope-fostering strategies. International Journal of Palliative Nursing 10:352–359

Farran C J, Herth K, Popovitch J M 1995 Hope and hopelessness: critical clinical constructs. Sage Publications, Thousand Oaks, CA

Felder B 2004 Hope and coping in patients with cancer diagnosis. Cancer Nursing 27:320–324

Flemming K 1997 The meaning of hope to palliative care cancer patients. International Journal of Palliative Nursing 3:14–18

Hegarty M 2001 The dynamic of hope: hoping in the face of death. Progress in Palliative Care 9:42–46

Herth K A 1990 Fostering hope in terminally ill people. Journal of Advanced Nursing 15:1250–1259

Herth K, Cutliffe J 2002a The concept of hope in nursing 3: hope and palliative care nursing. British Journal of Nursing 11:977–983

Herth K, Cutcliffe J 2002b The concept of hope in nursing 6: research/education/policy/practice. British Journal of Nursing 11:1404–1411

Hinds P S 1984 Inducing a definition of hope through the use of grounded theory methodology. Journal of Advanced Nursing 9:357–362

Hockley J 1993 The concept of hope and the will to live. Palliative Medicine 7:181–186

Klyma J, Vehvilainen-Julkunen K 1997 Hope in nursing research: a meta-analysis of the ontological and epistemological foundations of research on hope. Journal of Advanced Nursing 25:364–371

Kubler-Ross E 1969 On death and dying. Macmillan, New York

Lair G S 1996 Counselling the terminally ill. Taylor & Francis, Washington, DC

Lin C C, Lai Y L, Ward S 2003 Effect of cancer pain on performance status, mood states, and level of hope among Taiwanese cancer patients. Journal of Pain and Symptom Management 25:29–37

Lin H R, Bauer-Wu S M 2003 Psycho-spiritual well-being in patients with advanced cancer: an integrated review of the literature. Journal of Advanced Nursing 44:69–80

McIntyre R 2002 Nursing support for families of dying patients. Athenaeum Press, Gateshead

McIntyre R, Chaplin J 2001 Hope: the heart of palliative care. In: Kinghorn S, Gamlin R (eds) Palliative nursing: bringing comfort and hope. Baillière Tindall, Edinburgh, p 129–145

McIntyre R, Lugton J 2005 Supporting the family and carers. In: Lugton J, McIntyre R (eds) Palliative care: the nursing role. Elsevier Churchill Livingstone, Edinburgh, p 261–302

Nekolaichuk C, Bruera E 1998 On the nature of hope in palliative care. Journal of Palliative Care 14:36–42

Nekolaichuk C L, Bruera E 2004 Assessing hope at the end of life: validation of an experience of hope scale in advanced cancer patients. Palliative and Supportive Care 2:243–253

Perakyla A 1991 Hope work in the care of seriously ill patients. Qualitative Health Research 1:407–433

Post-White J, Ceronsky C, Kreitzer M J et al 1996 Hope, spirituality, sense of coherence, and quality of life in patients with cancer. Oncology Nursing Forum 23:1571–1578

Twycross R 1997 Symptom management in advanced cancer, 2nd edn. Radcliffe Medical Press, Oxford

Whyte D (ed.) 1997 Explorations in family nursing. Routledge, London. Chapters 1 & 3

Wright L, Leahey M 2000 Nurses and families. F A Davis, Philadelphia

Chapter 9

Supporting the family facing loss and grief

Janet Brown and Graham Farley

The aim of this chapter is to introduce the reader to some concepts about how a family experiences and copes with the loss of someone close and how the palliative care nurse can respond to and support them.

The chapter explores our previous personal and professional experiences, and reflects on how these can influence our approach to a patient's loss. It aims to identify skills that could be helpful to palliative care nurses when supporting patients and their families, and reviews some of the current models and literature that underpin good practice. The greatest opportunity to learn comes from the experience of working with families who teach us about their experiences, and we have included some narratives of people who have struggled with grief and discovered resources to help the healing process.

Each person experiences grief in their own unique way, yet they are usually part of a family and a community that will influence their thoughts, feelings and behaviours. Three areas are explored to help nurses increase confidence, knowledge and skills:

1. Exploring personal awareness of how we feel and behave when faced with loss
2. A review of theories and models of grief and loss to help make sense of the process and ensure evidence-based practice
3. Identifying practical skills that can be learned and practised to increase competence.

INTRODUCTION TO LOSS AND GRIEF

The grief that we feel when someone close to us dies is a universal experience that all human beings share. Sometimes the stress of the experience divides families and communities; at other times it brings them closer together. On the Indonesian island of Sumatra, where the north of the island was wracked by civil war, the aftermath of the 2004 tsunami, which swept away much of the community, enabled people to work together, sharing their grief to build a new and more peaceful community.

Most of us don't want to think about someone close to us dying. When families find themselves in this situation they are usually stunned and shocked into disbelief, unable to believe what is happening. As people struggle with the reality, they begin to feel the pain of grief and know that their lives are changed for ever. When friends and carers become involved they are touched by the sadness and gravity of the situation and want to offer support, but are often unsure about what to say or how they can be of most help. As a carer, I am reminded of the enormity of the task by John Bowlby (1991, p 7), in his work on loss:

> The death of a loved one is one of the most intensely painful experiences any human being can suffer. And not only is it painful to experience but it is also painful to witness if only because we are so impotent to help.

Bowlby acknowledges the depth of grief for an individual and the challenge that carers face. Knowing that we are not alone in feeling powerless and inadequate can be reassuring. If we have the privilege to be alongside a person, we might be able to make a small contribution to support them at this time of change and crisis.

WHAT DO FAMILIES WANT?

There are many factors that influence the way in which a family feels and responds to loss. Their previous experiences of loss, the circumstances of the death and social situation, the environment, genetic make-up, developmental age and personality will contribute to the uniqueness of the experience for each family member. Families interrelate, and sometimes this will be supportive and cohesive whereas other families experience conflict and isolation. Individual family members have different wants and needs, and these may not always be recognised by others in their family. Often people want to protect particular family members whom they believe to be very vulnerable and consequently unable to cope with the reality of the illness and death.

This can be especially true when children and young people are involved, but children also need to understand what is happening and feel that there is someone that they can talk to. Grace Christ, a profes-

sor of social work in Columbia, studied a number of families in which a parent was dying and found that the period before the death was the most stressful time for children (Christ 2000). Most commonly, children and young people want to talk about things that are happening in their families; they turn to their parents or other siblings for support but are worried about upsetting them (Brown 2006). Opportunities to talk with someone outside the family can help in this situation.

People usually want to feel in control and to be given choices; they may want to share their feelings and need someone to listen, or may prefer to express their grief privately. Their needs can change from day to day so that sometimes they may want support and at other times they want to be independent. This oscillation in behaviours has been well documented by Stroebe et al (1992), and is discussed in more detail later in the chapter. Asking the question 'What does this family/person want' can be a useful starting point. Nurses need to be tentative, sensitive and flexible so that the support fits with what is appropriate and helpful.

Why is working with loss difficult and uncomfortable for the carer?

Caring for families that are experiencing painful loss is a challenge because there is uncertainty about what is required and a risk of offering support which may be rejected.

Papadatou (2000) identified factors that make working with people who are dying and experiencing loss and grief stressful and challenging:

- Loss of a close relationship with a special patient
- Identification with family members if there are similarities to our personal situation
- Powerlessness at being unable to change the situation and make them better
- Loss of personal beliefs and a lack of control
- Reminds us of unresolved losses or anticipated losses for the future
- Reminds us of our own mortality

Who can help?

The emotional care of a grieving family is shared, and there may be some family members and friends who are very supportive and facilitative. Sometimes nurses feel that they do not have the time or depth of experience needed, and therefore specialist skills are required. Knowledge of who in the multidisciplinary team could best help the family and how to contact them can be reassuring in sharing the responsibility for emotional care.

Multidisciplinary teams will have expertise and skills in a range of services that can be accessed to support the patient and family or act as a source of information and consultancy for nurses. Making personal contact and finding out about the other members of the team can increase confidence and add a wider base of knowledge.

In your team you may have district nurses, palliative care medical consultants, general practitioners (GPs), Macmillan nurses, Marie Curie nurses, chaplains, occupational therapists, social workers, counsellors, psychologists, dieticians, complementary therapists, children and young people's therapists, and volunteer support workers. The list is quite long and it is important to access the services that will help families but not overwhelm them with a stream of professionals who will undermine their strengths and resources, leaving them feeling powerless and incompetent.

In addition there are a number of websites, books and articles that the family can use; some of these are listed at the end of the chapter.

THE PALLIATIVE CARE NURSE'S UNIQUE OPPORTUNITY

Patients are referred for palliative care when curative treatment is no longer possible and the focus of care is to create the best quality of life for them and their family. For the purpose of this chapter, the term 'family' includes all close family members, important significant relationships and the patient until they die.

When caring for these patients, nurses have an opportunity to develop an intimate relationship with both the patient and family members, and can help them express their fears and feelings about dying, the death and bereavement. If we can be emotionally alongside families at this time, we can help them prepare for the loss, support them in making choices and help them take some control in a frightening situation.

As the patient and their families think about the many losses caused by the illness, they begin to experience grief. This process starts with diagnosis of the illness when there is potential loss of the future, and continues for the patient until they die. For the family left behind, the grief continues into their bereavement. Palliative care nurses usually have contact with families before, during and for a short time after the death, so the focus of this chapter is on the grief during this period of time.

Sometimes patients and their families meet the palliative care nurse during the last few days or even hours of life and there is a very short time in which to get to know the family. This makes building the relationship a challenge, as a sensitive caring approach can be very healing and make a difference to the family during their bereavement (Rosenblatt 1993).

HOW CAN NURSES LOOK AFTER THEMSELVES?

If we are to work constructively with families that are experiencing loss, we need to be comfortable with our own experiences. We are all familiar with feelings of loss, from the irritation of losing a pen when we want to write something down to the experience of leaving friends or familiar surroundings when we move house or job. By the time we reach adulthood, most of us will know what it is like when someone in our family or a close friend dies. The way in which we have learned to manage smaller losses will have influenced the way that we cope with bigger losses and bereavements. For some of us, the experiences may have been profound and have left unresolved issues; others may have been left with both good memories and sadness that the person is no longer here.

Whatever your experience of loss it is important to acknowledge the risk of re-experiencing strong feelings when working in this area, either when in contact with patients and families or when reading about death and dying. By knowing and understanding your own feelings you can find ways to keep yourself safe and healthy. From this position of clarity and strength we can support others.

> ### REFLECTION POINTS
>
> - Who could I talk to if I become upset when working through this chapter?
> - Where do I get my support from?
> - What can I do for myself to keep myself safe?

These reflection points denote sensitive issues and you may consider talking about these to a colleague who is experienced in loss, grief and supervision.

Hopefully you will have already identified a good support system which includes family, friends and colleagues, as well as the support that you get from clinical supervision. You will have learned how to relax and recharge your batteries in a busy and demanding life.

WHAT DO NURSES NEED IN ORDER TO HELP OTHERS?

When asked what they need to help them care for families experiencing loss, most nurses want to feel more confident when in contact with a grieving family. They want to know what to say, and fear that they may say the wrong thing or become tearful and upset themselves.

Sometimes nurses lack confidence in their ability to support grieving families. This can stem from fear about their own experience of loss. Gaining insight into personal experiences increases awareness of how to respond and behave when caring for families of dying patients, and enhances confidence. A basic knowledge of current theories about loss and grief will help to make sense of the process, giving reassurance of what is normal in a sometimes chaotic situation. A knowledge of a range of practical skills in knowing what to say and how to support a family will increase competencies and confidence in difficult situations.

Personal awareness

It is important to know something about how we have managed our own losses in the past so that there are no surprises and we are aware of how we might behave when helping others.

> ### REFLECTION POINT
>
> Some of the losses that you have experienced in your life:
>
> • Can you remember any childhood losses and how they were different to your adult experience?
> • Can you remember the feelings that you experienced and how you behaved?

If you were aware of bereavement as a young child you may have felt curious about what was happening. The adults around you would probably have made decisions for you so that you may have felt included and secure, or you may have been frightened, confused, isolated or angry.

Your feelings as a young child will have been very different to those that you experienced as an adult,

although each loss will have been a different experience. Your awareness and understanding will have been based on your emotional developmental age as well as the circumstances of the loss.

As adults, the first feelings of loss are usually ones of disbelief and shock, even if the death is anticipated. Sometimes people carry on as though nothing has happened, trying to cling on to normality, before they allow the news to become a reality. Grief can be very frightening, with sadness, anger, a feeling of life being unfair, and guilt about what they could have said or done differently, fear about the future and loneliness without the person who has died. In the short term some people feel relief, if the person has had a long or painful illness, that they are no longer suffering. There may be a sense of relief and freedom that their responsibility to care is over, and then feelings of guilt about that. Using your personal experience wisely and professionally can help to increase confidence and enhance an empathic and caring approach.

Personal values and beliefs

It is easy to view grief and bereavement from the perspective we are most familiar with, yet other cultures have a lot to teach us and there are often many similarities.

People with strong religious faiths can find comfort from their beliefs, but for some people anger causes them to lose their faith. This is another loss to be suffered at a time when people most need support.

Our family upbringing will have influenced the way in which we respond. Some families want to share their emotions and express them openly, whereas other families cope by keeping busy or they want to keep their grief private. We may have very clear ideas about how we and others should behave, so it is important to be aware of our own ways of coping yet be flexible and accepting of the way others cope.

> ### REFLECTION POINT
>
> How some of your personal values and beliefs have influenced the way you have responded to loss. Think about:
>
> • your culture
> • religious beliefs
> • family upbringing

Sometimes, if patients and their families have experiences similar to our own, we can over-identify with them and this may elicit strong feelings in ourselves. If we can recognise this then we are able to acknowledge the differences as well as the similarities and have a more objective understanding. We need to be aware that this family is not our family but a separate and different family that is unique, with a different set of wants and needs from our own. It is also important to be aware that we may need some extra support when caring for this family, and it would be appropriate to discuss our feelings and how we can best help this family with our supervisor during clinical supervision.

REFLECTION POINT

The families you have cared for:

- Are there any families that you have found particularly moving or thought about a lot?
- Were there any similarities between your personal experiences and that of these families?

You may have been quite surprised to find some similarities and strong feelings. Sometimes this can go back a number of years (see Case Study 9.1).

So far, we have reflected on some of our personal experiences and how these impact on our work with families. However, in order that nurses can develop their competence, it is necessary to acquire a sound knowledge base of loss and grief. This can be achieved through a greater understanding of the theories that have developed through a variety of research methods. Such an understanding will enable nurses to apply these theories and models to their clinical situations. To facilitate this process, the following section reviews models and theories related to loss, grief and bereavement.

REFLECTION POINT

- What models of grief are you familiar with?
- Do you apply these in your practice?

Case Study 9.1   An example of work when the loss impacts on the helper's experience

A middle-aged woman was referred for bereavement counselling because her first grandchild had died at birth. She felt very angry about this but was unable to express her anger because her daughter was distraught with grief. She said that all the medical and midwifery care had been excellent and yet she felt cheated and desperately disappointed, and wanted to blame someone.

In our first counselling session together I encouraged her to express her angry feelings and she spontaneously punched the cushions and cried with anger. I listened quietly, accepting her feelings and allowed her time to tell the story from her point of view.

The next week she returned, feeling calm but very sad. She brought with her a photo album of her grandchild which had been taken at the hospital with the family. She told me how beautiful the baby was, and as we looked at the photos together I shared her sadness. I was aware that I felt tearful as I was remembering my own grief after miscarrying a baby many years ago. I did not share this with her as this would not have been helpful to her, but I was able to acknowledge my personal feelings internally and then focus on her experiences and support her expression of grief.

HOW DID THE EARLIER THEORIES EVOLVE?

Loss can be viewed from the extremes of a continuum. At one end would be the view of loss as a unique, personal and intensely private experience for each and every individual. At the other end would be the view of loss as a series of patterns that have a commonality. Both views, however diverse, are as credible as each other, but the study into each takes a different research approach. The former is usually through a qualitative approach that offers unique insights into the lived experience of grief, whereas the latter attempts to gain further knowledge and understanding by measuring and categorising behaviour.

Corr (2003) suggests that grief is the normal internal and external response experience to the perception of loss. Mourning is described as the process of adaptation to loss, which is governed by a range of cultural rituals and rules. Bereavement is described as that duration of time in which grief is experienced and mourning occurs. Reimers (2001) suggests that bereavement is a loss caused by the death itself, whereas grief is the emotional feelings that accompany the loss.

The earliest exponents of those attempting to categorise behavioural responses were Freud, Lindemann and Bowlby. Freud (1917), in his early theory of mourning in 'Mourning and Melancholia', began to identify specific patterns of reactions which included the painful emotional sadness, the loss of interest in the external world, the capacity to show affection and lack of volition for any activity. Payne et al (1999, p 59) encapsulated Freud's four characteristics of mourning thus:

- a profoundly painful dejection
- a loss of capacity to adopt new love objects
- a rejection in activity or a withdrawal of activity not connected with thoughts of the loved person
- a loss of interest in the outside world because it does not involve the dead person.

Lindemann (1944) was one of the earliest psychiatrists to carry out an in-depth study of grief. There was a fire in a Boston nightclub that killed 500 people. Eric Lindemann carried out extensive interviews with the survivors and relatives of the deceased and concluded that there were patterns in the behaviours and emotions experienced by these people. His work influenced other researchers into this psychological phenomenon. One criticism of his work, however, is that it concentrates on traumatic loss and bereavement in sudden death, and therefore his findings need to be considered in this context. Lindemann identified a significant pattern of behaviours and responses associated with loss, including:

- somatic disturbance
- preoccupation with the deceased
- guilt
- hostility
- disorganised behaviour.

The premise of all these theories is that emotional ties need to be severed from the deceased and investments into new relationships made in order that the person who is grieving can move on. This theoretical foundation stone has been challenged by more contemporary authors such as Walter, Klass & Silverman, and Stroebe, who suggest that rather than encourage the severing of ties recipients of grief should be encouraged to maintain a continuing bond with their loved ones. This was a major watershed in bereavement theory. These theories will be discussed later. The early theorists were predominantly psychiatrists and psychologists who pathologised the emotional reactions, whereas the later theorists (who included sociologists and anthropologists) moulded the original theories to include a more holistic/humanistic perspective.

Bowlby's theory relating to loss stemmed from his belief that children form close attachments to their mothers and that any premature separation could lead to behavioural manifestations later in life. Bowlby (1991) identified a range of behavioural responses associated with grief, encapsulated in the following model:

- numbness
- yearning and searching
- disorganisation and support
- reorganisation.

Parkes (1986), who was influenced by Bowlby, introduced a phase model:

- shock and alarm
- searching
- anger and guilt
- gaining a new identity.

One of the rather unfair criticisms levelled at Parkes' phase model of grief is that those who have been bereaved are expected to pass through the various stages as if there were a fixed sequence of events (Small 2001). This is a misinterpretation of the model proposed by Parkes, and in reality the bereaved will probably find that they move from one phase to another and back again until such time as they reach a degree of resolution. Small (2001) offers this word of caution when considering models of grief. In Greek mythology Procrustes would welcome guests and invite them to spend the night in a special bed that he proclaimed would fit any guest regardless of their size or stature. What Procrustes did not reveal to his guests was that if they were too long for the bed he would shorten their limbs and if too short he would stretch them! Small indicates through this analogy the dangers of attempting to fit everyone into neat models and theoretical frameworks.

It is also important to make a cautionary note of Parkes' original research, as the subjects used in this study were not selected from a broad population but from a narrow range. As Walter (1999, p 171) observed:

Parkes's (1972) work is classic: based largely on data about prematurely widowed women, his influential book is termed *Bereavement: Studies of Grief in Adult Life*.

This emphasises the need to acknowledge that grief models are not always transferable or applicable to other populations that may differ in culture. Valentine (2006) makes an observation that these traditional universal theories of grief have evolved in a Western society that represents only one-quarter of the world's population. In simple terms, how convinced can we be that this universal model is truly representative of that of the world at large?

Worden (1982), like Parkes, suggested that the phases of grief were a process and not a state, and that the bereaved need to work through a transition to achieve an adjustment. The 'tasks' involved in this process are:

- accepting the reality of the loss
- working through the pain of grief
- adjusting to life without the deceased
- emotionally relocating the deceased and moving on with life.

In contrast to the stage, phase and task models, Stroebe & Schut (1996) proposed the Dual Process Model of Grief (Fig. 9.1). Stroebe & Schut suggest that there is an oscillation between two diverse coping strategies:

- *Loss orientation* refers to the individual facing the grief and becoming preoccupied with the loss, which includes yearning for the deceased.
- *Restoration orientation* refers to the individual attempting to adapt, which includes learning tasks and acquiring roles previously undertaken by the deceased.

The key to this model is the oscillation that occurs from one coping strategy to another. This is not necessarily determined by gender, but by the context of the individual loss itself and whether there is a preference for one particular orientation over the other. It is suggested by the authors that as time passes less time is spent in the loss orientation phase and more in the restoration phase.

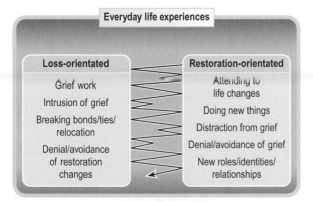

Figure 9.1 The dual-process model of grief.

Stroebe & Schut's model is based on seminal work carried out by Lazarus & Folkman (1984), who identified two coping strategies: emotion-focused and problem-focused coping. Emotion-focused coping relates to the individual's strategies that help to regulate the emotional outcomes resulting from stressful encounters. Problem-focused strategies are those that are employed actively to reduce the stressful nature of events.

It should always be remembered that, although we need to appreciate stages and patterns of grief responses, the experience of grief is an intensely unique experience for each individual. Kafka, in his book *Metamorphosis,* describes a young travelling salesman who awakes to discover that he has been transformed into a verminous bug. Kafka describes this transformation in minute detail, yet he is still a human being attempting to portray what it is like for a *human* to be an insect. This analogy serves to remind us that no matter how familiar we may feel about another's experience it is, in the end, *their* unique experience and not *ours*.

Attig (1991) draws an interesting distinction between the specific emotion of grief and the 'far more complex coping process which is *grieving*' (p 385). Attig argues that, while death and bereavement are choiceless events (based on their inevitability), the process of grieving itself can be subject to choice. Imagine falling into a river (this represents the death of a loved one), then imagine the river carrying the person along and eventually depositing them dead or alive at a certain point along the river bank (this symbolizes the longer, more complex, grieving process). In this scenario the recipient is passive and, because the situation appears hopeless, the victim does nothing to change the outcome. Imagine the same scenario where the recipient fights, struggles and eventually swims to safety on the other side. Here, the person does not take on the role of a helpless victim but actively works through the situation. There are reasons why the bereaved allow grief to overwhelm them, but it is this passive behaviour that prevents the active tasks of grieving that lead to resolution. Attig suggests there may be biological attachment, or that the passive behaviour offers a greater degree of comfort than facing the agonising reality of the death. Once the bereaved are able to overcome their debilitating need to yearn and search for the deceased, their deep sadness is gradually replaced with realistic memories of their life. Grieving is (ironically) the very barrier that prevents the bereaved from having true memories of their loved ones.

Kubler-Ross (1969) described the emotional stages of dying as denial, anger, bargaining, depression and acceptance. While this reflects a patient's lived experience of dying and identifies anticipatory grief, it has become a universally adopted model of bereavement. Many health professionals apply the model too rigidly, expecting the person to experience each stage. Earlier models that evolved from the psychology base suggest that the bereaved person who continues a bond with the deceased should be considered unhealthy. Silverman & Klass (1966, p 4) summed this up rather well:

> In this model the bond with the deceased is not part of the resolution of grief, but is an attempt to preserve the relationship by fighting against the reality that the person is dead. In this formulation such resistance to reality is doomed to failure, for eventually the person must accept that death is real and permanent, and the end of the bond must be relinquished.

In summary, what the earlier exponents of grief suggested is that there needs to be a severing of ties with the deceased, whereas more modern authors have suggested that there needs to be a continuing bond for a healthier resolution. Interestingly, in a recent study Stroebe et al (2005) concluded that the inevitable coping strategies that deal with the stress of bereavement are dependent on the nature of the attachment that had been developed with the deceased. These authors suggest that the coping strategies employed, that is to say the continuation of bonds with the deceased or the severing of ties, is dependent on the nature of the attachment between the deceased and the bereaved. Stroebe et al (2005, p 62) attest:

> Whether a bereaved person actually continues or relinquishes the bond with the deceased, and whether the strategy is sustaining or detrimental in the process of coming to terms with the loss, depends on the nature of the relationship to the deceased, which is influenced by the individual's learning style.

What Stroebe and colleagues are suggesting is that those who are securely attached would not normally require any interventions and that they would oscillate between orientation and restoration until their grief was resolved. Those who were insecurely attached, however, may require support in a variety of ways to help them confront their grief, and may benefit by severing ties completely.

A significant amount of nursing and medical research has employed quantitative methods to measure information about patients. However, it is often difficult (and inappropriate) to use this hard-science approach to explore human suffering and its expression. This approach runs the risk of destroying or damaging the very 'essence' of that which it is attempting to explore, because humans respond in a holistic and multidimensional way. Stroebe's model (see Fig. 9.1) demonstrates how individuals fluctuate from one coping strategy to another. What the nurse may be unaware of is that there may be some hidden benefits in the fluctuations, the duration spent in that orientation and the frequency at which these fluctuations occur. A qualitative approach attempts to keep that holistic phenomenon intact and tries to capture the unique individual response.

It would be interesting at this point to reflect on a case study and see how these theories and models apply in practice; see Case Study 9.2.

REFLECTION POINT

- How do the newer models you have read about change your thinking about grief and bereavement?
- Which models might you now consider applying to your area of practice?
- Why in particular do you feel this is the case?

The earlier part of the scenario in Case Study 9.2 reveals how the behaviours can be observed from the phase/task/stage models such as anger and denial. It also suggests that some of the bereavement behaviour can be seen from the Dual Process Model in that Joe would sometimes be enveloped in the enormity of the grief while at other times he displayed behaviour that suggested he was getting on with the practicalities of his brother's death. Yet later in this trajectory there is a suggestion that he showed behaviour that would fit with the more contemporary models of grief, in that he was able to establish a continuing dialogue with his deceased brother. These models offer useful frames of reference that identify particular modes of behaviour. From a phenomenological perspective, the holistic case history also offers a clear insight into the unique behaviour for this individual as well as attempting to capture the particular meaning and philosophy. It would therefore appear to be beneficial to be able to take both a reductionist and holistic perspective of grief. Being able to juxtapose (place these two approaches side by side) and view both at the same time helps to give a more three-dimensional view of what is a complex sequence of behaviours.

Case Study 9.2

Joe had lost his brother Mike, who had died from lung cancer aged 45 years. Joe had found this loss very hard to cope with. Within the first year, he started to develop a lot of pain in the shoulder and left arm. Joe went to see his GP and also complained of increasing shortness of breath, which he claimed came on both spontaneously and after exertion. Despite repeated assurances from the GP, Joe (who had not smoked for 15 years) was convinced that he too was suffering from lung cancer. Joe spent long periods ruminating and reminiscing about his younger brother. He also took a trip to where his brother had lived, and laid flowers on the grave. He visited his bereaved sister-in-law, nephew and nieces, and offered both financial and emotional support.

Joe had vivid dreams about Mike, and as his brother had lived some distance away Joe would sometimes pretend that Mike wasn't dead and that he would probably ring him at some point. Joe also had frequent mood swings and was emotionally labile. He became angry and irritated over quite trivial things. Joe was also suffering from insomnia and eventually returned to the GP, who referred him to a counsellor.

Joe disclosed to his counsellor how difficult he felt it was to 'let go' and that in doing so he would risk losing the precious memories of his brother. The counsellor asked Joe why he felt this was likely to happen; Joe replied that all that he had left of Mike were his memories and that as Mike had been taken from him there was always the danger that these would be taken as well.

The counsellor asked Joe what he missed most about his brother. Joe explained that he missed the weekly phone calls when they would talk about what each had been up to that week, such as the books they had read or the films they had seen. Through a succession of counselling sessions, Joe decided to write a letter to his brother explaining how he missed him but also including fond memories. At a later stage Joe would also include what books he had recently read and would suggest in his letters whether Mike would have liked them as well. Eventually Joe stopped writing the letters and just talked to his brother 'in his head' . . .

NEUROMATRIX THEORY AND GRIEF

People who have undergone the loss of an arm or leg can experience phenomena sometimes called 'stump hallucination', which manifests as an awareness that the lost limb is still present. For some, these aberrant sensations can be perceived as being painful and are termed 'phantom limb pain'. Remarkably there is no external trigger for these sensations and so they must be generated by the brain itself. In 1993 a psychologist called Ronald Melzack proposed what is now known as the neuromatrix theory to help explain these observations. This theory proposes that the brain constantly compares sensory information from outside and inside the body to what it considers should be normal. This 'normality' could be viewed as an anatomical map. For the amputee, the loss of sensory information due to the severed limb would create an 'unexplained' aberration which the brain would attempt to correct and in doing so produce the various phantom limb sensations. Eventually, in the majority of cases, the brain adjusts to the loss and the phantom limb pain dissipates.

It has been well documented that many bereaved people sense the dead person's physical proximity or believe they have heard, smelt, touched or even seen their dead loved one. These experiences tend to occur mainly in the acute period of grief. What the brain considers 'normal' may therefore extend beyond the anatomical and encompass all aspects of our sensory experience. It is quite common for a husband or wife to describe their spouse as their 'other half', and spending years in the company of another person quite often leads to the feeling that the friend or loved one is an extension of ourselves. From this it could be postulated that in the event of an acute emotional loss a similar pattern of events could ensue as with the amputee. In this case, however, instead of phantom limb pain the brain's compensations could lead to the phantom sensory experiences that have been described. In essence, it may be that the deficit between the new raw reality of the loss and the previous emotional 'normality' gives rise to the emotion of grief, yearning and sensory aberrations.

LINKING THEORIES TO PRACTICE

Reading about theory gives some structure to a changing and complex response to loss but linking our own practice to a theory is an exciting experience, which I call a 'Eureka moment'. When I (Janet Brown) had been working with bereaved families for some time I was struck by how people struggled with the physical loss of the person who had died even though cognitively they knew that they had died. Their extreme isolation and loneliness consumed them as they longed for the person to return. The hope was so strong that they would look out for them at certain times of the day. One man kept the teacup with a tea bag in it just where his wife had put it when she left the house on the morning she died. It stayed there for over a year. This fits with Melzack's theory postulated about grief in the previous section.

People would ask 'When will these strong feelings go?', so that they could lead a more normal life. I learned that this change occurred when there was an emotional acceptance that they would not physically return but recognised an internal relationship. I would tell them that although their physical relationship was lost they would come to know that they kept the person safe inside their hearts and that now they could never lose them. When I read about the work of Klass & Silverman (1996) on continuing bonds, I realised that I had come to the same conclusion – that was a Eureka moment for me. Abraham described this more succinctly in 1924 when he wrote: 'The loved one is not gone for now I carry it within myself and can never lose it' (p 437).

REFLECTION POINT

Your knowledge of theories:

- Are there any theories that link into your practice?
- Can you remember any Eureka moments?

SKILLS AND INTERVENTIONS

Ideally when a family is referred nurses will have a number of weeks or months to get to know the whole family and build a working relationship that is based on trust, liking, respect, a sense of common commitment, equality and mutual understanding (Horvath & Greenberg 1994). There is an opportunity for open honest discussion where fears and concerns are shared and choices made that include compromise and acceptance. In reality this is often not possible because there has not been time to get to know the family well and nurses need to work quickly, maximising any opportunities by being proactive and flexible.

Nursing is a practical profession which requires problem-solving skills to relieve emotional and physical discomfort. Relieving the physical discomfort in a practical way is often a more predictable process than attending to the emotional discomfort, which can be uncertain and less straightforward.

Although there are many skills, interventions and theoretical approaches for working with people to help relieve psychological distress, research suggests that it is the quality of the relationship between the helper and family that is the most healing aspect of the work (Gelso & Carter 1994). This is often referred to as the therapeutic relationship. Nurses have an ideal opportunity to build that relationship while attending to the practical needs of the patient, ensuring that their emotional needs are met.

Carl Rogers (1967) identified characteristics in a helping relationship that he said were necessary to form a healing relationship. These characteristics have been developed and are known as the Core Conditions that need to be conveyed by the helper; they are accepted as the basis for most positive therapeutic and helping relationships (Mearns & Thorne 1988). A distinction is made between effective caring support and becoming overwhelmed by the emotions. Families who are experiencing loss usually feel very sad, and nurses are often moved by this sadness. While being close to the family and sharing their feelings, it is also important to remain separate so that we keep strong enough to support and help. Boyle & Carter (1998, p 39) stated that the 'delivery of effective and efficient palliative care requires the nurse to have close personal contact with the dying patient and his family, thus encouraging open awareness of the patient's impending death'. Farley (2005) suggested that a possible paradox may arise between the nurse's wish for a close relationship and the possible risk of emotional turmoil. The nurse struggles with the emotional demands of the developing relationship and the ultimate realisation that the patient will die. This requires self-awareness and self-care, which can be facilitated by supervision.

Conditions that form the core of the relationship

Empathic understanding is the ability to imagine that you are the other person and therefore can see the situation from their point of view. It is different from imagining that you are in the situation yourself, as you then become lost in your own story and start to think about how you would feel. As mentioned earlier in the Kafka analogy, we can never fully understand what it is like to be someone else or know just how they are feeling, but if we take time really to listen then we may begin to understand something of what it is like for them. Rogers (1967, p 34) described a helpful relationship being characterised by 'A deep empathic understanding which enables me to see his private world through his eyes'.

Not judging, but accepting people with respect and equality, is another aspect of a healing relationship. It is all too easy to compare people's lifestyles, values and beliefs with our own and believe that our way is best. Accepting that people have different ways of managing their lives and that these choices have been made in response to the challenges and variety of their experiences goes some way to recognising their individuality. Valuing and celebrating differences are important attributes as well as trusting in people's strengths and personal resources, even when they seem lost and vulnerable.

Being genuine and honest with others and ourselves is a challenge, and we may be tempted to hide behind a 'professional facade'. In sharing our thoughts and feelings we become vulnerable but demonstrate that we are real people with genuine concerns. While maintaining professionalism we have also allowed the family to know our human side, so we are not the 'perfect professional' in a position of power but an equal human being. If families see us being open, honest and congruent they are more likely to share feelings that are difficult and painful for them. Nurses often debate the appropriateness of sharing their sadness and tears when a patient has died. Frequently families are moved by the genuine sense of caring that the nurse has demonstrated. They view this as a special aspect of the care which they treasure.

Counselling skills

These skills can be used by any helper to increase emotional contact in a supportive relationship. Using the skills does not amount to counselling, although they may also be used as part of a counselling relationship. Like any other skill, they need to be practised and there are many effective counselling skills courses that offer the opportunity to develop competence.

REFLECTION POINT

In your work with families:

* Which skills have you identified as helpful when offering emotional support?
* When you confide in someone else, what have they done that has enabled you to talk about something important and difficult?

You may have realised that you are a good listener and that sometimes people just want to talk to you. You probably notice that you say very little but give non-verbal clues that you are interested by nodding and encouraging them to talk. The following are examples of other skills that you may already use or could try.

Minimal encouragers

Making time to listen and offer privacy allows people the opportunity to talk. If we are aware of our body language, we might make some adjustments to appear even more open and available, such as sitting in a relaxed position and maintaining good eye contact. Tone of voice and facial expression often reinforce or belie what you are really thinking and feeling. Sometimes people are desperate to talk and may choose a difficult or inappropriate time when you are not able to give them full attention. Acknowledge the importance of their need and arrange a time when you can talk together. For example:

> 'I can see that what you have just told me is really important, I understand how worried you are about it and we need more time to talk about this. At the moment it is not possible for me to stay but when I come again this evening let's spend some time talking about this.'

Paraphrasing

This is the skill of repeating back to the person what they have just said. It may seem a little strange at first because we don't do this in normal conversation, but the effect is that the person you are supporting knows that you have been listening and that you have understood exactly what they are saying. For example:

Patient: I am finding it difficult to make decisions and my daughter keeps asking questions. She wants to know if she can go on a school trip in 6 weeks' time but I can only think of one day at a time.

Nurse: You sound as though you are having real difficulty in deciding what to do, especially with your daughter. You are finding it difficult to think about the future.

This response may encourage the person to go on and tell you more about their fears for the future. You will then understand more about how they are feeling; for them, the knowledge that someone really understands can be very healing.

Clarifying

Sometimes people want to tell you a lot of complicated information all at once or you may not be very sure if you have understood. Try to get them to stop for a moment so that you can check:

Nurse: Just stop for a moment because I'm not sure if I have got this right. You are worried about your daughter going on her school trip but your other daughter is away on holiday at the moment with your sister. Your mother has been helping you with your son but she has got to go into hospital next week. Is that right?

Reflecting feelings

The use of this skill demonstrates empathic understanding; the person feels less isolated because they know that you are trying to understand how they feel. When listening to the person, try to identify the feelings that are being expressed. These may be evident by their facial expressions, tone of voice or what they are saying:

Patient: Yes, everything is getting on top of me at the moment. Everyone is going away and I feel as though I'm being left to get on with it.

Nurse: You sound as though you're feeling very alone and abandoned at a time when you need your family around you.

Open questions

If we want to find out more, using questions can be a useful way of learning about the practical problem (e.g. the physical pain). As nurses, we often need to collect specific information: How long have you had this pain? Where is the pain? When did you last have any pain relief? These are closed questions because they require specific answers – 2 hours ... in my leg ... 3 hours ago. However, if the pain is emotional it may be more helpful to ask:

- 'Can you say what this pain is like at the moment, for you?'

This does not require the person to give a specific answer, but gives them the freedom to tell you what they want to. Other open questions could be:

- 'What was that like?'
- 'How do you feel now?'
- 'Can you say more about that?'
- 'How are things going?'
- 'What is the most difficult part for you right now?'

Using open questions gives the person the opportunity to talk about things you may not know about. Sometimes they may not have shared these with anyone else as they may not be fully aware of them themselves.

CARING FOR FAMILIES WHEN THE DEATH IS CLOSE

Armed with this knowledge and these skills we can feel more confident in facing families when they are at their most vulnerable and in need of support. As the patient's condition deteriorates, the family usually find this the most stressful time as they anticipate the worst possible outcome. There is fear and uncertainty about what the death will be like and how they will cope. Families need sensitive support which allows them the opportunity to take an active role in the care of the patient while offering help and guidance with the parts that they are struggling with.

Buckman (1988) offers some general guidelines:

1. See where you fit in
2. Expect variability
3. Expect repetition
4. Follow the patient's agenda, not your own
5. Do not equate activity with support
6. Become informed but don't become a world expert.

Nurses can pick up clues about how the family normally functions. Are they an open expressive family that shares feelings freely? Are they a family that normally experience a lot of conflict, and is this the normal way to function? Are they a close-knit family with a strong support system within the family?

Openness versus denial

One of the most difficult issues to confront is whether each family member knows that the patient is dying and how near the death is likely to be.

REFLECTION POINT

Families that have not accepted that a member of their family is dying and have denied their feelings:

- Did their feelings and behaviours change over time?

If families can be open about the reality of the death then focusing on the future can be a positive experience. They may be able to work together to make a memory box with children and other family members, organise photos and mementos, write down special recipes for a husband, make a will, plan the funeral and organise financial affairs. This will depend on how much energy the patient has, because there comes a point when the illness consumes all their energy and they start to withdraw emotionally.

The more difficult situation arises when some family members are denying the situation and do not want to talk about the death or the future. Family members try to protect one another, especially children or those with learning disabilities, as they do not want to upset them; they make excuses about them being unable to understand or cope, or that they need to get on with their lives.

Nurses have the opportunity to gently challenge this by approaching the subject:

- 'Have you had any thoughts about the future?'
- 'What do you imagine the children/other family members/patient are thinking?'
- 'Your wife/husband looks very weak now. Do you think the children have noticed this change?'
- 'Suppose we think for a moment about the worst that could happen, then we can think about the best outcome for you.'

Even if the immediate response is denial, given time the person may think about the question later and reflect on what has been said. This can lead to a change in behaviour.

Conflict and collusion

Sometimes families experience a lot of conflict when past unresolved issues surface at a time of stress. It can be particularly difficult for nurses to know how to respond when family members want different things, and nurses can be caught up in collusions with other members. Staying neutral and not being drawn towards one part of the family reduces the likelihood of members of the family feeling hostile. Being open and clear about professional loyalties and having awareness of the limits of the relationship so that all family members understand the nurses' position decreases the likelihood of being drawn into collusions.

> ### REFLECTION POINT
>
> Families you have known where there has been a lot of conflict:
>
> - How did this conflict affect you?
> - What strategies did you use to manage the situation?

A family's anger can sometimes be directed at nurses and it is important not to take this anger personally. Although it can be upsetting, it is sometimes better for the professional to bear the brunt of this misdirected anger instead of the family. However, there are limits to this in terms of physical safety, and the support of colleagues and clinical supervision is invaluable.

Religion and culture

This may be the time to check on any important religious or cultural needs that the family has and how

any arrangements can be effected. Communicating this important information to others in the caring team will ensure continuity of the spiritual care which may be very precious to the family.

In our multicultural society people have different faiths, and the rituals that are associated with dying are all very diverse. Even within one culture or religion there will be differences and it is therefore important to check with the family and close friends what is important to them and what they will need.

> ### REFLECTION POINT
>
> The different ethnic backgrounds, cultures and religious beliefs that are important in your area:
>
> - Have you encountered any particular difficulties in meeting these families' needs?
> - Where do you get information from, and with whom could you discuss these differences?

CHANGING CONSCIOUSNESS

As the death draws close there may be a decision to increase the sedation and analgesia. This often results in a changing of consciousness and the family need to be gently warned that communication could be difficult after this and given an opportunity to say anything that they feel is unsaid. Nurses can be proactive in suggesting that it may also be an opportunity for members of the family to come and say something special – remembering a treasured memory or time together, a thank you, telling the person how much they love them. These are all ways of saying goodbye.

Sometimes, even though the death is expected it happens suddenly before the family have time to gather round or say what they need to. If this is the case there may need to be a period of time to adjust to this, and the family could be encouraged to spend time together with the body and talk about the things that they would have told the deceased person. This opportunity provides part of the ending and reduces the likelihood of regrets and unfinished business during the bereavement; see Case Study 9.3.

AT THE TIME OF DEATH

To make choices about whether they want to be present at the death, family members need information about what it will be like. They may prefer to be

> **Case Study 9.3   Example of supporting families with an ending**
>
> When his mother was dying, her 18-year-old son Mark felt that he had not said all that he wanted to say to her. She had lapsed into unconsciousness after the insertion of a syringe driver giving her analgesics. He had withdrawn into his bedroom, but on questioning admitted that he was particularly upset because he felt that his two elder sisters had been more able in expressing themselves. He was encouraged to go and sit with his mother quietly on his own, and reassured that hearing was the last sense to go so that she would be able to hear what he said. After 15 minutes he left his mother's bedside, visibly relaxed and reassured that he had been able to communicate with her and said what he needed to.

> **Box 9.1   Example of using objects to bring comfort**
>
> A family friend discussed with two young daughters what they might do with their mother's fleecy dressing gown after she had died. They decided that it could be made into two cushions, which they could keep and cuddle. The dressing gown smelt of their mother. It brought back vivid memories of cuddling up to her, and made them feel close to her.

on their own, knowing that the nurse is close at hand, or feel supported by having a nurse present. As nurses we can try to encourage people to take their time and not feel rushed in any way. Time to sit with the body and cope emotionally with the enormity of the event allows the family to feel some control. Even if at first they make some hurried decisions, by being calm and reflective the nurses can slow the process down. If the close family member is alone then identifying who could be told next and who could give support can be the stepping stone to the nurse withdrawing.

THE FIRST FEW DAYS

During the first few days after the death there are usually a lot of practical things to do. This is often a focus and helps the bereaved family cope with their emotions as they feel that they are doing something for the deceased person. Knowing what to expect, for example what will happen when they collect the death certificate and personal belongings, reduces the shock of the death as they are faced with practical realities.

> **REFLECTION POINT**
>
> How different family members have reacted after the death of someone close:
>
> • Did you notice any gender differences?

BEREAVEMENT

After the funeral there is often a sudden drop in activity as family and close friends return to work; the intense activity that has been a part of the last few weeks of life has disappeared. There will still be practical tasks to do, such as sorting out financial affairs, the will, and dealing with possessions. Sometimes people feel that they should get all of this done quickly, and there may be pressure on them from family and friends to get on with these tasks. We can help the family slow down by suggesting that there is no rush and that they should take their time, making important decisions when they feel ready (Munroe 1998). Occasionally one family member feels it is their responsibility to deal with possessions and that other people would find it too upsetting or too much trouble. It may be gently suggested that other family members and friends may like to be included in decisions. Going through possessions usually brings back memories; taking time to talk through these memories will be sad and upsetting but also an opportunity to experience a positive and healthy part of grieving. Encouraging families to take time to think about using possessions to bring comfort can enhance the healing process (Box 9.1).

IDENTIFYING PEOPLE WHO ARE AT RISK AND MAY NEED EXTRA HELP WITH THEIR GRIEF

Most people who experience a significant bereavement cope with the support of their family and within their social network. Inadequate social support is the best predictor of a poor outcome in the bereaved. It is estimated that about 10–20% of bereaved people will need extra support from an outside source (UK Bereavement Care Standards Project 2001), but sometimes good but brief support by the palliative care team can prevent a lot of emotional suffering and reduce the likelihood of later problems. A review of the research that identifies factors associated with a poor outcome after the death of someone close is given in Box 9.2 (Payne et al 1999).

These factors can increase our awareness of families' possible needs. The palliative care team has an opportunity to identify these factors and follow up the death with an offer of extra support. Many hospices have bereavement services that provide bereavement support, counselling or psychology sessions in either individual or group settings. If there are any concerns then alerting the GP can ensure that a follow-up is made. There are also a number of voluntary organisations (e.g. Cruse) that offer bereavement support, and making contact with a local branch and finding out what they offer will identify resources if they are needed later on.

Some palliative care teams use assessment tools to identify those in need of extra help during bereavement. Others offer support to everyone in the belief that those who need it will take up the offer of support, whereas those who do not will refuse the service. The group most at risk may come from the community where a late referral diminishes the opportunity of

effective emotional support before the death. Awareness of those most at risk may best be assessed by the GP or practice nurse over a period of time, for it may be several months after the death that the family find themselves struggling with their grief.

Sometimes people are confused and frightened by their thoughts and feelings, and need to be reassured that what they are experiencing is normal (Case Study 9.4).

The example in Case Study 9.4 was very straightforward, but if the woman had not attended for the session there may have been some serious consequences of believing that she was abnormal. It is unlikely that she would have been identified as in need of support as she had a good social network and there were no known 'risk factors'.

Long-term grief support

There are those who need support with their grief and if they are not able to access it then the repercussions can have lasting effects on them and the family (Case Study 9.5).

Case Study 9.5 provides an extreme and difficult example of how grief can exacerbate existing problems and lead to family breakdown. Even though the GP was aware of the risk early on, it was only when Jackie had reached crisis point that she could accept help. Many professionals had been involved in caring

---

Box 9.2   Factors associated with a poor outcome (Payne et al 1999)

- *Age* – older widow(er)s suffer more distressing symptoms and younger people experience more health problems
- *Relationship with the deceased* – loss of a spouse, loss of an adult child or sibling, or bereavement in childhood
- *Nature of relationship* – ambivalence or dependence in the relationship and an unacknowledged or secret relationship
- *Personality* – people with low self-esteem, anxiety, extreme self-reliance, denial of emotion and clinging personality
- *Pre-existing health* – poor pre-existing physical or mental health
- *Circumstances of the death* – violent, unexpected, untimely deaths, stigmatized or long protracted illness
- *Initial grief reactions* – extreme distress initially and poor social functioning
- *Concurrent crisis* – people facing other losses and crisis in their lives; also low income and socioeconomic status

---

Case Study 9.4   Example of the need for reassurance

A woman was referred for counselling by her GP after the death of her husband from lung cancer. When she came to the first session she was agitated and told me that there was something of which she was very ashamed and that she could not talk about. During the session she began to relax, and towards the end found the courage to tell me about the thing of which she was so ashamed. She said that when she got into bed at night she reached out for her husband and talked to him. She felt that this was wrong and that she must be 'going out of my mind'. I reassured her that I thought that what she was doing was quite normal and that she must have loved him very much and missed him a great deal. When she heard that it was quite normal and healthy to talk to a deceased person, she smiled with a look of relief and we agreed that she did not need any further counselling. I suggested a book that she could read about grief which might reassure her of her normal feelings.

Case Study 9.5   Example of complicated grief

Jackie's husband died suddenly from a brain tumour leaving her with four children aged under 10 years. Although healthcare workers were alerted to her need for support, she refused offers of professional help. Four years later she had become drug and alcohol dependent and her children were in local authority care. At this point Jackie asked for some counselling to help her with her unresolved grief, her drug and alcohol dependency, and to help her get the children back.

Our weekly sessions were spasmodic; Jackie would often disappear for a few months, occasionally being admitted to hospital for drug overdoses. When she attended the session she was often vague and confused, so it was difficult to communicate with her. This pattern continued for 18 months, but with our occasional sessions I learnt more about her and slowly she began to trust me.

At first she said that the relationship with her deceased husband had been wonderful and they had shared everything together. He had protected her and he 'thought the world of her', and she could not accept life without him.

It took nearly 2 years for Jackie to trust me enough to allow herself to face the sad and terrible truth about the life that she had lived. After her marriage her husband had drunk heavily, had relationships with other women and had physically abused her. She was too frightened and ashamed to admit this to anyone as she felt it was what she deserved. The excessive use of drugs and alcohol were a way of numbing the pain.

Jackie had strong beliefs about herself – that she was worthless and deserved all the abuse that she got. I worked with her, reflecting back my thoughts and feelings, and challenging the negative beliefs she had about herself.

Gradually Jackie allowed me to see her vulnerability and I got to know the real Jackie. I understood how she had been rendered powerless by abuse, but slowly she found the resources and energy to change her life. I admired her strength, courage and determination to get her children back. She loved them very much and had a great sense of fun and love of life. She attended a drug dependency unit programme and stopped the drugs and alcohol. This improved the contact that I had with her, and her integrity and commitment became apparent.

Her children came out of care and returned home, giving her new joy and purpose to her life, but life was not always easy. We talked about how she could support the children with their loss and she learned new skills to build a better relationship with them.

for her but she needed enormous amounts of patience, time and empathy. This highlights the importance of building a trusting relationship in order that the client can feel safe enough to disclose intimate details.

CONCLUSION

Supporting families with grief is challenging but can improve people's quality of life and prevent complications of grief if those who may need extra help are identified and offered the appropriate support. Case Study 9.5 demonstrates that support needs to be available for a long time after the death, that specialist help may be required.

Nurses can help the bereaved more effectively if they are able to establish effective therapeutic relationships. These relationships require a range of attitudes and knowledge, including being non-judgemental, empathic and congruent. In addition, competence in the basic counselling skills gives a sound foundation for working with families and increasing confidence in the helper. These skills include listening, reflecting feelings, paraphrasing and clarifying; they need to be learnt and practised frequently.

There is a range of factors that influence how each person grieves and a sound theoretical knowledge will help to underpin the nurse's understanding of this. Whether individuals completely sever ties with their loved one or maintain a continuing bond depends on the nature of the attachment that existed prior to the death. Nurses need to accept and respect the individual's belief system and coping strategies, and respond sensitively and with flexibility.

A further requirement for nurses is self-awareness and an understanding of our own response to loss. Failure to do this can result in a lack of resolution and impede helping others. Making sure that we have good supervision and support ensures that we can keep some objectivity and a sense of balance in our work.

This is undoubtedly a challenging aspect of nursing that can impact on your personal resources. Therefore it is necessary to develop self-awareness and to harness support and guidance through supervision. However, despite these challenges, this area offers huge potential in palliative care delivery coupled with powerful personal learning experiences.

References

Abraham K 1924 Selected papers on psychoanalysts. Hogarth, London

Attig T 1991 The importance of conceiving of grief as an active process. Death Studies 15:385–393

Bereavement Care Standards Project 2001 Standards for bereavement care in the UK. Online. Available: http://www.bereavement.org.uk/ 1 Feb 2006

Bowlby J 1991 Attachment and loss.Vol. 3: Loss, sadness and depression. Penguin Books, London

Boyle M, Carter DE 1998 Death anxiety amongst nurses. International Journal of Palliative Medicine 4(1):37–43

Brown J 2006 Young people and bereavement counselling. What influences their decision to access professional help? Bereavement Care 25(1):3–6

Buckman R 1988 I don't know what to say. Papermac, London

Christ G 2000 Healing children's grief. Oxford University Press, Oxford

Corr C A 2003 Bereavement, grief, and mourning in death-related literature for children. Omega: Journal of Death and Dying 48:337–363

Farley G 2005 Death anxiety and death education. A brief analysis of the key issues. In: Foyle L and Hostad J (eds) Dimensions in cancer and palliative care education. Delivering cancer and palliative care education, p 73–84

Freud S 1917 Mourning and melancholia. Collected Papers, Vol. 4. Basic Books, New York

Gelso C, Carter J 1994 Components of the psychotherapy relationship: their interaction and unfolding during treatment. Journal of Counselling Psychology 41(3):296–306

Horvath A, Greenberg L 1994 The working alliance: theory, research and practice. Wiley, London

Klass D, Silverman P R 1996 Introduction: what's the problem? In: Klass D, Silverman P R, Nickman S L (eds) 1996 Continuing bonds: new understandings of grief. Taylor & Francis, Washington, DC, p 3–23

Kubler-Ross E 1969 On death and dying. Macmillan, New York

Lazarus R S, Folkman S 1984 Stress, appraisal and coping. Springer, New York

Lindemann E 1944 Symptomology and management of acute grief. American Journal of Psychiatry 101:141–148

Mearns D, Thorne B 1988 Person-centred counselling in action. Sage, London

Melzack R 1993 Pain: past, present and future. Canadian Journal of Experimental Psychology 47(4):615–629

Melzack R, Wall P D 1996 The challenge of pain, 2nd edn. Penguin Books, London

Munroe B 1998 Bereavement care. In: Oliviere D, Hargreaves R, Munroe B. Good practices in palliative care: a psychosocial approach. Ashgate, Aldershot, p 133

Papadatou D 2000 A proposed model of health professionals' grieving process. Omega: Journal of Death and Dying 41(1):59–77

Parkes C M 1972 Bereavement: studies of grief in adult life. Penguin, Harmondsworth

Parkes C M 1986 Bereavement: studies of grief in adult life, 2nd edn. Routledge, London

Payne S, Horn S, Relf M 1999 Loss and bereavement. Open University Press, Buckingham

Reimers E 2001 Bereavement: a social phenomenon? European Journal of Palliative Care 8:242–244

Rogers C 1967 On becoming a person. Constable, London

Rosenblatt PC 1993 Grief: the social context of private feelings. In: Stroebe M, Stroebe W, Hansson R (eds) Handbook of Bereavement. Theory, research and intervention. Cambridge University Press, Cambridge.

Small N 2001 Theories of grief: a critical review. In: Hockey J, Katz J, Small N (eds) Grief, mourning and death ritual. Open University Press, Buckingham, p 19–48

Stroebe M S, Schut H 1996 A model for coping with grief and its practical applications for the bereavement counsellor. Paper presented to the third St George's 'Dying, Death and Bereavement' conference, St George's Hospital Medical School, London, 6 March 1996

Stroebe M, Stroebe W, Hansson R 1992 Handbook of bereavement: theory, research and intervention. Cambridge University Press, Cambridge

Stroebe M S, Schut H, Stroebe W 2005 Attachment in coping with bereavement: a theoretical integration. Review of General Psychology 9(1):48–66

Valentine C 2006 Academic constructions of bereavement. Mortality 11(1):57–78

Walter T 1999 On bereavement: the culture of grief. Open University Press, Buckingham

Worden J W 1982 Grief counselling and grief therapy. Springer, New York

Further reading

Cruse Bereavement Care. Bereavement Care Journal. For information email: info@cruse.org.uk

de Board R 1998 Counselling for toads: a psychological adventure. Routledge, London

Marie Curie Cancer Care, Children and Young Peoples Support Service. Five booklets for families with children and young people: Talking to children when someone close is very ill; Teenage grief – things you might want to know; Helping children when someone dies; Questions children may want to ask when someone close to them has died; Books and cassettes for children, teenagers and adults about bereavement. Online. Available: http://www.mariecurie.org.uk/aboutus/helpandinformation/advice_for_families/children_and_young_peoples_support_service.htm

Mearns D, Thorne B 1999 Person-centred counselling in action, 2nd edn. Sage Publications, London

Oliviere D, Hargreaves R, Munroe B 1998 Bereavement care. In: Good practices in palliative care. Ashgate, Aldershot, Ch. 6, p 121–143

Useful websites and organisations

Bereavement Research Forum, Sir Michael Sobell House, Churchhill Hospital, Oxford, OX3 7LJ. Tel: 0186 522 5878

Childhood Bereavement Network, 8 Wakley Street, London EC1V 7QE. An umbrella organisation for bereaved children. Tel: 0207 843 6309. Website: www.childhoodbereavementnetwork.org.uk

Cruse Bereavement Care, Cruse House, 126 Sheen Road, Richmond TW9 1UR. Website: http://www.cruse.org.uk

Missyou. A memorial website for bereaved people. Website: http://www.missyou.org.uk

RD4U. Website for bereaved young people run by young people: http://www.rd4u.org.uk

riprap. Information for young people affected by cancer. Website: http://www.riprap.org.uk

Winston's Wish. Help for grieving children and their families. Website: http://www.winstonswish.org.uk

Chapter **10**

Evidence–based palliative care

Shaun Kinghorn, Kevin Donaghy and Jacqueline Howard

EVIDENCE-BASED PRACTICE IN CONTEXT

Developing palliative care based on the best available evidence has become an essential component of care delivery, commissioning and service design. The publication in 2004 of the National Institute for Clinical Excellence (NICE) guidelines 'Improving supportive and palliative care for adults with cancer' is an affirmation that evidence-based palliative care is here to stay. Bosanquet & Salisbury (1999) insightfully suggested that in the future there would be greater expectations for evidence-based care in a world of escalating care costs. The ethos of obtaining evidence to assure the healthcare community and the public that what we are delivering is effective is starting to surface in the provision of specialist palliative care (Hearn & Higginson 1998). The rise of evidence-based care has been dramatic within some specialties, whereas in others its development is patchy.

Palliative care embraces a person-centred approach that focuses on physical, psychosocial and spiritual care in progressive disease (Higginson 1999). Developing evidence-based practice within palliative care is not without its problems, such as the ethical and moral issues associated with involving patients at the end of life with a poor prognosis in research (Wilkinson 1998). Despite these difficulties, evidence-based guidelines have been developed to guide staff in the care of people who are dying, including guidelines for symptom control, psychosocial support and bereavement care (Ellershaw et al 2003). Some palliative care groups have rapidly adopted best evidence, whereas others have expressed concern that some of these interventions could blur the boundaries of palliative care. Many debates have arisen due to the lack of solid evidence on the role of different palliative interventions.

Practitioners engaged in the delivery of palliative care need to be familiar with the process of *finding the best evidence* and of *analysing the strengths and weaknesses of available evidence* and to have an understanding of *how you can put best evidence into practice*. It is these three phrases that epitomise evidence-based practice, and they are also used to frame this chapter. We do not aspire in this chapter to provide a resumé of best evidence. It is acknowledged that the reader will be exposed to a wide range of evidence in other chapters. The key emphasis is to enable the reader to develop an understanding of these three processes. It is suggested that, armed with the skills and knowledge to find, analyse and consider how the evidence can be integrated into clinical practice, the reader will be empowered and enabled to understand the nature of evidence-based practice more fully.

Therefore, the aims of this chapter are to enable the reader to:

- understand the nature of evidence-based practice
- appreciate the steps involved in obtaining various types of evidence
- develop an understanding of how they can discern the quality of a variety of types of evidence
- reflect upon strategies to ensure that best evidence becomes an integral feature of clinical practice.

It is acknowledged that this is very much an introduction to evidence-based practice, with entire texts devoted to the subject. The resources and principles contained in the chapter will enable the reader to develop an insight into the key issues and processes that need to be considered in ensuring that palliative care moves towards being an evidence-based discipline. A comprehensive range of supportive websites will provide added value to the issues covered in the chapter.

WHAT IS EVIDENCE-BASED PRACTICE AND WHY HAS IT EMERGED?

A variety of definitions have been presented to clarify the essential features of evidence-based care. These definitions appear to place differing emphases in specific elements. In one of the earlier definitions, the Department of Health (1996) defined evidence-based practice as:

> The extent to which specific clinical interventions, when deployed in the field for particular patients or population do what they intend. That is, maintain or improve health and secure the greatest possible health gain from the resources available.

You will note that the use of the term *health gain* is emphasised. The term 'health gain' within the context of cancer and palliative care is problematic as relief of symptoms and adaptation to the physical/psychosocial impact of the disease and support of the family are the aims of care rather than health gain. In a later definition Hamer & Collinson (1999) placed emphasis on the process of evidence-based practice by describing it thus:

> Evidence-based practice is finding, appraising, and applying scientific evidence to the treatment and management of healthcare.

This definition assumes that the practitioner may come from any one of a variety of disciplines and possesses the skills to find, appraise and apply evidence into everyday practice.

In what is seen as one of the most credible definitions, Sackett et al (1996, p 71) placed emphasis on a systematic approach to evidence-based practice by defining evidence-based medicine as:

> . . . the conscientious, explicit and judicious use of current best evidence in making decisions about the care of individual patients, based on skills which allow the doctors to evaluate both personal experience and external evidence in an objective and systematic manner.

Bradshaw (2000) suggested that evidence-based practice has three key characteristics:

1. It is linked to extracting information from the internet, databases and library links that provide details of current relevant research.
2. It places emphasis on practitioners reading research with a view to critical analysis of both qualitative and quantitative research.
3. It aims to bridge the gap between theory and practice by applying the findings of research to individual patients or groups of patients.

A common theme arising from all definitions is the fundamental need to find the evidence, critically review the evidence, and finally ensure that the best evidence becomes a feature of clinical practice. Trinder & Reynolds (2000) suggested that evidence-based practice is a product of our time that has emerged in part because we are increasingly living in a risk society. They suggest four factors that have led to the emergence of evidence-based practice:

1. *Research–practice gap* – because of the limited extent to which practitioners draw from research findings to base their practice.

2. *Poor quality of much research* – it is argued that a proportion of research is poorly designed and is not based on the 'gold standard' approach of a well conducted randomised controlled trial.
3. *Information overload* – the global output of research is difficult to keep up with. Practitioners may also not be able to distinguish between rigorous and poorly designed research.
4. *Practice that is not evidence-based* – the consequences of factors 1–3 are that practitioners may deliver care that may be ineffective or harmful, and may not be aware of interventions that are proven to be more effective. This situation clearly encourages variations of quality in practice.

Insisting that care should be based on best evidence can bring problems as well as benefits. Boyd & Deighan (1996) highlighted a selection of the benefits and problems of utilising an evidence-based approach, as described below.

The benefits of an evidence-based approach

- Could lead to redirection of resources towards more effective treatments
- Can ensure cost and clinical effectiveness of treatment/healthcare
- May help providers to make better use of limited resources and overcome rationing
- Provides a basis for clinical decisions in clinical practice
- May improve continuity and uniformity of care through common approaches and guidelines
- Can invalidate outdated tests and treatments
- Provides a common language for multiprofessional healthcare.

Some of the problems associated with the evidence–based approach

- Tends to be understood as evidence-based medicine, rather than as a multiprofessional approach
- Can deny the place of values other than efficiency and effectiveness (e.g. ethics, caring)
- Limited tools or suitable methods to evaluate use of evidence in clinical and managerial decision-making
- Will not necessarily reduce costs – the most effective treatment may not be the cheapest
- For full implementation, use of evidence will have to be incorporated into policy decisions
- May erode role of patient choice or patient preference. Does not necessarily tell you what will be best for an individual patient

- Those who develop guidelines and protocols might possibly be held legally responsible for their impact on health
- It is difficult to keep pace with the evidence that is produced
- Patients rarely present with a single one-dimensional problem

In essence, the central tenet of evidence-based practice is a care system where reasoning and clinical decision-making is based on the 'gold standard' evidence derived from best evidence emerging from randomised controlled trials (RCTs). Developing an evidence base derived from the RCT is problematic within palliative care, as informed consent, ethical issues, attrition from studies, and obtaining adequate sample sizes have been cited as difficulties within a palliative care context. Barker (2000) provides a sobering reminder that in this era of evidence-based practice the power of 'caring' should not be lost.

TYPES OF EVIDENCE ON WHICH WE BASE OUR PRACTICE

In delivering palliative care there are many sources of knowledge that provide the base upon which we practise and make decisions about the best course of action. Table 10.1 highlights these various types of evidence and their strengths and weaknesses.

SEARCHING FOR THE EVIDENCE

Searching for evidence can be time consuming and frustrating, but nevertheless an essential part of evidence-based practice. Without searching for the best current evidence how can practitioners ensure they are making the right decisions that will benefit patient care (Hatcher et al 2005).

Performing a literature search involves a number of different stages, all of which are necessary. Box 10.1 highlights the different stages involved once you have identified your question.

Box 10.1   Stages involved in a literature search

1. Identify and choose resources to be accessed.
2. Identify keywords that can be used to search electronic resources.
3. Undertake the actual search.
4. Obtain the full text of short-listed references.

Table 10.1   Source of evidence on which care can be based

Source	Strength of source	Weakness of source
Literature review	Can summarise current research and other types of evidence	Can be diffuse and non-committal, unless reviewer has a specific aim for the search
Expert opinion	May summarise succinctly much knowledge and experience	May not be based on much knowledge and experience, and may be intuitively based. What are the criteria for being classed as an expert?
Systematic review	Collates in a systematic manner current and past research relating to a specific healthcare intervention	Sometimes difficult to implement the findings of systematic reviews in complex patient scenarios
Randomised controlled trial	Objective, quantitative results (assuming methodology is sound)	May provide evidence for only one or a small number of aspects of a complex scenario
Critical incident review	Can provide rich, detailed, qualitative information	Refers only to a particular instance (or instances); may be difficult to disseminate to a wider audience
Audit of practice in own clinical area	Encourages scrutiny of own practice in a way that accommodates unique practice circumstances	Ascertains value of care intervention only at local level; results often not shared widely and may not be applicable to a wider audience
Clinical guidelines	If based on best evidence can make a real difference in encouraging consistency in practice. If designed well they often give clear guidance on how best available can be delivered	May be based on local opinion with little or no evidence to base practice

Table 10.2   Skills required for internet searching (Fitzpatrick 2004)

Question	Answer
How can I improve my computer skills?	If you are not confident at using a computer, searching the internet or electronic resources, it may be beneficial to: • Enrol on an introductory IT course • Improve your internet search skills by completing one of the many free tutorials available on the Internet
What if I don't have access to a computer at home?	Find out whether you can access a computer at work or contact your local library to check availability.
How can I manage my time better so that I have the time to do a literature search?	Discuss your needs with your family or employer and negotiate time, where possible, to do your search at a time when you are less likely to be disturbed. Negotiate protected time to do your search, where possible.

Before you begin

Access to the internet has made finding the evidence much easier, but has introduced a new tier of skills that need to be developed in order to find the evidence. Table 10.2 provides answers to some common questions.

Common problems experienced with searching

There is a variety of common problems that may be experienced when searching for the literature. Table 10.3 displays answers to the most common questions.

Table 10.3   Common problems encountered when searching

Question	Answer
How do I ensure that I have enough time to complete a search?	Plan your search well in advance. Have dedicated dates and times to concentrate on doing your search where possible.
Where can I find out about information resources available?	Contact a healthcare librarian, who will be able to advise you.
How can I search databases and the internet more effectively?	Refer to the help screens or search tips available within the resource for guidance. Contact your librarian for advice and guidance with searching.
How can I reduce the number of records I retrieve when searching a database?	Review your search strategy. For example, use the focus function or narrow the date range you are using.
I have retrieved too few records using a particular database. How can I extend my search to retrieve additional records?	Depending on the topic chosen, there may simply not be many records in the database. If you think there should be more information available, review your search strategy. For example, have you chosen the most appropriate database(s) to search? Use the explode function or extend the date range you are using.
How can I ensure that books and photocopies of articles I order arrive by the required deadline?	Order photocopies of articles or order books well in advance and allow plenty of time for them to arrive. For example, a photocopy of an article ordered via your local library document delivery service may take up to 2 weeks to arrive from the ordering of the item to delivery if it can be delivered only in paper format. Your librarian or the organisation from which you order items will be able to advise you. Many organisations provide guidance on their websites.
How do I ensure that I record the bibliographical details of items properly?	Identify the system of referencing that is to be used and become familiar with it. Devise a method of recording bibliographical details of references that suits you, such as index cards or referencing software programs. Record bibliographical details of references as you come across them; this will save you time having to trace items.

Identifying and choosing resources

There is no single resource available that can be used to search all of the literature. Therefore, a number and variety of resources, including print and electronic resources, need to be accessed (Bird 2003). Resources available will differ from country to country and from organisation to organisation; they may be available at work, via a further education college or university, or freely available via the internet. The resources you use will depend on your search question, resources and time available. Table 10.4 provides general guidance and tips about different resources available.

Searching electronic databases

Electronic databases such as the Cumulative Index to Nursing and Allied Health Literature (CINAHL), Medline and PsychInfo can usually be searched in two different ways. Keyword searches, sometimes referred to as free searches, involve entering individual words and result in the retrieval of records containing the words entered. Databases can also usually be searched by subject heading, also known as thesaurus mapping. Each database may use different names for subject headings, the most commonly known one being MeSH (Medical Subject Headings), used in Medline.

Databases also use a number of operators, commonly known as boolean logic, to aid searching. These operators are instructions that help interrogate the database and retrieve the relevant records. Tables 10.5 and 10.6 give answers to questions about boolean logic and provide information about other operators commonly used to aid searching.

Searching the web

There are a number of different search engines available that can be used to find evidence on the web. Examples include Google (http://www.google.com), Alta Vista (http://www.altavista.com) and Yahoo (http://www.yahoo.com). Search engines index vast amounts of information available on the web. Some

Table 10.4   Guidance and tips about resources available

Resource	Tips
Internet	Use the internet to find and access many recommended evidence-based websites including guidelines. Search engines such as Google or Yahoo can be useful. If you do not find what you want using one search engine, try another.
Electronic databases	There are a number of databases available to help with the retrieval of evidence-based information, of which some are particularly relevant to cancer and palliative care. Although they may differ in coverage and target audience, databases may contain bibliographical details of journal articles, conference proceedings, books, dissertations, theses and other publications. Many also contain abstracts and references of item(s), and some may even contain links to the full text. Access to databases is usually via a personal or institutional subscription. Increasingly, pay-per-view services are being made available. Contact a local library to find out about databases available and your eligibility for access.
Journals	There is a wide range of journals available related to cancer and palliative care, with many available electronically as well as in print. The table of content pages of many journals is also freely available on the world wide web (WWW) and bibliographical details of many journals are also indexed on databases, although many are not. To overcome this problem and to ensure that you do not miss important information, it is beneficial to hand-search current journals. It will also be beneficial to contact your local library to identify what full-text electronic journals you may have access to.
Books and reports	May be available in electronic format as well as in print. Searching library catalogues such as the British Library catalogue at http://catalogue.bl.uk or your organisational library catalogue can help to identify books and reports available, as can searching both publishers' and organisational websites, which also have the added benefit that they quite often display details of forthcoming publications.
E-mail discussion lists	A number of email discussion lists that allow individual healthcare professionals to communicate with one another can be found at http://www.jiscmail.ac.uk/index.htm
Organisations	Organisations may have undertaken research that is kept in-house, the details of which will not be readily available on databases or the WWW. Contacting an organisation directly may lead to the identification of further information that you may find useful, but note that if you are not a member of the organisation a charge may be incurred for any information. It is also worth noting that some organisations often collate relevant information and provide useful links on the WWW.
Librarians	If you need assistance with your search contact a librarian in your clinical field for help (Pond 1999).

index more information than others so, if you do not retrieve what you are looking for using one search engine, it may beneficial to use more than one search engine. Similar to electronic databases, some search engines allow basic keyword searches, advanced searches, and the limiting of information by date and language, in addition to other options such as searching for pictures and video footage. There is much evidence-based information available on the web, but the volume of information retrieved by a search engine may be huge. In order to ensure that the information you retrieve is credible you will need to evaluate the websites. Check them against basic criteria such as:

- authorship
- publisher
- date of publication or date of last update
- bias
- referral to supporting literature

Further guidance for evaluating websites can be found on the Johns Hopkins University website at http://www.library.jhu.edu/researchhelp/general/evaluating/ or by doing a general internet search on the subject of evaluating websites.

Other points to consider

Whether searching the internet or databases, there are additional pointers that you should be aware of that can help you with the retrieval of evidence and save you time. These are summarised in Table 10.7.

Obtaining the full text of short-listed references

Once suitable references have been identified, the next step is to obtain the full text of the item(s). These may be:

Table 10.5   Use of common operators to aid searching

Question	Answer	Example
How do I combine terms?	Use the operator AND	Entering the terms terminal AND agitation will retrieve records containing both the words terminal and agitation.
If I enter two or more keywords, how can I retrieve records that contain any one of the terms I entered?	Use the operator OR	Entering the terms palliative OR terminal will retrieve records that contain either the word palliative or terminal or both.
How do I exclude records containing specified words?	Use the operator NOT	Entering the terms hospice NOT adult will first retrieve records containing the word hospice but then exclude the records that contain adult.

Table 10.6   Additional operators

Operator	What will this allow me to do?	Explanation
EXPLODE	This function allows you to explode the thesaurus term and its more specific headings.	If you choose to explode a thesaurus term, records with that term or the more specific associated term(s) will be retrieved. This helps to widen a search and retrieve more references.
FOCUS	This function allows you to limit the number of records retrieved.	If you choose one thesaurus term and select focus, records retrieved will be those for which the thesaurus term is the main focus of the record.
TRUNCATION	This function enables you to search for words with the same beginning but different endings. The sign for truncation is often the $ sign, but this may differ between resources.	Entering the term palliat$ will retrieve records containing palliative and palliation.
LIMITING	This option enables you to limit a search, thereby helping you to reduce the number of records retrieved.	Searches can usually be limited via year of publication, language, age range and type of publication.

Table 10.7   Additional pointers to help in the retrieval of evidence

Pointer	Tip
Spellings	Be aware of the differences in the spellings of the same word in different countries.
Synonyms	In relation to multidisciplinary record keeping, the keywords interdisciplinary, multiprofessional or interprofessional record keeping relate to the same topic but would produce very different results if used as individual keywords. This would also apply to technical jargon and drug names.
Singular and plural words	Entering the keyword tooth will result in a different number of records retrieved compared with using the keyword teeth. Therefore, you would need to search using both keywords.
Keywords that have different meanings	Entering the keyword AIDS (acquired immune deficiency syndrome) would retrieve irrelevant records relating to items such as hearing aids and walking aids in addition to acquired immune deficiency syndrome.

- in stock at a local library
- available on the world wide web
- available via a link to the full text from the electronic database to which you have access
- available via pay per view – an increasing amount of information is being made available electronically via this method, which involves pre-payment before the full text of the items can be accessed and viewed
- purchased from a bookshop or professional organisation
- purchased directly from organisations such as the British Library, which provides a document delivery service throughout the UK and internationally
- obtained via an interlibrary loan from your local library. Contact your librarian for further information.

It is important to remember that it can take time to obtain items, so allow plenty of time for their ordering and receipt. For example, you may have access to the full text of an article via a database at your place of work and so can easily print off the article. On the other hand, an item may be accessible via a local library but if it is out on loan you may have to wait a couple of weeks for it to be returned by the current borrower.

Recording bibliographical details

Referencing is simply a way of recording the bibliographical details of items used in your work. Throughout your search, record details of works as you use them. You could use a manual method such as writing bibliographical details on index cards and storing them in alphabetical order by author. If you are undertaking an electronic search, obtain a print-out of your references. There are also electronic referencing software products available such as Endnote or Reference Manager, which could be used. Further information about these products can normally be found on the web. There are several systems of referencing, such as the Vancouver, Harvard and British Standard systems. Whichever system is used, it is essential that you take the time to record the bibliographical details of all the item(s) that you have used as you may need to cite references in your works, at the end of a chapter or as part of a bibliography. If you do not record sufficient detail, you may have to spend additional valuable time backtracking to retrieve missing details. When recording bibliographic details there is some key information that should be included wherever possible such as author, title, year of publication, edition, page numbers, publisher, place of publication, ISBN or ISSN. Remember to include volume and issue numbers of journal issues and, if using the web, remember to record the website and the date you accessed it.

Remember copyright

Copyright legislation relates to the copying of items in print and other media without either the permission of the copyright holder or an appropriate licence. Copying items above the allowed limitations of a licence or without permission of the copyright holder is a serious matter that can lead to legal proceedings, fines and even imprisonment. Find out about copying limitations before you start copying to ensure that you do not breach the law. Further information and guidance can be obtained by contacting the appropriate copyright licensing agency.

Top tips for a successful literature search

- Brush up on your computer, internet and database search skills before you begin your search.
- Allow yourself plenty of time to do the search. Have dedicated dates and times, where possible, to do your search and avoid being disturbed.
- Make a list of the resources that are to be accessed and work through the list systematically.
- Refer to the help sections of electronic resources for guidance on how best to search the resource.
- Be prepared to review a search strategy if you are retrieving too much or too little information.
- Record the details of items as they are accessed.
- If you need to order the full text of items, allow plenty of time for the receipt.
- Do not forget about copyright limitations.
- If you need help at any stage during a search, ask a librarian for help.

Case Study 10.1 gives an example of search on best practice in palliative care undertaken by a nurse on an acute medical unit.

ANALYSING THE EVIDENCE

The second stage of evidence-based practice is analysing the evidence. This section discusses why we need to question what is published and highlights

Case Study 10.1   Searching for the evidence – an example

Jean is a 39-year-old registered nurse who currently works on a busy 30-bed acute medical unit that deals with a wide range of conditions. The team thus has to provide end of life ward care for patients with cardiac failure, lung cancer and diabetes. Jean qualified 20 years ago and has become increasingly interested in palliative care. She has identified that, as a unit, the staff are unsure about what constitutes best practice for managing terminal agitation/terminal restlessness and breathlessness.

• Where would Jean need to search for best evidence in this area? What sorts of skills and help might she need to find the best evidence to help guide staff to deliver the best care possible for those who are agitated in the terminal stage?

As part of her search, Jean could include the following databases, both of which are internationally renowned and contain bibliographical records specific and related to palliative care:

1. Cumulative Index to Nursing and Allied Health Literature – contains bibliographical records of more than 1200 publications from 1982 onwards, including records of healthcare journals and books, dissertations and conference proceedings.
2. Medline – the US National Library of Medicine database contains bibliographical records of 5000 journals from 1950 onwards.

Jean could also use other resources such as the internet, related organisations and other information sources (see Table 10.6).

Keywords that could be used to help interrogate the databases and the internet include: terminal agitation and terminal restlessness; breathlessness, breathless, dyspnoea and dyspnea.

To help retrieve records specific to her question, Jean could restrict her search to include: publication date, research articles, articles relating to adults, articles in English.

As an example, using the above terms and limits, the following number of records were retrieved during a search:

Database – CINAHL

Keyword search	No. of records retrieved
Terminal agitation or terminal restlessness	41
Breathless or breathlessness or dyspnoea or dyspnea	3270
Combined keyword searches	14
Limit to previous 5 years, research articles relating to adults and available in English	10

Database – Medline

Search by subject (using MeSH terms)	No. of records retrieved
Dyspnoea	2334
Terminal care/palliative care	50 966
Combined subject searches	106
Limit to previous 5 years, research articles relating to adults and available in English	63

the skills required to analyse evidence. This section also introduces frameworks that can be used to critique different types of evidence as well as providing resources to direct you to other supportive resources.

For many healthcare professionals, reading the professional literature, especially research, is daunting. It is tempting just to skim-read the title, abstract, introduction and results. For most, however, the methodology, results and discussion sections are pretty much unknown territory and considered to be for the attention of other researchers! Do these habits sound familiar and do you wish to understand the processes involved with appraising literature? If you answered 'yes' to either question, you should know that you are not on your own and should find this section helpful to begin improving your skills in this area.

REFLECTION POINT

ANALYSING THE EVIDENCE
• Do you know how to find or evaluate this evidence?
• Are some types of evidence more valuable than others?
• Are you aware of the range of frameworks that can help you evaluate different types of evidence?

Why do we need to analyse?

As healthcare professionals we need to weigh up the robustness of the evidence we have retrieved and how this evidence best suits the needs of the patients we care for. This 'weighing up' is the process of

> **Box 10.2   Overview of the critiquing approach in practice – some benefits and considerations**
>
> - Analysing evidence allows the reader to quickly assess the usefulness of various types of evidence.
> - Analysing reminds us of the importance of considering the local context when deciding how to introduce best evidence into practice.
> - Analysing brings good-quality research to where it is needed most in clinical practice.
> - Analysing promotes objectivity in all decisions.
> - Analysis of the underlying skills can be learned and developed.
> - Analysing may not produce all the answers. You may not always get a definite or easy answer as the evidence may simply not be available to meet your specific question or situation – lack of evidence does not prove a care.

analysis that is more commonly called 'critiquing' (Box 10.2). The consequence of not analysing literature is that you are never truly in a position to judge the worth of the evidence, its applicability to clinical practice, or whether it makes a real difference to the care provided.

On what evidence do you base the care you deliver to patients and families?

Consider the following case scenario: Peter, a 74-year-old man, has been receiving chemotherapy, which has led to the development of oral thrush. As a nurse working in a medical unit, you have assessed his condition correctly and the team wishes to treat him appropriately. What do you do?

1. Continue to provide oral hygiene and medication as you have always done?
2. Check out the literature to see whether there is anything new?
3. Follow the unit's guidelines for this condition?
4. Discuss with a colleague what is the best option in the circumstances?

If you opted for 1 or 2, you need to ask yourself how up-to date this information is. For example, are you basing your practice on what you were taught 10 years ago or on something you read in the last month? Equally, when were the guidelines last updated? If you choose to ask somebody for advice, how sure are you that the information they have is

any better than what you consider to be the right course of action?

Guides to aid critiquing

According to Sackett & Haynes (1995) the three aims of analysis are:

1. To appraise the individual piece of evidence (i.e. to weigh it up)
2. To assess its validity (closeness to the truth)
3. To assess its usefulness (to clinical practice).

Other organisations have come up with very similar overview questions to help guide the process of critiquing (Table 10.8). These questions have been devised to allow evidence to be analysed in a standardised way. However, although this provides an effective starting point, evidence is rarely presented in a manner that might allow these questions to be answered using a simple 'yes' or 'no'. In fact, 'results *may* be valid, *perhaps* demonstrate an important effect, and they *might* improve patient care' (Oxman et al 1993, p 2093). To the person looking for answers to clinical situations, this still means analysing the evidence systematically. In acknowledgement of this problem, a branch of the National Health Service Public Health Resource Unit known as the Critical Appraisal Skills Programme (CASP) has designed some user-friendly tools to help practitioners analyse evidence.

Evidence levels

The formalised use of 'levels of evidence' and 'grades of recommendations' was first announced in 1979, and since then a team of practitioners and researchers has put together a chart that has become very popular and widely used in evidence-based practice circles (Belsey & Snell 2003, p 2):

I. Strong evidence from at least one systematic review of multiple well-designed randomised controlled trials.
II. Strong evidence from at least one properly designed randomised controlled trial of appropriate size.
III. Evidence from well designed trials such as non-randomised trials, cohort studies, time series or matched case-controlled studies.
IV. Evidence from well designed non-experimental studies from more than one centre or research group.
V. Opinions of respected authorities, based on clinical evidence, descriptive studies or reports of expert committees.

Table 10.8 Overview questions to help guide the process of critiquing

Organisation	Website	Questions
Centre for Health Evidence (CHE) – a multidisciplinary initiative that provides walkthroughs of a large variety of evidence types. Each one is based on papers published in the Journal of the American Medical Association and includes detailed descriptions of the analysis process	http://www.cche.net/usersguides/main.asp	Are the results of the study valid? What are the results? Will the results help locally?
Centre for Evidence Based Medicine (CEBM) – an Oxford-based organisation aiming to promote evidence-based healthcare. Provides blank worksheets to aid analysis of common types of published evidence	http://www.cebm.net/downloads/ worksheets.pdf	Is it valid? Is it important? Is it applicable to the patient?
Critical Appraisal Skills Programme (CASP) – has helped to develop an evidence-based approach in health and social care since 1993. Has produced a number of useful directive guides to help the user analyse different types of clinical evidence	http://www.phru.nhs.uk/ casp/critical_appraisal_tools.htm	Is the study valid? What are the results? Will the results help locally?

By organising evidence into a ranked system, users can quickly weigh up one type of evidence against another, and by assessing the types of study used in a meta-analysis, a grade of recommendation can be derived to help the reader decide on the overall validity level. This type of approach for assessing quality and validity of supportive evidence has also found its way into many clinical guidelines, such as those produced by the Scottish Intercollegiate Guideline Network (http://www.sign.ac.uk). The limitation of this tool is that it is used primarily for empirically based research and can help indicate only the general validity level.

Process of analysing

The steps involved in analysing different types of evidence are very similar to those we use in our everyday lives to solve problems. For example, working out the best route to a place you have never visited before necessitates a certain degree of questioning and piecing together relevant facts to help decide on the best route and mode of getting to the venue.

There are five discrete layers within the whole critiquing process (Fig. 10.1). The first three layers are generally covered by the type of guide found in some traditional texts on research, which provide you with

The 5-Step critique		
Layer	1	Background
	2	Methodology
	3	Analysis
	4	Local applicability
	5	Comparison

Figure 10.1 Analysing research reports.

a 'script' of questions to aid in appraising each section of a single study. These first three layers can be seen to question the study itself, whereas the last two layers go further by judging applicability to the local situation and making comparisons with other similar evidence.

If you need an *aide mémoire* for the five-step critique, you could try 'Better Make A Local Comparison'.

Note: As with all tools, the purpose of this guide is to help you get a logical feel as to what is most important to question and why this might be so. Moreover, you should be mindful that the stages listed here, as layers 1–5, do not always need to be worked through in order, as quite often something listed as layer 4 or 5 may strike you initially and dissuade you from furthering your critique. Knowing this may help to save you time in the long run.

Layer 1 – Background Typical questions found here tend to be highlighted by the less experienced appraiser; however, the answers to these questions, although important to your overall perception of the paper, will probably not be sufficient in themselves to sway your opinion one way or another.

Typical questions include:

- Are the authors appropriately qualified to study the subject material?
- Is the publishing journal peer reviewed or does it have international readership?
- Has a full review of available literature been undertaken?
- Are specific aims or research questions clearly stated?

Layer 2 – Methodology If the engine is finely tuned the research should progress correctly, but if not all sorts of problems may ensue. Using research terminology, it is here that problems with reliability and validity are most likely to be uncovered (together known as 'rigour'). It is imperative that the authors are clear about all aspects of the methodology including the research approach (such as whether the study is qualitative or quantitative), the tools employed to collect data and the sample from which data were collected.

Typical questions include:

- Have all the research processes been described in detail so that the study could easily be repeated?
- Are all aspects of the sampling technique clearly described?
- Is the sample clearly representative of the population under study?
- How well matched is the study design to the purpose?
- Are methodological strengths and weaknesses listed or acknowledged?
- Using your own clinical experience, is there anything else in the methodology that might be seen as a limitation?

Layer 3 – Analysis This finalises appraisal of the coherence of the study by focusing on how the data were analysed to form results and conclusions. It should be noted that at this level bias can very easily creep in. Remember that in almost all studies only a summary of collected data will be presented for practical purposes. This summary should accurately reflect what has been collected in the raw data, using either a statistical or systematic method for data abstraction. Of course, more than one set of summary data can be derived from a single set of raw data depending on how the data were summarised. This is vital to appreciate, as conclusions are drawn from results, which in turn are just a summary of the raw data. Knowledge of the method used to produce the results summary can help to indicate how well this reflects the raw data, or indeed whether bias might be an issue. In essence, if you have any reason for questioning the rigour of how the data were collected or analysed, you must also question the results and conclusions based on these data.

Typical questions include:

- Is the process of analysis consistent with the research design?
- Are the tests used appropriate to the sample, design and purpose?
- Are statistical significances, confidence levels and ranges clear?
- Are absolute numerical values used in addition to percentages (relative values)?
- In qualitative research, is the process of analysis fully described?
- Were the summary results or emergent themes checked in any way?

It is worth noting that this area of analysis is the most daunting and more often than not requires the input of a statistician or someone who has been trained in statistical analysis.

Layer 4 – Local applicability At this point of the critiquing process you should have judged the overall rigour of the study in terms of your confidence in the way in which the authors have interpreted and presented the results and conclusions. Nonetheless, the value is only academic unless you personalise the results you have so far considered valid. In other words, knowing the study has been rigorously undertaken does not necessarily make it applicable to your situation. For this, local factors need to be introduced into the equation so that you can determine how well the research matches your actual clinical situation. Reflecting back to the original scenario for a moment, this process can be carried out for each of the citations originally selected from your literature search.

Typical questions include:

- Is the study sample comparable to my own patient(s) in terms of sex, age and disease?
- Are there other pertinent sample influences, such as cultural background, beliefs or medical history?
- Does the clinical setting described in the study differ from my own, and is this important?

- Do I have the required resources to implement the findings?

Layer 5 – Comparison (with other related sources of evidence)

The single most important aim of analysis of evidence is to attempt to determine whether there is enough suitable evidence available to develop an aspect of your palliative care practice. This decision can often be that there simply is not sufficient evidence upon which to base a practice change confidently – or, indeed, the opposite might be true. What do we do when we find more than one study that appears both rigorous and relevant, but they offer conflicting or differing conclusions? This final stage of weighing up the full extent of the evidence selected seems often to be neglected or poorly managed, with the potential consequence of continuing with a non-evidence-based procedure.

Typical questions include:

- How does this study compare with other similar studies in this area?
- Consider methodology and sampling differences to help judge rigour and validity.
- Consider methodological approach/study design to compare evidence levels.
- Consider which sample best matches your own patient(s) to help judge suitability (i.e. generalisability and transferability).

What stops us from analysing?

As a healthcare professional you are expected to maintain a familiarity with advances in your field of practice. This is challenging in terms of keeping pace with the constant flow of evidence that needs reviewing, and can be seen as an added work pressure. There are many reasons why practitioners find it difficult to analyse literature, but most tend to be related to the need for certain skills and/or resources. Some of these are listed in Table 10.9. The best way to overcome this fear or procrastination is to make efficient use of all available resources including colleagues, librarians, friends, internet sources and advice articles published in journals.

Table 10.9 summarises feedback from a small informal investigation of nurses undertaking further study in the area of evidence-based practice within a hospice setting. Can you identify with anything here?

From time to time we might wonder why we need to question what experienced researchers have written, especially when the research has been edited and peer-reviewed. Sometimes we may feel that if its in print it must be right! Thus, the mindset we may take leads us to fail in probing or questioning the content of published evidence. What should be borne in mind, though, is that the authors of a research article, book or other literature source may have strong opinions that they might like to see supported by a set of results (Adams 1999). Of equal importance for the reader is that the sample used in any piece of research is unlikely fully to reflect your own patient group, and so you must satisfy yourself as to how far you can reasonably apply conclusions or recommendations (Gonzales et al 2002). Finally, your involvement in any practice change should first consider the evidence fully and be in line with specific local resource factors within your clinical setting.

Mindset and skills necessary for analysing evidence

Preparing to engage in critical thinking

Critical thinking underlies the ability to analyse sources of evidence. Critical thinking results in the

Table 10.9	Results from a small survey on barriers to analysing evidence
Perceived barriers to analysing evidence	**Possible solutions**
Time constraints Boring	Wise use of all available resources can help select what is most suitable for you and save time in all areas of pursuing evidence-based practice.
Complicated or confusing terminology Don't know enough about research	Persistence and questioning those who are more research literate, coupled with the use of reference material (such as a research dictionary), soon leads to better understanding and a personal desire to learn more in your area of interest.
Difficulty getting literature Fear/inability to use library	Librarians are a fantastic resource – even when you learn the basics of IT-related or manual searching, they will always have more to teach.
Happy with current practice Same old content again Leads to more change	Change is inevitable and must be accepted. What should not be accepted is either maintaining an outdated practice or implementing an unproven one. It is also wrong to think that one piece of evidence merits implementing a change.

formation of conclusions based on the reasoned and systematic consideration of evidence. It can be applied to a variety of situations and can be both taught and learned. Within practice, the skills underlying this process can even be used to help bring clarity to many awkward situations in everyday clinical practice. Critical thinking forms part of evidence-based practice (Richardson & Detsky 1995). It should be noted, though, that critique should be an objective activity (Polit & Hungler 1991). For these purposes, objectivity can be considered a deliberate detachment from the content under review. This can be difficult for both the reader and the investigator, as we are rarely without bias, and should therefore be remembered when deciding whether to accept another's conclusions or not (Smith et al 2000).

Reading actively

Another skill required is that of reading actively (or 'interactively' according to some authors; Brown 1999). This is where the reader engages in what is being read to the point of constantly questioning whether he or she has understood and made sense of what is being reviewed. It is the opposite of skim reading and is necessary owing to the concentration of information present in the literature. Every sentence of a research report should contain information that is neither superfluous nor unimportant. Deliberately reading in this manner means that, as soon as you are aware of becoming bored or no longer understand what is being read, you can choose to re-read, go to another part of the paper for enlightenment or seek advice from a different source altogether. Adopting this approach takes practice and, like any other skill, will improve only with experience, but gradually you will realise that you yourself are the central component in the process of deciding the relevance to your practice of any piece of academic evidence. The tools at your disposal are your experiences, skills and knowledge, as well as the array of critique frameworks that can be used to analyse a variety of types of evidence, including audit, research, systematic reviews and clinical guidelines.

Developing knowledge of the research process

Part of any analysis is to question how the researchers dealt with the practicalities of undertaking the study. The logical implication is that a more substantial and meaningful critique can often be revealed as one's overall knowledge and understanding of research develops. However, it is this lack of confidence in research understanding that often promotes fear or disheartenment in critiquing (Ax 2001). You should remember though that only through probing for answers will you increase your understanding and in turn make the task easier over time. Thus, a basic awareness of the different types of research will undeniably help in forming judgements on a particular paper. Understanding the difference between qualitative and quantitative approaches will help in uncovering or accepting limitations in issues of design and rigour. Knowing whether a statistical test was appropriate or whether its result was interpreted correctly may uncover flaws in a study. In addition, using levels of evidence to compare different sources can be a very efficient method of comparison. This area is covered further in other areas of this chapter.

Don't overlook the statistics

Quantitative research often requires statistical analysis and presentation of results, which should be carried out using an appropriate test. Although you may not feel confident or able to assess to this level, you should at least attempt to make logical sense of the results and bear in mind that all statistical tests take us one step away from the original data and by necessity involve some sort of averaging of the results. Important and normal information may be considered irrelevant or erroneous and therefore be ignored; reflect on any textbook indication of physiological or anatomical normality such as height or heart rate to get a feel for how this averaging could mislead.

Types of evidence that need to be analysed

Essentially, any and all evidence that will have a bearing on your practice decisions should be analysed. Although this might range from colleague opinion through to systematic reviews, the basic process of questioning and judgement described above remains the same. However, as the average practitioner in palliative care is likely to encounter primary research, narrative reviews and clinical guidelines most often, these will be focused on here. Primary research usually has the tell-tale sign of being based on experiment, survey or clinical trial; secondary research uses primary studies as the basis for discussion or further analysis, and can take the form of a systematic or narrative (i.e. non-systematic) review. Table 10.10 describes some of the more common types of evidence and lists some resources that may be useful in helping to understand and analyse them. A comprehensive list of evidence

Table 10.10 Resources for analysing common types of evidence

Type of evidence	Definition	Example	Further information
Systematic review	A clearly defined and repeatable method to search and analyse a group of studies that relate to a specific question. Statistical analysis is generally used to help draw conclusions.	Cochrane Library (http://www.cochrane.org)	Greenhalgh T 1997 How to read a paper: papers that summarise other papers (systematic reviews and meta-analyses). British Medical Journal 315: 672–675. Available: http://www.bmj.com/cgi/content/full/315/7109/672 Higgins J P T, Green S (eds) 2005 Cochrane handbook for systematic reviews of interventions 4.2.5 (updated May 2005). In: The Cochrane Library, Issue 3. John Wiley, Chichester. Available: http://www.cochrane.dk/cochrane/ handbook/ hbook. htm
Randomised controlled trial (clinical drug trials)	An experimental approach in which the central variable is carefully controlled so that comparisons can be made within two or more matched samples. The experimenters and subjects should be unaware of intervention details to avoid bias.	For an updated list of 'double blind' drug trials see: http://www.controlled-trials.com/isrctn/ Galantino M L, Shepard K, Krafft L et al 2005 The effect of group aerobic exercise and t'ai chi on functional outcomes and quality of life for persons living with acquired immunodeficiency syndrome. Journal of Alternative and Complementary Medicine 111(6):1085–1092	http://www.answers.com/topic/randomized-controlled-trial
Meta-analysis (quantitative data)	A system of collating and combining results from related research using statistical methods in order to try to uncover an effect not able to be determined from a single study.	Berlin J A, Colditz G A 1990 A meta-analysis of physical activity in the prevention of coronary heart disease. American Journal of Epidemiology 132(4):612–628	http://www.evidence-based-medicine.co.uk/ebmfiles/WhatisMetaAn.pdf
Cohort study	Research, generally in the fields of medicine and social science, focusing on a group of people with one or more common demographic variables (e.g. specific to birth or exposure to a particular factor). These studies	Swiss HIV Cohort Study (see http://www.shcs.ch/)	http://www.socialresearchmethods.net/tutorial/Cho2/cohort.html

Table 10.10 Resources for analysing common types of evidence – cont'd

Type of evidence	Definition	Example	Further information
	tend to be longitudinal (i.e. carried out over a certain time period to record shared emerging similarities).		
Qualitative research (general)	Qualitative research examines concepts and phenomena. Sample sizes are typically smaller than in quantitative studies and data collection generally involves a series of probing or exploratory questions. The technique of participant observation is also commonly used. Data are analysed by the researcher uncovering themes and patterns to produce a rich summary of the area under investigation. Objectivity and validity are maintained by checking accuracy of summaries with original participants. Qualitative research involves many methods to promote insight and understanding; the most common in healthcare are: • Ethnography – studies culture or ethnicity • Phenomenology – examines the lived experience • Grounded theory – develops theory through theoretical sampling and constant comparative methods.	Davies B, Collins J B, Steele R et al 2005 Children's perspectives of a paediatric hospice program. Journal of Palliative Care 21(4):252–261 Iredale R, Brain K, Williams B, France E, Gray J 2006 The experiences of men with breast cancer in the United Kingdom. European Journal of Cancer 42(3):334–341	Morse J M, Field P A 1996 Nursing research. The application of qualitative approaches, 2nd edn. Chapman & Hall, London For a list of comprehensive resources and links see: http://www.qualitativeresearch.uga.edu/QualPage/ http://www.nova.edu/ssss/QR/qualres.html

Table 10.10 Resources for analysing common types of evidence – cont'd

Type of evidence	Definition	Example	Further information
Review (narrative reviews or updates)	This is a non-systematic summary of a body of work focusing on one particular area of research. Selection and inclusion of primary articles as well as extraction and summarising of critical data from these studies need not be carried out using any formalised approach. Although these papers provide important overviews and updates, their evidence level must be considered in light of the potential bias involved in the generalisations and conclusions drawn. For this reason, it is advisable to access and assess the primary article(s) from which an interesting summary point has been made in the review.	Mills M E, Sullivan K 1999 The importance of information giving for patients newly diagnosed with cancer: a review of the literature. Journal of Clinical Nursing 8(6):631–642 Burns T L, Ineck J R 2006 Cannabinoid analgesia as a potential new therapeutic option in the treatment of chronic pain. Annals of Pharmacotherapy 40(2):251–260	Siwek J, Gourlay M L, Slawson D C, Shaughnessy A F, Pharm D 2002 How to write an evidence-based clinical review article. American Family Physician 65(2):251–258. Available: http://www.aafp.org/afp/20020115/251.html
Quantitative research (general)	Traditionally describes any study based primarily on strictly controlled empirically based data collection that is analysed statistically. In the health sciences, the distinction between quantitative and qualitative approaches is more difficult to discern, however, as almost any form of data including qualitative can be treated numerically. Equally, quantitative studies need results to be described and	Munch T N, Zhang T, Willey J, Palmer J L, Bruera E 2005 The association between anemia and fatigue in patients with advanced cancer receiving palliative care. Journal of Palliative Medicine 8(6):1144–1149	http://en.wikipedia.org/wiki/Quantitative_research

Table 10.10 Resources for analysing common types of evidence – cont'd

Type of evidence	Definition	Example	Further information
	contextualised through which demands going beyond statistics and forming more qualitative material. Therefore, it may be simpler to consider the aim and nature of the research rather than the methodological design alone. Using this approach, a typical quantitative study would be experimental in design with a focus on hypothesis or deduction and with a general intent to test, form predictions, or help explain observable phenomena.		
Clinical guideline (clinical protocol, clinical practice guideline, medical guideline)	These documents systematically identify, assess and summarise key evidence relating to an area of healthcare practice. Their purpose is to help guide practitioners make judgements in line with current best evidence and in a way that allows local factors to form part of the decision tree. The adoption and use of clinical guidelines is thought to promote standardisation and quality of care as well as potentially reducing cost and risk. Many countries maintain guideline clearinghouses which stock high-quality clinical guidelines.	Some clinical guideline clearinghouses: http://www.nice.org.uk/ http://www.guideline.gov/ http://www.cbo.nl/english/default_view http://www.mja.com.au/public/guides/ guides.html	The Guidelines International Network is a fantastic resource that collates and links organisations interested in promoting quality healthcare through the use of clinical guidelines. Most countries are represented. http://www.guidelines-international.net/

sources has been collated by the Critical Appraisal Skills Programme (CASP) and can be accessed online: http://www.phru.nhs.uk/casp/sources_of_evidence.htm

Analysing clinical guidelines

A guideline is a systematically developed set of statements that can assist practitioners in making clinical decisions (Hutchinson & Baker 1999). Benton (1999) mentions that, in many ways, pathways, guidelines and protocols are one and the same thing in that they map out a treatment or care process but may place emphasis on specific aspects. For example, the care pathway ought to include statements regarding services and expected patient outcomes, whereas clinical guidelines tend to be state-of-the-science in relation to a treatment or patient problem, and are more dependent on using the best possible evidence. Pathways, guidelines and protocols are designed to be vehicles for the promotion of clinically efficient and effective practice through the use of the best available evidence. Clinical guidelines should be used to assist in clinical decision-making, promote common practice, and put into question the management 'routines' that many practitioners develop over time (Sackett et al 2000).

A European Union collaboration (Appraisal of Guidelines Research and Evaluation – AGREE) has coordinated the development of an assessment instrument for clinical guidelines based upon an earlier framework (Cluzeau et al 1999). This tool prompts users to question under six domains, each of which is intended to capture a separate dimension of quality (The AGREE Collaboration 2001, p 4):

Scope and purpose is concerned with the overall aim of the guideline, the specific clinical questions and the target patient population.
Stakeholder involvement focuses on the extent to which the guideline represents the views of its intended users.
Rigour of development relates to the process used to gather and synthesise the evidence, the methods to formulate the recommendations and to update them.
Clarity and presentation deals with the language and format of the guideline.
Applicability pertains to the likely organisational, behavioural and cost implications of applying the guideline.
Editorial independence is concerned with the independence of the recommendations and

acknowledgement of possible conflict of interest from the guideline development group.

Sackett et al (2000) describe guidelines as being divided into two components: the evidence component and the detailed instructional component. The first component can be judged by whether all relevant up to date literature has been used and whether validity has been assessed. The second component needs to be judged on its practicality for implementation and potential benefits, risks and costs. Guidelines are exactly what they say they are – guidelines – and therefore should not be implemented blindly but only after careful assessment in relation to evidence levels, validity and correspondence to local factors. In some cases, national guidelines can be used as the basis for local guideline development (Feder et al 1999). However, in all cases, 'guidelines should provide extensive, critical and well balanced information on the benefits and limitations of various diagnostic and therapeutic interventions so that the physician can carefully judge individual cases' (Broughton & Rathbone 2003, p 1).

More on qualitative research

Little distinction has been made so far between the two main branches of research – qualitative and quantitative – although the general approach described above (see Process of analysing) should work equally well for both. That said, there are aspects of each branch that may demand particular attention when critiquing and, as before, this appreciation will develop only with time and experience. What is most important, however, is to understand how methodology can influence both reliability and validity. For example, an interviewer may inadvertently lead the interviewee to respond in a certain way and thus upset the reliability of the responses; a poorly developed questionnaire may not allow the respondent room for a complete explanation, and this may pressure the researcher to make assumptions later, thus reducing validity; or a group of social workers not trained in using a tool designed to measure dimensions of grief are likely to produce inconsistent (unreliable) results. As shown in these examples, bias at all levels is always something to be wary of when critiquing. Practising the techniques of active reading and critical thinking will help you to recognise and question inadequacies or oversights in methodology.

Nursing research tends to use qualitative methods more commonly because this paradigm enables the researcher to explore experiences in a holistic manner. However, because most high-quality evidence is derived from quantitative approaches, evidence-based practice focuses on quantitative methods. It is important to spend some time focusing on what specific questions should be asked when appraising qualitative studies. CASP has developed a 10-question assessment tool for qualitative research that covers the areas of rigour, credibility and relevance.

Rigour

Definitions of 'scientific' research usually highlight that the whole process be carried out systematically and rigorously (Parahoo 1997). It should be quite evident that use of a systematic approach will help to produce a consistent approach based on centuries of inductive and deductive thought development. Rigour, on the other hand, demands that every facet of the research process be carried out in a precise and measured manner. Burns & Grove (1997, p 41) describe it as 'the striving for excellence . . . and involves discipline, scrupulous adherence to detail, and strict accuracy'.

In this sense you should see that when you critique a research article you are actually judging rigour. All investigators should therefore pay particular attention to their research design, checking for coherence between aims, methodology and conclusions, measurement procedures, and sampling. Of utmost importance at every stage is an attempt to plan, measure and conclude using complete objectivity. The use of a systematic research process does much to reduce subjective involvement, but you should always remain alert for any clue of possible breaches.

However, qualitative research quite often uses a less systematic approach and by necessity directly involves the researcher's own interpretations and ability to guide and probe areas being explored with the sample participants. It would therefore be wrong to judge rigour in qualitative studies in the same way as in quantitative ones. The important considerations should be in relation to openness of methodology, thoroughness and consistency in data collection, considering all the data equally when checking for emerging themes, and an assessment of how well the paper increases our understanding of the phenomenon under investigation (Giacomini & Cook 2000). The following questions may help as a general guide:

1. Are the aims clearly described?
2. Are the methodology and data collection procedures appropriate to meet the aims?
3. Is sampling fully described and congruent with the approach?
4. Is data analysis described in sufficient detail to indicate rigour and objectivity?
5. Are findings clear and supported with quotations where available?
6. Have conclusions been interpreted logically?
7. Are the results and conclusions clinically useful?

Relevance

When research is carried out rigorously, it should follow that it is both reliable and valid. This means that if you yourself were to carry out the same study under the same conditions then you should obtain comparable results. Taking this a bit further, it should also indicate that you can trust the results to be representative of any sample type studied; thus, if the sample type matched your own patient(s), you are now in a position to put into practice what has been recommended by the study. The extent to which the study sample meets your own patient group is termed its transferability (also generalisability or external validity). Even with the introduction of easily accessible and readable evidence-based practice summaries (Barton 2001), the question of whether the original is a match needs to be asked.

Finally, one of the most important points to remember about evidence-based practice is that the specific clinical question you are trying to answer has only one true answer. Realising that this one answer can be true only for the unique situation and patient(s) that gave rise to the question in the first place raises the problem of ever getting to the answer. The information provided by a research study must be taken on board only after judging both the rigour and the extent to which the sample, setting or conditions match the sample, setting and conditions of your local situation (Fig. 10.2). You may need to go over this in your mind a few times before it becomes clear. In other words, knowing that you can never carry out a specific research study for every single clinical question that you have, your only alternative is to find a study that fits the bill as closely as possible whilst proving itself to be worthy of belief (rigorous). In reality, you may need to find several such studies to help you piece together different aspects of the answer you are seeking, and this again underscores the importance of first undertaking a clear and systematic literature search (see above).

ENSURING THAT BEST AVAILABLE EVIDENCE BECOMES A COMPONENT OF PALLIATIVE CARE PRACTICE

The prime aim of evidence-based practice is to promote the constant evolution of practice, which is driven by the needs of the patients we care for. The

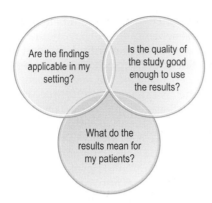

Figure 10.2 Analysis of any study must finally assess the relevance to your specific patient or group. (From Research Centre for Transcultural Studies in Health 2006. Online. Available: www.mdx.ac.uk/www/rctsh/ebp/3aspects.htm)

assumption is often made that if we make the best evidence available to practitioners then changing practice is a natural consequence. Dopson et al (2001) caution against such an assumption by suggesting that there is much research pointing to the fact that dissemination of evidence is insufficient to persuade practitioners to change. Kennedy & Lockhart Wood (2005) provide a timely reminder that transferring research-based knowledge into practice is a complex process. There are a number of factors that contribute to the integration of best evidence into clinical practice:

1. The palliative care team have *easy access to best available evidence,* which is presented in a way which practitioners can understand.
2. Palliative care practitioners have the *information technology skills* to extract best evidence.
3. Practitioners have *access to databases and other high quality web-based resources* in order and have the skills to confidently and efficiently extract various types of evidence.
4. The confidence and competence to *discern the quality* of a variety of types of evidence and have the skills to reflect on implications for local practice.
5. That as a palliative care team we embrace the importance of referring to best available evidence and that evidence-based practice is everybody's business.
6. Local mechanisms and leadership are in place to ensure the palliative care team are able to *regularly discuss best evidence* in the context of the palliative care needs of the patients and families they support.

7. Actively *evaluate the effectiveness of best evidence* within a local context to ensure that the evidence can be affirmed/limitations identified locally.

Practitioners, of course, refer to a wide range of sources to decide what the best course of action is. Malone et al (2004) go so far as to suggest that 'evidence' has become a fashionable term in healthcare and suggest four sources of knowledge on which we base our care:

- knowledge from clinical experience (e.g. practical know-how)
- knowledge from patients and carers (e.g. the views and experiences of service users)
- knowledge from local context (e.g. audit).

Looking at the evidence in isolation will result in a failure to ensure that best evidence becomes a component of everyday practice. Haynes (2002) notes that we can be confident in making better use of research evidence in clinical practice, especially if the wishes of the patient are taken into account. Therefore it is necessary for the practitioners to merge existing best evidence with appropriate sources of knowledge.

The reflective activity shown in Box 10.3 intimates strongly the notion of the theory and practice of change. Ensuring that best evidence becomes an integral component of practice is very much dependent on high-calibre clinical leadership and an intimate understanding of implementation and evaluation of change.

Davies (1999) suggests that we need to ask ourselves a number of questions before initiating a change. These questions might include the following:

- What do you want to change?
- What do you hope to achieve by the proposed change?
- Over what timescale?
- What will it cost to bring about the change?
- What resources will be required to initiate the change?
- Is there any evidence that the proposed change has worked/not worked elsewhere?
- What is the status of the evidence that is being used to stimulate the need for change?
- What process and outcome measures will need to be used to know that the change has been successful?
- Will another aspect of practice be affected by the proposed change?
- What other staff will need to be involved in supporting the proposed change, and are they likely to be cooperative?

- What are the ethical implications of the proposed change?
- Are the available resources and personnel capable of initiating and sustaining change?
- Is the proposed change feasible?

Box 10.3   Reflecting on putting the evidence into clinical practice

In this activity you are invited to select a recent research paper or systematic review on a topic that is relevant to the area in which you practice, and to undertake a two-stage review of the paper.

STAGE 1
- What are the strengths and weaknesses of the paper?
- What are the main findings of the paper?
- What is the current approach to care in the area you practise your chosen topic?
- Identify one area of practice that you feel needs to change in your area of practice as a result of reviewing the piece of research or systematic review.

STAGE 2
- What are the likely reactions of your colleagues to the recommendations of the systematic review?
- What might be the main obstacles to putting the evidence into practice?
- How do you propose that this intervention could be sensitively and appropriately used in your unit/colleagues' practice?
- What strategies would you use to ensure the evidence is integrated into practice?
- How would you evaluate that the change in practice had been implemented?

Those practitioners whose role it is to augment care based on best evidence should have both an expressed interest in where they can find the best evidence, and a confident grasp of change processes. We are fortunate, as a result of the development of bodies such as the National Institute for Health and Clinical Excellence (http://www.nice.org.uk) and the Cochrane Collaboration (http://www.cochrane.org/) that we have easy access to the latest evidence via the world wide web. This permits us to devote more time and attention to developing strategies for putting best evidence into practice. Taylor (2005) offers a cautionary note by intimating that change of practice is not easy, that effective change comes about through choice, and that there is no change without loss and no loss without change.

Wherever there is a team of practitioners involved in delivering palliative care it is essential that they are of the attitude that the evidence base of palliative care is constantly changing and that it is essential to maintain openness to new and emerging evidence. This will ensure that the team is accepting of a reality that we need to be open constantly to the possibility that the care our team delivers may be either ineffective or, at worst, significantly outdated.

In Table 10.11 you are invited to review a number of strategies that may be worth considering as practical ways in which you can, in your unit, ensure that change is initiated and followed through. You are invited to reflect personally on how these suggestions would be relevant to where you practice.

CONCLUSION

This chapter has tried to identify clearly the three interrelated components of evidence-based practice, namely finding, analysing and putting into practice. As a discipline, palliative care presents a number of complex challenges in ensuring that care is based on

---

Table 10.11   Implementation of evidence-based practice

Approach	Helpful	Not helpful	Comments
Present and discuss the findings of best evidence at a team/unit meeting or teaching session			
Use clinical supervision as an opportunity to discuss taking forward a piece of best evidence			
Develop or review a set of clinical guidelines in consultation with other members of the team			
Discuss your individual responsibility in taking forward best evidence within your individual performance review			
Other approaches – can you think of any more?			

the best possible evidence – not least building a comprehensive evidence base to inform practice. It is essential that practitioners be empowered with the skills to find the best available evidence and be able to discern the quality of the available evidence. If such competence is developed, it provides only part of the solution, because best evidence needs to be rooted firmly in change management, which is based on transformational leadership. It is at this point that leading change comes into its own, and is a crucial yet often overlooked step in the whole component of evidence-based practice.

Evidence-based practice needs to be an integral component of the education and training of nurses and other professionals in a way that provides a common ground for professionals to integrate their skills and knowledge to ensure that palliative care is administered both effectively and sensitively. Education about evidence-based practice needs to be supported within the culture of an organisation that delivers palliative care, whether it be in the community, nursing home, hospice or hospital. It is such an endorsement that encourages the free flow of best evidence in everyday practice.

It is acknowledged that little has been written in this chapter on the role of the patients and their family within an evidence-based care system. The underlying ethos of patient choice means that patients theoretically have the option of opting out of care based on the best available evidence, even though we know that it might be the most effective option. Haynes (2002) provides a timely reminder that evidence doesn't make decisions, people do. This leads to the conclusion that care based on the best available evidence needs to be acceptable to the patients. Such tensions illustrate that the future of evidence-based palliative care needs to have an ethical code to underpin the rolling out of best available evidence.

References

Adams C 1999 Clinical effectiveness – part 3: interpreting your evidence. Community Practitioner 72(5):289–292

Ax S 2001 Nursing students' perceptions of research: usefulness, implementation and training. Journal of Advanced Nursing 35(2):161–170

Barker P L 2000 Reflections on caring as a virtue ethic within an evidence-based culture. International Journal of Nursing Studies 37:329–336

Barton S 2001 Using clinical evidence. British Medical Journal 322:503–504

Belsey J, Snell T 2003 What is evidence-based medicine? Evidence-Based Medicine 1(2):1–6.

Benton D 1999 Clinical effectiveness. In: Hamer S, Collinson G (eds) Achieving evidence-based practice: a handbook for practitioners. Baillière Tindall, Edinburgh, p 87–108

Bird D 2003 Discovering the literature of nursing: a guide for beginners. Nurse Researcher 11(1):56–58

Bradshaw P L 2000 Evidence-based practice in nursing – the current state of play on Britain. Journal of Nursing Management 8:313–316

Bosanquet N, Salisbury C 1999 Providing a palliative care service: towards an evidence base. Oxford University Press, Oxford

Boyd K, Deighan M 1996 Defining evidence based healthcare: a health-care learning strategy. Nursing Times Research 1(5):332–339

Broughton R, Rathbone B 2003 What makes a good clinical guideline? Evidence-Based Medicine 1(11):1–8

Brown S J 1999 Knowledge for health care practice: a guide to using research evidence. W B Saunders, Philadelphia

Burns N, Grove S K 1997 The practice of nursing research: conduct, critique and utilization. W B Saunders, Oxford

Cluzeau F A, Littlejohns P, Grimshaw J M, Feder G, Moran S E 1999 Development and application of a generic methodology to assess the quality of clinical guidelines. International Journal for Quality in Health Care 11:21–28

Davies P 1999 Introducing change. In: Dawes M, Davies P, Gray A, Mant J, Seers K, Snowball R (eds) Evidence-based practice: a primer for health care professionals. Churchill Livingstone, Edinburgh, p 203–218

Dopson S, Locock L, Chambers D, Gabbay J 2001 Implementation of evidence based medicine; evaluation of the promoting action on clinical effectiveness programme. J Health Service Research Policy 6(1):23–30

Ellershaw J, Ward C, Neuberger J 2003 Care of the dying patient: the last hours or days of life. Commentary: a 'good death' is possible in the NHS. British Medical Journal 326:30–34

Feder G, Eccles M, Grol R, Griffiths C, Grimshaw J 1999 Clinical guidelines: using clinical guidelines. British Medical Journal 318:728–730

Fitzpatrick J 2004 How to surf the internet. Nursing Times 100(10):46–47

Giacomini M, Cook D J 2000 A user's guide to qualitative research in health care. Journal of the American Medical Association 284(4):478–482

Gonzales J J, Ringeisen H L, Chambers D A 2002 The tangled and thorny path of science to practice: tensions in interpreting and applying 'evidence'. Clinical Psychology: Science and Practice 9(2):204–209

Greenhalgh T 1997 How to read a paper: papers that summarise other papers (systematic reviews and meta-analyses). British Medical Journal 315:672–675

Hamer S, Collinson G (eds) 1999 Achieving evidence-based practice: a handbook for practitioners. Baillière Tindall, Edinburgh

Haynes B 2002 Physicians' and patients' choices in evidence based practice: evidence does not make decisions, people do. British Medical Journal 324:1350

Hearn J, Higginson I J 1998 Do specialist palliative care teams improve outcomes for cancer patients? A systematic literature review of the evidence. Palliative Medicine 12(5):317–332

Higginson I 1999 Evidence based palliative care: there is some evidence – and there needs to be more. British Medical Journal 319:462–463

Hutchinson A, Baker R 1999 What are clinical practice guidelines? In: Hutchinson A, Baker R (eds) Making use of guidelines in clinical practice. Abingdon: Radcliffe Medical Press, Abingdon, p 1–13

Kennedy K M, Lockhart Wood K 2005 Evidence based palliative care. In: Lugton J, Mcintyre R (eds) Palliative care: the nurse's role. Elsevier Churchill Livingstone, Edinburgh, p 367–411

Malone J R, Seers K, Tichen A et al 2004 What counts as evidence in evidence based practice? Journal of Advanced Nursing 47(1):81–90

National Institute for Clinical Excellence 2004 Improving supportive and palliative care for adults with cancer. NICE, London

Oxman A D, Sackett D L, Guyatt G H 1993 Users' guides to the medical literature. I. How to get started. Journal of the American Medical Association 270(17):2093–2095

Parahoo K 1997 Nursing research: principles, process and issues. Palgrave Macmillan, Basingstoke

Polit D F, Hungler B P 1991 Nursing research: principles and methods, 4th edn. J B Lippincott, Philadelphia

Pond F 1999 Searching for studies. In: Brown S J (ed.) Knowledge for healthcare practice. W B Saunders, Philadelphia, p 41–58

Richardson W S, Detsky A S 1995 Users' guides to the medical literature. VII. How to use a clinical decision analysis. A. Are the results of the study valid? Journal of the American Medical Association 273(16):1292–1295

Sackett D L, Haynes R B 1995 On the need for evidence based medicine. Evidence-Based Medicine 1:5–6

Sackett D L, Rosenberg W M C, Gray J A M, Haynes R B 1996 Evidence based medicine: what it is and what it isn't. British Medical Journal 312:71–72

Sackett D L, Straus S E, Scott Richardson W, Rosenberg W, Haynes R B 2000 Evidence based medicine. How to practise and teach EBM. Churchill Livingstone, Oxford

Smith L A, Oldman A D, McQuay H J et al 2000 Teasing apart quality and validity in systematic reviews: an example from acupuncture trials in chronic neck and back pain. Pain 86:119–132

Taylor B 2005 Personal change. In: Hamer S, Collinson G (eds) Achieving evidence based practice: a handbook for practitioners, 2nd edn. Baillière Tindall, Edinburgh, Ch. 8, p. 155–170.

The AGREE Collaboration 2001 Appraisal of guidelines for research and evaluation: AGREE instrument. Online. Available: http://www.agreecollaboration.org/pdf/agreeinstrumentfinal.pdf 1 Aug 2006

Trinder L, Reynords S 2000 Evidence based practice: a critical appraisal. Blackwell Science, Oxford.

Wilkinson S 1998 The importance of evidence based care. International Journal of Palliative Nursing 4(4):160

Further reading

Forchuck C, Roberts J 1993 How to critique qualitative research articles. Canadian Journal of Nursing Research 25:47–56

Grade Working Group 2004 Grading quality of evidence and strength of recommendations. British Medical Journal 328:1490–1498

Greenhalgh T 2006 How to read a paper: the basics of evidence-based medicine, 3rd edn. Blackwell Publishing, Oxford

Hamer S, Collinson G (eds) 1999 Achieving evidence-based practice: a handbook for practitioners. Baillière Tindall, Edinburgh

HealthLinks. Evidence-based practice. Online. Available: http://healthlinks.washington.edu/ebp 1 Aug 2006

Higginson I 1999 Evidence based palliative care – there is some evidence and there needs to be more. British Medical Journal 319:462–463

Hill A, Spittlehouse C 1998 What is critical appraisal? Evidence-Based Medicine 3(2):1–8

Hutchinson A, Baker R 1999 What are clinical practice guidelines? In: Hutchinson A, Baker R (eds) Making use of guidelines in clinical practice. Radcliffe Medical Press, Abingdon, p 1–15

Netting the Evidence. Online. Available: http://www.shef.ac.uk/scharr/ir/netting/ 1 Aug 2006

Ploeg J 1999 Identifying the best research design to fit the question. Part 2: qualitative designs. Evidence-Based Nursing 2(2):37

Polit F, Beck C T 2003 Nursing research: principles and methods, 7th edn. Lippincott Williams & Wilkins, Philadelphia

Useful resources

Databases

AMED (Allied and Complementary Medicine)
CancerLIT

CINAHL (Cumulative Index to Nursing and Allied Health Literature)

Embase
Medline
PsychInfo

Websites

The Cochrane Collaboration. http://www.cochrane.org

Bandolier. Evidence based thinking about health care. http://www.jr2.ox.ac.uk/bandolier

Centre for Reviews and Dissemination. http://www.york.ac.uk/inst/crd/index.htm

National Cancer Institute. http://www.cancer.gov/search/cancer_literature/

NHS Public Health Resource Unit. Critical appraisal tools. http://www.phru.nhs.uk/casp/critical_appraisal_tools.htm

Netting the Evidence. http://www.shef.ac.uk/scharr/ir/netting/

Search engines

Google. http://www.google.com

AltaVista. http://www.altavista.com

Yahoo. http://www.yahoo.com

Alltheweb. http://www.alltheweb.com

Chapter **11**

Choice at the end of life: ethics and palliative care

Simon Chippendale

CHAPTER CONTENTS

INTRODUCTION

Since the initial publication of this book there has been a marked increase in the interest in ethical issues towards the end of life, particularly surrounding the capacity of a person, choices at the end of life and, specifically, the debate surrounding euthanasia. Ethics continues to provide a basis whereby the multi-professional team, patients, their carers and society in general can consider challenging circumstances and continue to discuss the acceptability and permissibility of actions and their respective outcomes within contemporary society, and within the professional and clinical environment.

Ethics may be considered by some to be a dry, theoretical subject that has little relevance to, or at best is remote from, patient care. On the contrary, I would suggest, and hope to illustrate within this chapter, that ethical issues are extremely relevant to palliative care. The chapter commences with a discussion about contemporary issues and their impact on palliative care, demonstrating how relatively simple aspects of patient care may find challenges focusing on ethical permissibility of actions, and how such decisions can depend on values held by the carer. The reader is invited to reflect on this and, drawing from their personal experiences, to identify similar occasions where ethical dilemmas arose in clinical situations. The chapter sets out two key philosophical approaches, consequentialism and deontology, that have influenced the values and morals of Western-based societies and cultures. Key ethical principles related to healthcare are introduced, and provide the basic building blocks from which the ethical permissibility of potential dilemmas may be explored. These principles, together with other tools used in ethical clinical decision-making, enable healthcare professionals to determine whether clinical actions or decisions about care are ethically justifiable. Finally, current issues in palliative care are explored, focusing particularly on the subject of extraordinary and futile care towards the end of life. The reader is encouraged to reflect actively on the ethical component of these issues and on their personal views. By removing emotional reactions to issues and by reflecting on both personal values and the ethical principles involved in the issue, the reader should be able objectively to examine the ethical permissibility of clinical actions within palliative healthcare. Far from being a dry subject, it is anticipated that the reader will be drawn into constructive, informed, critical argument and debate, bringing alive the ethics within palliative care.

The provision of healthcare is becoming increasingly complicated by the expectations of a society that is better informed about current treatment options, has high demands and high expectations about the healthcare provided. The focus of palliative care, by its very definition, looks towards multiprofessional holistic care provision following the recognition of no potential cure. This places an emphasis upon individual preferences in determining the quality of life. The subjective issues that arise should be considered on an individual basis, and should be recognised as reflecting values that are the essence of individualised care. In attempting to provide appropriate care, healthcare professionals may find conflict between their assessment of the needs of the patient and their family, the interventions deemed necessary by both parties, and in determining objectively the general subjective priorities that individuals place on their own value and quality of life.

In general, ethics can only provide an indication of the general ethical permissibility or acceptability of actions. If carers respect even the most fundamental principles of ethics, then the autonomy of the individual patient should be respected; this is balanced by the principles of beneficence and nonmaleficence. However, decisions that are arrived at will result in implications for our society in general, and as such the ethical permissibility of care for individuals needs to be tapered by the implications for the ethical implications of similar situations within our society and for all similar clients or patients – the notion of the principle of justice.

Ethical issues that arise in palliative care may be recognised as being similar to those in other specialities. Common examples include issues affecting the professional–patient relationship, resource allocation, truth-telling, confidentiality, respect of individual and professional autonomy, consent and refusal to treatment, the withholding and the withdrawal of treatments at both the macro- and micro-level within palliative care.

Palliative care has had a major review of its planned service provision, indicating clear recommendations and guidelines for contemporary clinical practice (National Institute for Clinical Excellence [NICE] 2004). Clinical service provision has had to become increasingly evidence-based and, as a consequence, the management of palliative care services is in danger of becoming overcome with the insipid invasion of identifiable audit trails strangling the evolution of innovative clinical care. Although such 'evidence' provides a welcome indication of the standards and quality of care, the emphasis on providing such information for auditing bodies detracts clinicians away from the focus of care on the patient and their family. Hospices whose focus needs to be on patient care provision are increasingly having to divert their charitable funds to meet the paper-oriented 'evidence base' arising from work provided from their partners within the National Health Service (NHS). On the one side this is by no means a bad thing: hospices need to account for the care they provide and it quantifies the amount of specialist palliative care that is provided outside the NHS. This in turn provides the basis for appropriate requests for increased funding from the NHS to support the care provided, with current initiatives focused on tariffs for the provision of aspects of palliative care. On the opposite side are the increased demands on staff time to qualify the care provided, detracting from the time available for patient care. A balance is required, and in many places achieved. Such issues regarding resource distribution (particularly financial support) can add a further dimension to the ethical debate about palliative care – alongside the debate about what clinical services and treatments ought to be provided compared with what services are available to be provided and what can realistically be provided within the financial resources available.

In the first edition of this book I argued that defining palliative care maintains a focus on the quality of life until death, and should not include euthanasia, which, at best, can be regarded as the intentional ending of life or otherwise killing. Events have since moved politically and legally. There is significant current debate over the acceptability of euthanasia and personal choice at the end of life.

Ethics is about understanding where, if and when these decisions may become ethically permissible. The Mental Capacity Act 2005, due to come into effect in April 2007, applies to people aged over 16 years and suggests that:

a person lacks capacity 'if he is unable to' make a decision for himself by reason of an impairment or disturbance of his mind or brain, whether on a temporary or permanent basis.

(National Council for Palliative Care [NCPC] 2005a)

The issue of capacity is additionally unrelated to a person's behaviour, age or appearance, and the ability to make a decision relies on a person being able to understand, retain and utilise relevant information, and to communicate their decision. In palliative care this becomes one of the challenges facing 'decision-making' towards the end of life. A person who has been previously competent (i.e. they have capacity) can becomes less competent as a result of the disease process, drugs or decreasing consciousness, particularly during the later stages of palliative care. The Mental Capacity Act will enable people legally to identify another person with Lasting Power of Attorney, enabling them to make decisions for the client not just over their estate (as is the current situation), but also over their welfare, which will include health decisions. This will in effect continue to provide a clear indication of what would personally continue to be acceptable care for the person whose capacity diminishes. Advanced decisions (replacing advanced directives) will hold greater legal sway in providing an indication of the client's wishes, which will have to be respected by care providers. Although advanced decisions cannot include a request to end life, they can indicate preferences of care given choices of care options and available clinically indicated treatments. Equally the advanced decision may indicate on behalf of the patient a wish to refuse as well as to accept interventions and care. Such decisions will have to be respected. This has implications for the palliative care team in that the team will need to determine whether clients have advanced decisions and what the advanced decision indicates.

The Act will continue to promote the respect for autonomy of the individual after the point at which they are unable to communicate their wishes. However, clients will need to place implicit trust in those whom they give Lasting Power of Attorney. The Mental Capacity Act is likely to ensure that medical teams continue to act in best interests of clients. When a person is unable to make a voluntary decision (where they lack capacity), this is unlikely to allow the ending of life where the client has not previously, or is currently unable, to make a recorded decision.

The final development recently discussed by parliament was when Lord Joffe presented the Assisted Dying for the Terminally Ill Bill to the House of Lords for its second reading. This resulted in great debate on 12 May 2005, but was subjected to challenge by Lord Carlile of Berriew, who moved to make an amendment to delay the reading for 6 months, effectively delaying the Bill and killing it. The result was that the Bill ran out of time within the parliamentary session and was effectively put aside, but not without passionate and well reasoned debate from both sides as to whether it is ever permissible to end a life at the wishes of a client (voluntary) through active means. Perhaps the benefit of this Bill has been to encourage open debate about euthanasia within our society. There has been much opposition towards the Bill from within palliative care (NCPC 2006), as well as discussion regarding the implications for care (Finlay et al 2005).

The focus of this bill is on the voluntary, active elements of euthanasia, where a patient who has capacity makes a voluntary decision to take or request actions that would end their life. Individuals have the right to refuse treatments if aged over 17 years in England (children under 18 years cannot refuse a life-saving intervention if their parents wish them to have it). Such refusal of treatments by the competent patient may result in death of the patient. However, if this is the accepted situation for a terminally ill patient, this may result in prolonged suffering, which raises the question of whether assisted suicide could ever be an alternative in these circumstances, particularly where a patient is unable to activate measures that would end their own life.

The concept of euthanasia raises two contributory factors in the ethical debate, primarily that of the sanctity and value of life, and secondarily the resource issue debate. It is against this background that the issue of euthanasia needs to be considered. The perception of the euthanasia debate seen from a classical ethics viewpoint relies on whether it can ever be acceptable to hasten the death of a person, to kill them through either actions or omission, reflecting fundamentally on the value of 'human' life.

In our society and culture we find ourselves with the 'luxury' of determining when and what clinical services we access, the luxury of choice, and the image that we have control over our lives (and how we live them) – and the expectation that healthcare services are there to support us. Some even have the expectation that we have a right to expect all available services. The reality is rather different. Local services reflect past commitments to maintaining clinical services and developments of new services. In some areas palliative care has evolved at differing rates. Clinical services available in some parts of the country are more advanced and developed compared with others who are learning from the success of other providers.

Palliative care purists may argue that with the appropriate services, fully funded and functioning, there ought to be no need for euthanasia: a superb individual service would support the patient and their family through the spectrum of clinical need across differing service providers, enabling the client to die in their preferred place of death. The majority of palliative care services strive to attain this utopian goal. The reality for some clients may be quite the opposite. It is where palliative care fails to meet the expectations of clients, where palliative care is unable sufficiently to alleviate the holistic spectrum of pain and anguish, that clients are faced with the option of choosing not to continue with their suffering, but of dying. The debate within the House of Lords on the Assisted Dying for the Terminally Ill Bill on 12 May 2005 recognised the need for adequate funding of palliative care services to ensure appropriate provision for all those who require palliative care (Lords Hansard 2006). The reality of whether such funding becomes readily available is an issue for resource distribution, with further ethical considerations.

What is often omitted from the debate around euthanasia is the perception of determining the subjective issue of the quality of an individual's life – whether that life has a worthwhile quality and, if deemed not to have such quality, then whether it is acceptable to end it. If the ending of a life becomes an ethically acceptable premise then there is the issue of dying: what would be an appropriate manner of dying and death (again a subjective choice) and whether in palliative care the duty of care should extend to ensuring the quality of the actual dying process? Finally, if death becomes an ethically acceptable quality of care – equitable to the palliative care provided during the last few months and weeks of life – then the original definitions of palliative care will need to be revised.

Whether palliative care services are limited, accessible, or whether just due to the increasing complexity of the patient's needs during the disease progression, the reality for some patients and their carers is that the services are unable to meet their needs. Clinicians will recognise instances where dying is not a peaceful process, and that some aspects of care, physical as well as spiritual, social and psychological, are just not universally available. Where inadequate service provision detracts from the continued acceptable quality of living for clients, then circumstances arise whereby, for some, passive voluntary euthanasia becomes a desirable option, but others may choose to seek an active end to their life – active voluntary euthanasia – either through pharmaceutical means or otherwise. In such instances, where the quality of living has been reduced to a point where death becomes a desirable alternative, there is the question that deserves to be addressed: What about the quality of dying? Ought palliative care be just as willing to concede care for those who are dying as well as the earlier interventions, not forgetting the ongoing support for a family where a person who has capacity chooses to end their life?

Currently individuals making such difficult personal decisions to end their lives need to be able physically to travel to Switzerland. This choice may deny that person those last few days or weeks of living at home (or other clinical setting), in effect shortening their lives. Palliative care services ought to be ensuring a focus on maintaining a person's quality of life during this time. The lack of legalised active euthanasia denies those few people a period of their lives that they might have had if the Assisted Dying for the Terminally Ill Bill had been passed.

Conversely, individuals ought to be equally concerned that, if palliative care follows the path to accepting active voluntary euthanasia (if assisted suicide were to be legalized) then there may be scenarios where palliative care treatment interventions become too costly to provide within the financial limitations of health care provision compared with the costs of the option of ending life. This may be of increasing relevance where a patient permanently lacks capacity to indicate the choice. In such circumstances the danger of limited finances may adversely influence how the best interests of the patient is determined.

Internationally the acceptance of limited aspects of euthanasia would appear to be increasing. In Holland euthanasia was decriminalised in 1991 and eventually legalised in 2002. Belgium similarly legalised euthanasia in 2002. In France clients can refuse treatment, as in England, but euthanasia is not legal. Current focus seems to be on Switzerland where legalised doctor-assisted suicide is permitted but not full euthanasia. The State of Oregon legalised the process of enabling the provision of medication that would end life for people who were terminally ill in 1997 – with specific conditions built in to safeguard clients and professionals before satisfying the circumstances that allow clients to request this. There is an indication that, although increasing numbers of terminally ill people in Oregon are requesting medication to end their lives, the proportion actually choosing to take the medication has not increased as much (Oregon Department of Human Services 2006). One hypothesis for this is that enabling people to have the power to end their lives legally might actually contribute to the quality of their last few days, knowing that, for them, if it gets worse tomorrow they can then end their life, but for today it makes issues more bearable. Alongside the demographics, the report highlighted complications for three people in 2005 for whom death was not instantaneous, raising further concerns about the appropriateness of this style of euthanasia.

Additional consequences remain with those professionals involved with the care of their clients during this stage at the end of their life. Kade (2000, p 506) provided a challenging account of his reflections, as a doctor in Oregon, when caring for a client for whom he had legally prescribed medication to end the client's life, describing his personal psychological conflicts in respecting his client's choice to end her life:

> I am grateful for the great disruption in my emotional stability that this experience precipitated. This act should never be easy, never routine. It should be among the most difficult and disquieting acts we embark upon.

The undiscussed side of the euthanasia debate is that of the consequences and support for those who would be directly involved with the decision-making and in furthering the actual ending of life.

The current situation in the UK appears to accept that, where a person has a terminal illness, retains capacity and is mobile, they can travel from their home to a different country and culture to die. This raises the question of whether palliative care may be failing clients in caring for them up to and including their death. English law currently does not allow the active ending of life. Similarly the palliative care approach reflects the position of neither hastening death (equivalent to euthanasia) nor unnecessarily prolonging dying. The emphasis on 'no killing' stance in palliative care while acknowledging the need to respect an individual's choice has been refleted by many professional bodies concerned about the standards of palliative care. Several professional bodies promote this through emphasis on clauses of 'doing no harm' within their professional codes of conduct. Currently people receiving palliative care, and the support that gives them, may lose that clinical support when they have to leave the country seeking an active end to their lives, perhaps just when they need such support following what has to be for them a most difficult decision. This appears to be the situation for a small number of families, but the numbers seeking euthanasia abroad may increase if the NHS and palliative care fail to meet the expectations of people dying from life-threatening diseases.

So, legally and professionally, carers face difficult circumstances with impending alterations in the law regarding euthanasia. Challenges for professional practice will need to be clarified. Can clients be harmed, perhaps psychologically, if their wishes are not met? If in palliative care we seek to provide holistic care, ought this to extend to include the dying phase? And where clients request assisted suicide, would it ever be ethically acceptable for professionals to perform this last act for them, where the clients wishes to be, with those whom they want around them?

There would also need to be discussion on the outcome and implications of the effect of assisted suicide on those who will perform the final act. If these are health professionals, issues are raised regarding trust between health professionals and clients. Further concerns may arise where treatment resources cost too much, resulting in a potential for weak coercion on clients to accept voluntary assisted suicide in preference to a lower anticipated quality of life than they had hoped for. Finally, where will clients go for the ending of their lives? If health professionals do not perform the ending of life (killing) then who will, and where and what quality controls will need to be in place to prevent potential abuse at the end of life?

Who holds the moral high ground? – It is easy to accept or challenge the ethical permissibility of such actions leading to euthanasia, even in voluntary passive instances. Add to this the challenges of prolonged mental and physical suffering without the sense or hope of relief, and it becomes easier to understand why some challenge for the acceptance of voluntary forms of euthanasia where a person is terminally ill. But where might this end – if acceptable for a person who is terminally ill, why not for a person who has a long-term medical condition, or who just does not want to live?

Frequently palliative ethics is solely considered – mistakenly – to be focused on the debate surrounding euthanasia. The reality is that the nature of the very concept of palliative care, particularly within the hospice network, excludes the euthanasia debate in that palliative care by its very definition does *not* intentionally hasten, shorten or unnecessarily prolong the end of life of those in receipt of quality palliative care. Palliative care cannot therefore include the deliberate ending of life within its objectives, whether it is actively or passively sought, either voluntarily or non-voluntarily. However, palliative care needs to provide care up to, including, and beyond the point of death. The provision of specialist palliative care intervention requires a holistic approach to care. The consideration of psychological, emotional, social, and spiritual care interventions in addition to meeting physical needs is a basic requirement. Palliative care professionals are able to provide this for the great majority of clients. However, realistically, there will be infrequent circumstances when, as specialists we are unable to meet all of the needs of clients, physical or otherwise. In these circumstances clients may make the choice not to continue with their low quality of life and may wish to hasten their death. Where does this leave palliative care professionals?

Palliative care continues to be challenging in recognising the extent and alleviating the spiritual, psychological and social symptoms in addition to the ongoing relief of physical needs. Regrettably, at times, carers and families become the reluctant observers of inadequate symptom control, where suffering, distress and fear become unmanageable by the multiprofessional team. At these times it is possible to begin to understand the view of some who hold enough value on their lives not to wish to experience such distress, and would prefer to shorten their natural lives. This brings up the emotive subject of passive voluntary euthanasia.

Ethical debate focuses on the sanctity of life and the value of life, whether it could ever be ethically permissible deliberately to end a life, whether by deliberate action (killing) or by non-actions (omissions) of care that result in the client being allowed to die.

person. Circumstances at the end of life may result in ethical dilemmas being further complicated by issues concerning the competence of the dying person, their right to refuse or accept care, and in maintaining their personal integrity over their own death. Ethical dilemmas may arise from differing values placed upon the value of life by patients and their carers. Dilemmas may also extend to circumstances surrounding resource distribution: Do dying people have the right to access every possible treatment whatever the cost in terms of finance, time and available resources? It would appear that palliative care has a unique set of ethical situations that challenge the multiprofessional team, the patient and their family to determine ethically permissible courses of action.

In bringing comfort and hope to patients and their families who are in need of quality palliative care, multiprofessional healthcare teams are frequently challenged by decisions that need to be made depending on the circumstances at a particular time. Potential influences on these decisions can be seen in Box 11.1.

In addition to these influences, there exists a cycle of trust and expectation between the client, their family and health professionals (Fig. 11.1). The interaction between each relies on respect between all parties.

REFLECTION POINT

- Can you recognise instances in your professional career where you were faced with a professional dilemma about one or more of the issues already identified?
- How did you come to the decision you made?
- What influenced you at that point in time?
- On reflection, would you make the same decisions now?
- If not, what circumstances might influence your current values?
- If you had to make similar decisions outside your professional life, would your decisions reflect similar outcomes to your professional decisions?
- How might the Mental Capacity Act 2005 influence your professional care?
- If active voluntary euthanasia were to become legal, how might this influence your personal views and professional care?

Although these issues may be similar in different health specialties, there exists a unique edge to some ethical dilemmas in the specialty of palliative care. The very nature of palliative care focuses debate about ethical issues on the inevitable death of the

Box 11.1   Potential influences on ethical decision-making

- Societal and cultural values
- Personal values and beliefs
- Law
- Professional codes of conduct

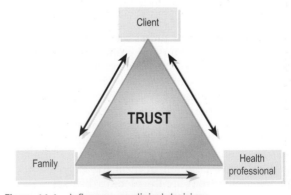

Figure 11.1   Influences on clinical decisions.

Those who work in palliative care may understand the wishes of patients who want to die peacefully and with a quality of life whose acceptability can be determined only by the patients themselves. In some situations patients may *value* an early *end to their lives*. While perhaps not agreeing with some practices it is the compassionate nature and understanding of a patient's circumstances that reflects empathy with their patients.

For a simple example of an ethical dilemma in palliative care, consider the concerns about truth-telling. Consider the hypothetical scenario in Case Studies 11.1 & 11.2.

Consideration of ethics may not provide the answer to all of the difficult questions that can arise in palliative care. Frequently there is no clear right or wrong, black or white side to a clinical situation, only a greyish state of affairs that appears to change depending on the way the overall picture is perceived.

What ethics does allow for is specific argument to be made about the circumstances surrounding individual cases that looks to answer the question, not of whether the result is essentially right or wrong, but whether it is *ethically permissible*. In ethics the emphasis must be regarded and thought of in terms of the ethical permissibility of actions or inactions. An awareness of ethical issues and arguments enables practitioners to come to informed decisions about their actions and to help clarify situations for patients and their families.

Challenges faced by healthcare professionals within palliative care are frequently focused around specific ethical issues at the end of life (Fig. 11.2), such as decisions relating to the continued provision of artificial hydration, certain drugs and artificial feeding. These are in addition to the general issues that commonly affect most clinical specialties, as well as palliative care. Ethics can provide a basis to determine whether decisions made about care,

---

Case Study 11.1

A patient, A, has been sensitively informed by the palliative consultant, B, that treatments for her disease have not been successful and that her prognosis is very poor, with perhaps less time to live than had previously been expected. However, the medical expectation was that she would experience few symptoms requiring treatment until the last few days of life. The consultant also tells her that he will inform her general practitioner, C, of the appropriate palliative care that she is likely to require and make referrals to the community specialist palliative care team, D and E. A then informs B that, for personal reasons, she does not under any circumstances want her partner, F, to know of her shortened life expectancy. She wants this wish to be passed on to all professionals involved with her care. C is also the GP for her partner F.

This may seem an appropriate request by A, particularly if we are to respect her autonomy and that she meets the criteria competently to make such a request. But what happens when her partner asks for details from B, C, D or E? Familiar situations may suggest the use of a variety of communication skills in such situations, focused on encouraging A and F to be honest with each other. But there exists a professional dilemma, particularly for C, in such situations as the GP has a professional duty of care to both A and F.

Pause for reflection: if you were C, what would you do if, during a consultation, F asked you for assurance that A had a long time to live? How would you justify your decisions?

• If you hold strong *deontological* views then you would have to tell F the truth – this would be ethically permissible as it holds to the universal laws, and you would not be responsible for actions that F then carried out as a result of receiving that information. It would be preferable to inform A of those views.

Alternatively
• If you hold a *consequentialist* view, you would have to determine the greatest good and least harm for the potential consequences in justifying your actions. A partial lie may do harm later on but be of greater benefit to the patient in coping with their disease. This has to be weighed against the potential benefits and harms that may be incurred from the consequences of truth-telling.

Case Study 11.2

Patient B is generally well. He has no family. B fears hospitals, but otherwise has had an excellent relationship with his GP, who retired recently. On finding that B has an advanced stage of an incurable disease, the new GP wants to inform B of his prognosis and choices. B replies, 'No, I don't want to know. I've always trusted you to make the right decisions for me – I'll still trust you'.

On one hand, the GP can choose to respect B's wishes and act in his best interests – but how will he determine these? The lack of information for B will make it increasingly difficult to determine B's views and wishes.

Alternatively, the GP might insist that B listens to his prognosis, so that further decisions can be made in the confidence that they respect the autonomy of B. This runs the risk of the potentially protective denial of B being eroded.

How might you handle similar circumstances?

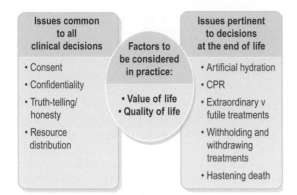

Figure 11.2 Ethical issues in palliative care. CPR, cardiopulmonary resuscitation.

treatment or withholding treatment can be ethically permissible.

Decisions are complicated further when a patient's personal autonomy is reduced. This can occur when the patient may no longer be able to indicate their personal preference as a result of drugs, a progressive deterioration of consciousness, or any disease process that restricts their ability to understand, deliberate or communicate their wishes (or any combination of these). In such circumstances, consideration of actions that would be in the best interests of the patient needs to be determined. This can be facilitated through discussion with close family members or, in their absence, the multiprofessional team providing care. Difficulties can arise because of conflict amongst immediate family or team members when, as individual people, they have differing values about issues at the end of life.

Even with palliative care during the early stages of a disease process there are difficult decisions to be made about the provision of expensive treatments. Such resource allocations are not linked just to individual treatments but to the decisions made by healthcare Trusts about the provision of certain long-term treatments, for example a particular drug treatment for patients with multiple sclerosis that may not be available in all parts of the country. Equally the preferences of patients to die within their home environment may be restricted by the local availability of appropriate care in the community, or the availability of local palliative units within remote rural areas that necessitate family members travelling long distances at a time when they may be increasingly vulnerable.

The Calman & Hine report (1995) went some way to recognise the need to achieve equality in the availability and provision of cancer care, and, as a conse-

quence of this, palliative care, across the country. Such initiatives are to be applauded, but must be acted on continually in order to maximise the benefit to patients who require palliative care regardless of the nature of the cause. Decisions increasingly need to reflect guidance from NICE (2004) regarding palliative care services and provision. The challenge for palliative care providers is how to provide and meet these recommendations within the limited clinical and financial resources available.

The ethics around euthanasia can be debated from many angles, both in support of and against euthanasia. Individuals need to decide what they feel is ethically appropriate. However, while defending the right of individuals to self-determination, it may not be ethically appropriate to request that someone assists in the death of a person if they are not willing to do so, nor if it challenges the professional code with which they work, nor if it challenges the legal circumstances in that country. The concept of euthanasia takes many forms, voluntary or non-voluntary, passive or active. In the utopian world, all symptoms in palliative care could be addressed, not just the physical but the psychological, social and spiritual. In reality healthcare is able to meet only some of these admirable goals, but in striving for them practitioners should never lose sight of the individual patient and their family. Guidelines from the National Council for Palliative Care (NCPC), formerly the National Council for Hospice and Specialist Palliative Care Services (NCHSPCS), have previously focused on the non-acceptance of voluntary euthanasia (NCHSPCS 1992, 1997a). These guidelines have since been withdrawn, but practitioners should be aware of the ethical arguments that underpin both sides of this emotive issue and, as the NCHSPCS guidelines used to, *recognise the right of the individual to request* to be allowed to hasten death, or to refuse treatment that results in the hastening of death, indicating that in these circumstances health professionals should acknowledge and respect the values and wishes of patients uncritically.

ETHICAL THEORIES

Two differing but highly influential ethical theories have influenced the morals of current society. Together with key ethical principles that influence current healthcare provision, these factors form the basis on which the ethical permissibility of clinical decisions across healthcare, and palliative care in particular, are based. An ethical approach to determining whether actions or inactions are ethically permissible, which includes consideration about the quality and the value of life and death, should in turn bring comfort and hope to patients and their families.

In considering clinical decisions or dilemmas there are several ethical approaches that can be used. The two key theoretical approaches introduced in this chapter reflect a duty-based approach, deontology, and a consequence-based approach, consequentialism.

These approaches may involve basing decisions according to a duty that follows certain rules that should always be adhered to, whatever the circumstances. This particular approach is known as *deontology*. Deontological approaches to resolving ethical dilemmas rely upon individuals adhering to specific 'rules'. Actions or inactions are considered to be ethically unacceptable if these rules are contravened. The rules are recognised as categorical imperatives that must apply in all situations: they are universal and include rules of 'not killing' and of 'telling the truth'. Problems for deontological approaches to healthcare arise, for example, when the truth can cause harm to the patient or their family, or when provision of treatment that might have a foreseeable side-effect of harming or ending the life of a patient.

Alternatively, decisions may be based on the potential consequences of one's actions – *consequentialism*. Consequence-based ethical approaches are concerned solely with making decisions according to the consequences that result from the actions of the decision. Consequentialist approaches to ethically permissible decision-making focus on maximising the benefit and minimising the harm of actions or inactions. As such, certain actions may become ethically permissible even if it means that certain 'rules' have to be broken. For example, a consequentialist could argue that it is ethically permissible to hasten the end of the life of a person if the consequences of that action would be to maximise the benefit for the person involved and perhaps for many others. Two forms of consequential style approaches occur: act-utilitarian and rule-utilitarian. The former involves consideration of the good and bad consequences for each individual set of circumstances; the latter involves following actions based on determining the overall consequences in similar circumstances, which then applies to all similar situations.

Although consequentialist approaches to decision-making can appear advantageous to some, the difficulty with determining the ethical permissibility lies in deciding what constitutes 'happiness and harm'. For some people, happiness may be derived from harm. The actual measure of the amount of happiness may cause difficulty in determining the overall consequence of our actions. What may maximise benefit to one person may be only a minor happiness to another, so how can you allocate and distribute a given amount of benefit for the maximum good? Should one person have it all and consequently have a maximised benefit, or should that given benefit be distributed amongst the many to maximise the overall benefit for everyone? Equally, what happens when an individual's happiness is dependent on the harm caused to another person?

These difficulties with a consequential approach to resolving whether actions are ethically permissible are inherent in the manner in which healthcare is distributed amongst populations, the allocation of resources to particular healthcare specialties, how individual healthcare professionals allocate their time to meet the needs of individual patients. However, the goal of all healthcare professionals should be to maximise the benefit of their care for individuals, reflecting a very consequential approach to healthcare delivery.

Other ethical theories exist and have their own particular approach to resolving moral difficulties. However, it is the above two approaches that healthcare professionals frequently encounter in determining the ethical permissibility of their actions.

RIGHTS AND DUTIES

There is an argument that the healthcare professional has a 'duty of care' to the patient. This would include respecting the individuality of the patient and their privacy, preventing harm from occurring to the patient, and consulting and giving information to the patient to enable informed consent to treatments. Professional bodies are required by law to maintain professional registers of those 'licensed' to practise; the Nursing and Midwifery Council (NMC 2004) additionally set a professional code of conduct that outlined the expectations placed on the professional nurse, more or less determining the duty of care that the nurse should provide. Registers for other professionals identify similar 'duties' within their codes of practice.

Such codes of practice reflect a duty-based approach to the provision of healthcare, setting the parameters by which professionals are duty bound to provide care for their patients. When clinically based dilemmas result in conflict between these duty-based guidelines and the consequential approaches of others to care, individual professionals may feel confused. At least this confusion indicates an awareness of the potential for conflict, indicating a questioning profession ready to challenge the sacred cows of practice for practice's sake. The duty of care appears to suggest that there is an ethical obligation to provide the best care, but how can the best available care be determined? Is the caregiver more obligated ethically to provide care that benefits patients or not to provide care that might do them some harm? Is there a greater obligation to remove a hazard that would otherwise certainly cause a harm to your patient, or to provide care that does the patient some good? One may feel ethically obliged to do both, but what if one has the time and resources to do only one thing – which is the greater ethically permissible action?

Recent developments in the Court of Appeal (R [on the application of Burke] v. the General Medical Council 2005) have indicated the continued status quo for competent patients wanting to continue life-sustaining treatments (or refusal of such treatments): for a doctor to go against such a competent expressed wish would be a breach of the doctor's duty of care, and a deliberate interruption or intervention to stop life-prolonging treatment against a patient's expressed wish to be alive would be a breach of the duty of care. This supports the GMC's propositions that a doctor's obligation towards a competent patient is to determine the treatments that are clinically indicated in those circumstances, offering them to the client while explaining the risks, benefits and side-effects. The competent client can then accept or refuse the treatments for reasons that may be totally irrational, or for no reasons at all. Where treatments have not been offered, in circumstances where they are clinically inappropriate, the doctor should discuss the reasoning for this with the patient. There appears to be no legal obligation to provide treatments that are deemed to be clinically inappropriate.

This indicates that the level of duty of care the doctor has in similar circumstances is limited to providing appropriate medically indicated care, in as much that there does not appear to be a duty to provide treatments where they are considered to be clinically inappropriate. Within palliative care the implications are that care needs to be provided where it is clinically indicated, but patients are unable to demand interventions where they are deemed to be inappropriate – that decision is likely to remain with the medical doctors in consultation with the multi-professional team.

PRINCIPLES OF HEALTHCARE ETHICS

Within healthcare there have been widely accepted principles from which the ethical permissibility of actions may be determined. Individual and collective actions are considered in terms of how they respect the four principles and in doing so assist in determining whether the actions or inactions are ethically permissible. Beauchamp & Childress (1994) identified the four ethical healthcare principles as:

- autonomy
- beneficence
- non-maleficence
- justice.

It is these principles that underpin the ethical permissibility of healthcare provision. In addition to these accepted principles, Randall & Downie (1996) originally argued for the inclusion of two further principles that warrant consideration in palliative care:

- compassion
- utility.

These latter principles were in recognition of the ethical problems faced by professionals in resource allocation, where utility is concerned with maximising of outcomes or preferences. Compassion, they argued, enables practitioners to gain insight into the needs and situations of others. In discussing this, they concluded that compassion could not take precedence over other principles but it remained an essential supplement to them. The problem in accepting Randall & Downie's additional two principles, while acknowledging their desirability in palliative care ethics, is that they tend to confuse the moral picture being argued. Compassion may well supplement the principles and provide insight to others' feelings; however, this should be accounted for in the principle of respect for autonomy, while the principle of utility is encompassed by the principle of justice. To consider the two as fundamental healthcare ethical principles in their own right, equating them with other perhaps stronger principles, may lead to added confusion in determining the ethical permissibility of actions.

These principles of healthcare ethics provide the foundations on which clinical palliative care issues can be discussed. The reality of ethical decision-making from such a principle-based approach is that a balance needs to be found between respect for an individual's autonomy and justice, and between doing good and doing no harm; see Figure 11.3.

CLINICAL DECISION-MAKING IN PALLIATIVE CARE

Consideration of ethical principles may indicate the ethical permissibility of actions or inactions, which should be respected by the multiprofessional team.

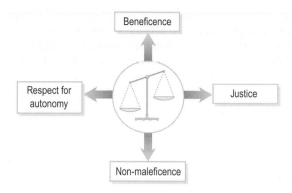

Figure 11.3   The balance of healthcare ethics.

The importance of making ethically permissible clinical decisions can often lead to conflict, depending on the particular philosophical viewpoint held by individuals. Within palliative care, difficult decisions are made that could be considered to result in the foreseeable consequence of hastening the death of the patient, or even of prolonging it unnecessarily. Actions within these decisions need to be ethically permissible. Clinical decisions at the end of life can involve ethical considerations of actions and omissions; killing and letting die; heroic and extraordinary means of treatment; futile treatment, withdrawing treatments, withholding treatments and the Doctrine of Double Effect (DDE). This is in addition to the duty to provide basic care that is required of all healthcare professionals.

A consequentialist clinician may consider that a greater good might come from the premature death of a person as a result of an action intended to benefit the individual in the short term, if this was what they wanted and where continued living would incur further harm to that individual and to others involved in their daily care. This would pose difficulties for deontologists, whose maxim of not-killing prevents notions of early death, regardless of the consequences that may inflict.

In ethical decision-making, the DDE can assist deontological clinicians who need to take actions that they can foresee will cause a harm to a patient (e.g. the use of palliative chemotherapy or radiotherapy where a benefit for a patient might be obtained but with some unpleasant side-effects). The DDE is a *tool*

that determines that, when four specific criteria are met, the foreseeable consequences of some actions are ethically permissible. Twycross (1999) summarises the tool effectively, but in doing so loses some of the significance and implications of the third and fourth conditions.

THE DOCTRINE OF DOUBLE EFFECT

The Doctrine of Double Effect suggests that, given certain conditions, one may not be responsible for the foreseeable effects of actions if they are not intended. The doctrine sets out four conditions that have to be met in order to determine whether the intentional actions are morally permissible despite some foreseen consequence (Campbell & Collinson 1988, p 155):

1. What is done must be, at the least, morally permissible.
2. What is intended must only include the good and not the bad effects of what is done.
3. The bad effects must not be the means whereby the good is brought about.
4. There must be proportionality between the good and bad effects of what is done.

The responsibility of one's actions would appear to depend on the particular arguments that one utilises, particularly with respect to the original intention and to the proportionality of the consequences. Although the DDE indicates moral permissibility for a particular action, it does not suggest whether a particular course of action should be followed at all times. The argument favouring the prescribing of these treatments is that it becomes morally acceptable as long as the intended effect of the treatment is solely to treat the symptom, reducing the suffering. A foreseeable consequence of the treatment is a potentially undesirable effect that may result in the premature death of the patient, but this is not the intention of the original action. This is a classic example of the use of DDE morally to justify what others may argue is the intentional killing of a person.

Issues that influence the balancing of right and wrong at the end of life require consideration of what makes life meaningful and purposeful, and hence valuable. If life is valuable then it becomes wrong to end it prematurely. Recognition should be given to the fact that in palliative care the process of dying combines the concept of an acceptable quality of living with the impending prospect of one's death. That which makes life valuable for the individual can become increasingly worthwhile towards the point of death. The aims of palliative care encompass this.

What contributes to the quality of life for some people may be seeing a distant member of the family, for others attending a performance of an artistic piece of work, for some it is to set their affairs in order and for others it is being able still to walk to the toilet unaided. The aspects that contribute to a quality of life are of subjective individual determination. At some stage in palliative care a decision has to be reached about the care that should be provided. Decisions should involve, whenever possible, the patient, healthcare professionals from the multidisciplinary team and the relatives. Each individual has information and opinion that inform the best possible course of events for the person concerned in order to provide the best possible circumstances that meet the individual's quality of living as they are dying. Healthcare professionals often want a predetermined checklist of quantifiable factors that suggest an appropriate standard of living. Consequently, where the quality of life appears to be minimal or where total suffering becomes unbearably protracted, the issue of death appears to be an increasingly attractive proposition for some. These decisions are, at best, difficult to make, but the resultant actions should always be ethically justifiable.

In the current climate of advancing medical technology and the associated escalating costs of providing treatments, an added complication might be that death could be an appropriate option if the cost of continuing treatments would deprive others of healthcare that enables them to live fuller lives. In the ideal financial healthcare service this should never be a consideration in determining the ethical permissibility of decisions. Decisions that result in hastening the point of death must be challenged by a strong universal prohibition of the killing of patients that stems not only from the duties and responsibilities of healthcare professionals but from the legal and moral values that are held within society.

In circumstances where there are difficult issues that need resolving or further clarification, there could be a case for employing clinically based healthcare ethicists who would be available to consult and advise over particular issues.

ACTS AND OMISSIONS

Traditionally it would be considered morally preferable to omit to provide a care that resulted in harm, rather than acting in a manner that invokes a harm. Rachels (cited by Glover 1977) contends that there is little difference between actions and omissions. He illustrates this using an example of two cousins who stand to inherit substantial amounts on the demise of a third cousin. They plot to end the life of the third cousin. In the first scenario, one cousin enters the bathroom with the intention of drowning the third cousin, and subsequently does so – the action. In a second scenario the other cousin enters the bathroom with the same intention but sees the third cousin slip, knock himself unconscious and disappear under the bath water (it was a deep bath!). He remains in the room but takes no action to intervene, with the result that the third cousin dies. Rachels contended that there is no moral difference between the action or the omission and that we are equally responsible for both actions and omissions. There is no difference between the ethical permissibility of actions or omissions to care.

This has particular relevance to palliative care, especially where treatments are gradually removed towards the end of life (NCHSPCS 1997b), and in particular is applicable to the situation of providing hydration at the end of life by either withdrawal or non-commencement of interventions. More recently such removal of inappropriate interventions at the end of life has been supported within the care of dying pathways advocated by Ellershaw & Wilkinson (2003) and NICE (2004), and is now beginning to be recognised as good practice. Perhaps the greatest significance of this argument is that, if what Rachels contends is acceptable, similar argument suggests that if there is no difference between actions and omissions then there can be no arguable difference between killing and letting die. In palliative care this suggests that it would be equally ethically permissible not to give treatments knowing that the patient will die, and there would be no moral difference between this and deliberately ending the life of the patient. This lays a serious challenge to palliative care principles where carers are unable to take actions or omissions that hasten death, but who work in a culture where it is accepted in specific situations just to provide basic care and allow (let) the patient die.

THE ROLE OF THE NURSE IN ETHICAL DECISION-MAKING

In making ethical decisions the nurse needs to be aware of key ethical principles, of the values that influence the approach to ethical issues and the tools used to justify decisions. Nurses have a role to ensure that there is common understanding and respect of the ethical principles affected by actions, and constructively to debate against issues that would not otherwise be ethically permissible. While doing this, the nurse has a key role in promoting the autonomy of the patient if they are unable to do this for themselves, or if part of their competence is eroded, and in keeping patients informed about decisions involving them if they wish to know. Nurses need to utilise their knowledge about the principles of ethics, awareness of their own values and those imposed on healthcare practitioners, and to give consideration to nursing interventions only where the justification of the care offered is ethically permissible. Being aware of different theories, the nurse is better prepared to come to a balanced and informed decision. Nurses are accountable for their actions: ignorance would not be a defensible justification should harm be incurred by the patient when action or omission was caused by nurses. It becomes a question of whether care given or care omitted is ethically justifiable; this is instigated by the issues raised by extraordinary and futile care.

The nursing role as a member of the multiprofessional team in palliative care will be increasingly involved in approaching difficult decisions towards the end of life, and in supporting those who are having to make such decisions for themselves. The involvement in discussions with clients is evident in local Care of Dying Pathways advocated by Ellershaw & Wilkinson (2003) and Thomas (2003), and in Preferred Place of Care documents (NHS Modernisation Agency 2004 – originated by Lancashire and South Cumbria Cancer Services Network) and Department of Health initiatives such as 'Building on the best: end of life care initiative' in 2005, and indicates a need for all palliative care team members to be aware of the ethical issues that face clients towards the end of their lives.

ORDINARY, EXTRAORDINARY AND FUTILE CARE: THE WITHHOLDING AND WITHDRAWAL OF CARE

As patients come to the end of their lives, the care offered may be seen to be ordinary, in terms of the provision of basic comforts, extraordinary in the continued provision of care and treatments beyond that which might be expected (sometimes described as heroic means), or futile in the sense that it is neither doing the patient any harm but equally it is not benefiting the patient. As previously indicated, determination of the significance of these degrees of care can be perceived as a quality of living/dying on an individualistic basis. What might be seen as futile care for one patient and their family may well be consid-

ered essential to another. The previous section considered the moral significance of acts and omissions, and whether the end result of killing or letting die has a moral significance. The indication was that there could be considered to be little moral significance between letting patients die and killing. Both actions or inactions, the ending of life or allowing to die are similar in their outcomes and there is little arguable difference between these ethical outcomes. However, carers recognise that the deliberate ending of the life of the patient would be morally and legally unacceptable. There could, however, be individual cases where the withholding or withdrawal of treatments, allowing the patient to die, becomes morally permissible when it respects individual autonomy or the futility of continuing to provide care that has no benefit or harm for the patient.

This section considers whether it is appropriate morally to continue to provide ordinary or extraordinary means of treatment for those in receipt of palliative care, and seeks to clarify the position of the clinical debate in palliative care regarding the benefits and harms of hydration and nutrition, and the information healthcare professionals and individual patients require in order to make an informed decision about the needs of the patient. Finally, the issue of whether there is a moral significance between food and hydration as basic need or as therapy is explored.

Rachels (1975) suggests that there is no moral difference between letting someone die and killing them; this is important in healthcare, particularly when healthcare professionals have the knowledge and ability to save the patient. In palliative care, though, patients have diseases that are incurable and eventually result in the patient dying. However, Rachels' position depends on the assumption that one could save the life. If the life cannot be saved then there is little ethical difference between letting the patient die and killing them. This must depend on the quality of the patient's life. The prohibition of killing is strong, but often patients are allowed to die peacefully without the need for active cardiopulmonary resuscitation at all costs. Rachels' argument suggests that the omission of actions is similar to killing the patient – something most professional carers would challenge.

Campbell & Collinson (1988), however, identify two positions where it could be suggested that it may be better to let patients die passively. One is that patients severely damaged by illness and who have poor future prospects in the quality of their lives (however measured) should be allowed to die if that is what they want, or if it is deemed to be in their best interest if they are unable to express their opinion. The second is that 'it may be permissible to let someone die if there is little or no hope of saving them' (p 143).

ORDINARY, EXTRAORDINARY AND FUTILE CARE

An illustration of a patient with little future prospect of a good quality of life and being allowed to die supported by ordinary means can be observed from the current state of the law, identifying the case of *R v. Arthur* in 1981 (cited by Gillon 1986). Dr Arthur provided only ordinary treatment in prescribing analgesics and nursing care after the parents indicated that they did not want their child with Down's syndrome. The baby in his care died shortly afterwards, and Dr Arthur was acquitted of attempted murder. This is an illustration of perhaps what ordinary care is and what it is not. Not to have done anything for the child would have been the equivalent of infanticide, so basic care was provided. The contentious issue in this example is that it was assumed that the baby with Down's syndrome was unable to have a future quality of life, whereas many older people with Down's syndrome live a productive life in the community. The case is used here to illustrate the provision of 'ordinary care' as what one might reasonably expect in order that the patient is kept comfortable. The level of ordinary care would be expected to vary depending on the particular circumstances in which the patient was being treated. In a coronary care unit it would be appropriate for basic care to include the provision of cardiac resuscitation facilities; in palliative care, reasonable ordinary care would be at the level of ensuring the comfort and symptom control of the patient and their family.

The second position offered by Campbell & Collinson (1988) suggests that in letting a person die one may only reasonably cease treatments that could be considered extraordinary or artificial, and that one could not morally deprive a person of the basic necessities of food, water and analgesics. In palliative care one can imagine where it would be entirely inappropriate to allow a patient in terminal stages of their dying process to be operated on to remove a tumour. Even if it were argued that this treatment was what the patient wanted, it would be a case of futile treatment and not of benefit to the patient. However, actions would be taken to provide a holistic basis of care, as the person was dying.

Examples of extraordinary care would include the provision of care beyond that which would be reasonable. If a patient who was expected to live for 6 months was discovered to have a bowel cancer with massive secondary spread that was not responding to any drug-based therapy, it might be considered appropriate to operate to remove some of the cancer if that might relieve some discomfort, but this would be inappropriate if the patient had a prognosis of only 1 week. How far might extraordinary treatment continue to be obliged to be offered if after the operation he suffered a pulmonary embolus, then a heart attack, followed by a chest infection treated with antibiotics, then another heart attack during which he sustained a flail chest, then, while on the ventilator, another severe chest infection? At what point does treatment and intervention during each progressive stage change from being extraordinary and beneficial to being futile and harmful? This depends on individual circumstances – but these are highly subjective, frequently relating to perceptions of quality of life. This series of treatments and interventions may be appropriate if there is a good chance of survival, and the age of the patient may be important, but not necessarily so. What becomes relevant is what the patient wants and balancing their requests for treatment and interventions with the medical indications for the treatments and the potential benefits or burdens that the patient might experience.

Whether care can be described as ordinary, extraordinary or futile depends on the individual nature of the patient, their condition and diagnosis, and their current circumstances. What in palliative care counts as ordinary and extraordinary means? Palliative care should provide ordinary care, but is ordinary care considered to be the same level of provision for all patients and for all types of care? For example, although most patients would want safety, analgesia, water and food, some may prefer aromatherapy, some reflexology, and each patient would consider their treatment ordinary. What some people want in the form of treatment may not be the choice of others. This individualism makes it difficult to determine exactly what constitutes ordinary care, and needs to be discussed with the patient along with the implications of the interventions. In such cases is it easier to consider ordinary treatment as being required or indicated treatment, and extraordinary treatments being beyond that of basic care. It is difficult to quantify this for individual patients. A course of radiotherapy may be considered to be ordinary treatment for a particular patient with a tumour that responds well to radiotherapy (reducing its mass), whereas it may become extraordinary for the same patient at a later period in their dying when the difficulty of transportation and lack of mobility mean that travelling to the radiotherapy centre becomes too hard for the patient. The benefit would become outweighed by the suffering. What does become apparent is that it is the individual perception of the quality of the care that gives it importance, and not whether healthcare professionals perceive the care to be ordinary, extraordinary or futile. The moral significance is the perceived benefit or burden of the care or treatment, and this is related to the quality of life/dying as perceived by the patient.

Patients at the end of life often require medical intervention through drugs and physical treatments such as peripheral intravenous hydration and nasogastric feeding. Such treatments may arguably prolong unnecessary suffering and extend a period of dying. The converse argument is one where the value of life is deemed to be so high, even up to the point of death, that all treatments are justified. It is difficult to determine whether ordinary, extraordinary or futile care is individually of moral significance; what does become apparent, and is perhaps of moral importance, is the benefit or the burden of the treatment or care for the patient.

THE MORAL SIGNIFICANCE BETWEEN LEVELS OF CARE AND WITHHOLDING AND WITHDRAWAL OF CARE

Withholding treatment would be the non-provision or omission of treatment that might be of benefit to the patient or that might prolong their suffering. The latter example would indicate a moral obligation to provide basic care, as withholding analgesia would be morally wrong for a patient in pain. Conversely, withholding antibiotics from a terminally ill patient in a coma at the end of their life who then develops an infection that is unlikely to cause further suffering, may arguably be morally acceptable in that the treatment is futile because the antibiotics are unlikely to change the course of events.. The two differ in that, while one treatment is essential, the other could be futile. Neither treatment by itself is morally inappropriate. What becomes important is whether 'this treatment is likely to provide this patient benefits that are sufficient to make it worthwhile to endure the burdens that accompany the treatment' (Lynn & Childress 1986, p 223).

ARTIFICIAL HYDRATION VERSUS DEHYDRATION; NUTRITION VERSUS STARVATION

When determining the level of benefit and burden for the patient, healthcare professionals need to decide on the level of obligation that the care will have. It is likely that the provision of food, water and analgesia will be of benefit to the majority of patients. This determines the level of obligation to provide basic care. However, there may be situations where the treatment may be so rare or costly, so complex or invasive, that the balance between the benefits and the burdens becomes less clear. In such instances there should be adequate reasons to justify the withholding of such treatment to the competent patient, and to those who are acting in the best interests of the incompetent patient. As basic care there appears to be a moral obligation to provide nutrition and hydration where the benefit for the patient outweighs any disadvantages.

In the recent medical past artificial hydration was not possible; it then became cost-effective and is now accepted as standard care, being less costly than some other more invasive treatments or interventions. The same pattern of reducing cost may well occur with the overall cost of transplantation in today's healthcare service, or the supply of costly drugs to patients in palliative care. Artificial treatments may currently be withheld because of present costs, but in the near future they may become standard care with the benefits (for the patient) of the costs outweighing the burden to healthcare providers.

The provision of nutrition and hydration may be appropriate to maintain the comfort of the patient in palliative care. This may well extend their life by a small amount, but if this is the patient's wish then provision of care is appropriate. In other cases hydration and nutrition do not appear to be needed (except to satisfy family needs), and may be contraindicated if they become an unnecessary burden for the patient; at this point the care may appropriately be withheld.

Where a course of treatment has been commenced it may be difficult to withdraw it and stop this particular aspect of care; this appears to be different from withholding care. Should a peripheral intravenous infusion be re-established if the line has become blocked? – If it extravasates; or if it is accidentally pulled out by the agitated patient in terminal care; or should the peripheral infusion be withdrawn? There appears to be a difference in direct actions that result in withdrawing care than not commencing, or omitting to commence, aspects of care in the first place. The moral significance of acts and omissions has been discussed above; however, what is perhaps important to note is the benefit/burden analysis in determining the patient's best interests. The problem in attaching a great deal of moral significance to continuing a treatment at all costs would be the temptation not to commence the treatment (withholding it) so as not to become legally obliged to provide treatments that were not of long-term benefit to the patient.

IS THE WITHHOLDING AND WITHDRAWAL OF ARTIFICIAL CARE MORALLY SIGNIFICANT?

The maintenance of homeostasis is important in maintaining the normal cellular functioning of the body. Once dehydrated and with no ability or opportunity to hydrate, the physiological response of the body is frequently that cellular metabolism becomes anaerobic, this in turn leading to increasing toxicity of waste products in the patient's blood, and to cerebral confusion, drowsiness and eventual death. What has to be asked is whether that manner of death is preferable to one that may be painful, drawn out, prolonging the psychological and physical suffering of both the patient and their family. The effect of the intervention could be perceived to be either a benefit or a burden.

In palliative care, issues that arise from the question of the potential beneficial aspects of artificial hydration are similar to those of basic oral hydration. Is there is an advantage that overrides the burden of artificial hydration? Following medical sedation in terminal care, should patients be allowed to become dehydrated and should basic comfort be maintained? The effects of hydration in palliative care are argued to be inconclusive: while benefiting some aspects of care, there is equal evidence suggesting that hydration may be detrimental to palliative care (Fox 1996, Malone 1994, Musgrave 1990, Roberts 1997, Stone 1993). Dehydration may improve the analgesic effect by relief of oedema, reducing need for opiates and reducing the risk of constipation that results from opiate usage. In dyspnoeic patients, the benefits of dehydration include a lowering of pulmonary secretions, reducing the feeling of drowning and discomfort of suctioning. Problems with dehydration include dry mouth and increased risk of pressure sore formation, which can both be cared for by implementing basic nursing care. Equally there are the psychological and emotional aspects of hydration that need to be considered as well as the physiological benefits.

Craig (1994), while focusing on the aspects of artificial hydration during sedation, addressed these issues by recognising that in oncology and palliative care there are patients who are unable to maintain their own hydration. Some who, as a result of their disease process, became unable to swallow might with artificial hydration have been able to derive some benefit from the remaining period of palliative care. Realistically, however, the medical intervention of providing artificial hydration would only prolong the inevitable death of the patient. Craig postulated that care must be taken to avoid certain mistaken diagnoses that may lead to an omission of hydration, as when the cause is rectified the patient may make a full recovery. She acknowledged that some patients will wish to eat and drink as long as they can, but where patients decide they no longer wish to eat or drink as a natural consequence of the disease process it would be inappropriate for them to continue to be artificially hydrated. She focused on the question of whether long-term artificial hydration is beneficial and whether the treatment is seen by the patient to be a benefit or a burden in sustaining life, concluding that this is an individual situation that requires individual assessment. In maintaining the comfort of the patient Craig recognised that their physical and psychological needs are paramount and that intravenous infusions need not hinder the provision of basic care. Patients who experience the effects of sore mouths or pressure sore formation can receive individually assessed care to improve their comfort. Craig suggested that there is a moral obligation to provide artificial hydration when patients have been sedated for a long period, but that this might not necessarily be so during the last few hours or even day(s) of life.

Differences with some of Craig's opinions have been expressed in a response by Gillon (1994), who indicated that there is no moral significance between killing and letting die (supporting the arguments of Rachels)

> withholding or withdrawing non-beneficial or positively harmful medical interventions would or might result in the patient's death earlier than would have been the case if the medical intervention had been instituted or maintained does not, it is widely agreed, demonstrate that such withholding or withdrawing is either wrong or illegal.
>
> (Gillon 1994, p 131)

Dunlop et al (1995) argued that, while Craig focuses on medical conditions that rightly require nutrition and/or hydration, there exist in palliative care indications that decision-making processes should be made on a risks and benefits balance of care and that there is no clear evidence that comfort is affected by artificial hydration. Again in support of the non-provision of artificial hydration due to assessment of the relevant benefits/burdens, the care for terminally ill dehydrated patients is discussed by De Ridder & Gastmans (1996), who, while pointing out the potential benefits and ill-effects of dehydration, suggest that treatment does not necessarily support the commencement of intravenous hydration, and that the overall management of such patients is required by the multidisciplinary team and not just the medical team who, in this later paper, acknowledges that in certain instances withdrawal of hydration is acceptable, citing, amongst others, the legal aspects of Bland (see below).

THE SIGNIFICANCE OF ARTIFICIAL NUTRITION AND HYDRATION AS BASIC REQUIREMENTS OR THERAPY

Artificial hydration may be morally withheld and withdrawn where it is in the best interests of the patient. This situation is illustrated by the case of Airedale NHS Trust v. Bland (1993). Anthony Bland was kept alive by artificial nutrition and hydration through a nasogastric tube. Following a protracted legal case it was decided that as the prime object of medical care was to benefit the patient, and that given there was a body of responsible medical opinion, continued treatment of provision of artificial nutrition and hydration was not beneficial to the patient in this instance, that the principle of the sanctity of life was not challenged by the cessation of medical treatment, particularly as the patient had been in a persistent vegetative state for more than 3 years. The argument used was that since the patient had no further interest in being kept alive (this was helped by Anthony Bland's father agreeing to this as it had been his son's wishes not to be kept alive) the justification of continued medical invasive treatment was no longer required. Therefore the doctors were no longer under an obligatory duty to continue treatment to keep Anthony alive, and cessation of the invasive medical treatment would not be unlawful. The judgement made two points that feeding artificially was therapy and that therapy can be withheld or withdrawn if it is not in the patient's best interests.

The issue of whether hydration or nutrition is or is not provided appears to be of less consequence than the issue of how that decision has been arrived at. What is significant is the assessment of the benefit or burden for the patient. In some instances it can be argued that medical indications require the intervention of hydration; in other circumstances medical indications do not support the continued hydration of patients at the end of life. If a patient indicates that they wish to continue to be hydrated at the end of their life, and there are no potential medical complications as a result of this treatment, then the patient's autonomous wishes should be respected as, for individual reasons, the patient may wish to maximise the value of their life by prolonging their moment of death. This may be important for them for emotional or spiritual reasons, or because they fear dying. The basic nursing care within such situations should be directed towards the provision of physical comfort and psychological support of the patient and their family. The converse aspect is that patients may fear a prolonged painful death; while appropriate symptom control should be provided as the basis of palliative care, this may not necessarily entail the provision of hydration or nutrition, particularly when after consultation with the patient, the patient and the medical team agree not to continue or to commence hydration, resulting in the eventual death of the patient. Such an arrangement should always be in the best interest of the patient. The Bland case illustrates the moral significance of regarding artificial hydration and nutrition as therapy, and that therapy may be legally withdrawn only if permitted by the legal system when it is judged to be in the patient's best interests.

The moral significance becomes that, for either competent or incompetent patients, the withholding or withdrawal of treatments and therapies must always be made in the best interest of the patient. Dunphy & Randall (1997, p 127) summarised the relevant issues appropriately:

> It seems reasonable to assert that the unilateral wholesale rejection of artificial hydration is as inappropriate in the care of individual patients as the assertion that all patients should have drips . . . It is no more defensible to provide or omit a drip purely on the basis of the wishes of the relative than it is on the basis of the culture of the admitting unit . . . The issues of primary ethical or legal significance will be the wishes of the competent patient, the previously expressed competent wishes of the presently incompetent patient . . . and clinical judgements of 'best interest'.

Hydration and nutrition would appear to be deemed to be medical interventions that may be morally withdrawn should competent dying patients indicate that this respects their wishes. The withholding or withdrawal of treatments of patients who are not competent to make decisions should be made in the best interests of the patient, taking note of any previous indications of previously stated preferences. The withdrawal or withholding of treatment does not, however, relate to the basic provision and duty of care towards the patient; there are occasions when hydration or nutrition is medically indicated that can enable the dying patient to maintain or even improve their quality of life.

Indications for good practice in palliative care regarding the artificial hydration for people who are terminally ill were recently identified by the National Council for Palliative Care (2005b). The recommendations focus on the individual nature of each case, and reflect the opinion that as artificial hydration in the terminally ill has little if any influence on the survival or symptom control of patients (Musgrave et al 1995) then the responsibility lies with the clinical team to decide the benefits and burdens indicating the appropriateness of hydration on an individual basis. Where hydration is not deemed to be appropriate, the NCPC recommends the use of frequent oral care to prevent unpleasant side-effects of a sore mouth, and that relatives are provided with the necessary information to address their anxieties. Such decisions are made on the understanding that competent patients have a right to refuse artificial hydration, even where it may be medically indicated, and that advanced indicators from incompetent patients enable them to retain similar rights. Similar guidelines have been issued for the debate surrounding cardiopulmonary resuscitation (CPR) in palliative care (NCHSPCS 1997c), about which similar ethical debates surrounding the ethical permissibility of withholding or acting to provide CPR can be made.

CONCLUSION

Ethical decisions are made daily within all aspects of healthcare. The uniqueness for the individual in receipt of palliative care requires carers to place emphasis on appropriate professional care. Active consideration must be given to the respect of the four key healthcare principles and to the manner in which decisions are justified. Consideration of ethics enables the care provided to be ethically permissible. This becomes significant in maintaining the quality of palliative care provided by the multiprofessional team.

With the changing nature of healthcare, the advances in medical science and the limitations of finances and resources placed on palliative care, there has to be specific provision for ensuring that the permissibility of actions or inaction are based on sound ethical principles. As the member of the team who liaises with all other team members, the patient and their family, it would be appropriate for the nurse to have an increasingly important role in ensuring that there is a sound ethical basis for care decisions reached by the multidisciplinary team. An increasing professional awareness about ethics and the influence and application of ethics to clinical practice has become a common theme in both pre- and post-registration nurse education. Consequently nurses should be in a position to recognise when key ethical principles are being respected and, perhaps more importantly, when clinically based decisions do not respect ethical principles. All professional carers should be active in raising their personal awareness about the ethical issues at the end of life. These issues are likely to become increasingly complex, and this will continue to challenge the position of both personal and professional codes of conduct and the actions that carers may wish to take.

The dissatisfied dead will not be able to question our ethical reasoning. On reflection, nurses and all health professionals have a duty of care to their patients, particularly where they are placed in a vulnerable state and increasingly depend on professionals to assist in decision-making processes, that all care and interventions are based on good practice that can be ethically justifiable. Ethical justification of actions or omissions in providing or withholding or withdrawing care are influenced by the law, by professional codes of conduct, by personal individual and societal values, and by our cultural and religious beliefs. The uniqueness of palliative care requires an honest appraisal of decisions, particularly on the behalf of patients whose autonomy is compromised. In ensuring that our decision-making is ethically justifiable, professional health carers can ensure that they can provide consistency, and bring comfort and hope to patients and their families.

The recent developments with the Mental Capacity Act 2005, influencing and determining capacity and the status of advanced decisions, combined with rulings resulting from Burke v. GMC and its subsequent appeal in July 2005, and taken together with the current focus on the potential for moving towards legalisation that allows for voluntary active euthanasia for people who are terminally ill, will continue to present ethical challenges for clinical decisions in palliative care, particularly for those where the end of life is imminent. Clinical initiatives such as the Care of Dying Pathways and Preferred Place of Care initiatives will work to enable difficult discussions to be held and recorded by the multiprofessional palliative care team. This should enhance the ethical decision-making process.

However, at the centre of all the prolonged deliberating and ethical and legal arguing, professionals should not take their focus from the person at the centre of all this debate – the patient, their situation and the manner of their dying. The professional needs to focus on supporting a dignified quality of living, and ensure that dignity continues alongside the dying, and beyond the point of death.

At some point we will all have to ask ourselves, albeit hopefully in the far-off future, 'What is it that I want? . . .', and hope that the professionals involved in our care will be understanding and enabling.

References

Airedale NHS Trust v. Bland 1 All ER 821 1993 4 Med LR 39–75

Beauchamp T L, Childress J F 1994 Principles of biomedical ethics, 4th edn. Oxford University Press, Oxford

Burke R (on the application of) v General Medical Council & Ors (2005) EWCA Civ 1003

Calman K, Hine D 1995 A policy framework for commissioning cancer services. Department of Health, London

Campbell R, Collinson D 1988 Ending lives. Blackwell, Oxford

Craig G M 1994 On withholding nutrition and hydration in the terminally ill: has palliative medicine gone too far? Journal of Medical Ethics 20:139–143

Craig G M 1996 On withholding artificial hydration and nutrition from terminally ill sedated patients. The debate continues. Journal of Medical Ethics 22:147–153

Department of Health 2005 Building on the best: end of life care initiative. Deparmtne of Health, London

De Ridder D, Gastmans C 1996 Dehydration among terminally ill patients: an integrated ethical and practical approach for caregivers. Journal of Nursing Ethics 3(4):305–316

Dunlop R J, Ellershaw J E, Baines M J, Sykes N, Saunders C M 1995 On withholding nutrition and hydration in the terminally ill: has palliative medicine gone too far? A reply. Journal of Medical Ethics 21:141–143

Dunphy K, Randall F 1997 Ethical decision-making in palliative care. European Journal of Palliative Care 4(4):126–128

Ellershaw J, Wilkinson S 2003 Care of the dying: a pathway to excellence. Oxford University Press, Oxford

Finlay I G, Wheatley V J, Izdebski C 2005 The House of Lords Select Committee on the Assisted Dying for the Terminally Ill Bill: implications for specialist palliative care. Palliative Medicine 19:444–453

Fox E T 1996 IV hydration in the terminally ill: ritual or therapy? British Journal of Nursing 5(1):41–45

Gillon R 1986 Philosophical medical ethics. John Wiley, Chichester

Gillon R 1994 Editorial: Palliative care ethics: non-provision of artificial nutrition and hydration to terminally ill sedated patients. Journal of Medical Ethics 20:131–132, 187

Glover J 1977 Causing death and saving lives. Penguin, London

Kade W J 2000 Death with dignity: a case study. Annals of Internal Medicine 132(6):504–506

Lords Hansard 2006 Assisted Dying for the Terminally Ill Bill (HL) Vol. 681:60512–01

Lynn J, Childress J F 1986 Must patients always be given food and water? In: Weir R F (ed.) Ethical issues in death and dying, 2nd edn. Columbia University Press, New York

Malone N 1994 Hydration in the terminally ill patient. Nursing Standard 8(43):29–32

Musgrave C F 1990 Terminal dehydration; to give or not to give intravenous fluids? Cancer Nursing 13(1):62–66

Musgrave C F, Bartal N, Opstad J 1995 The sensation of thirst in dying patients receiving IV hydration. Journal of Palliative Care 11(4):17–21

National Council for Hospice and Specialist Palliative Care Services 1992 Key ethical issues in palliative care: evidence to the House of Lords Select Committee on Medical Ethics. Occasional Paper 3. NCHSPCS, London

National Council for Hospice and Specialist Palliative Care Services 1997a Voluntary euthanasia: the Council's view. NCHSPCS, London

National Council for Hospice and Specialist Palliative Care Services 1997b Changing gear – guidelines for managing the last days of life in adults. NCHSPCS, London

National Council for Hospice and Specialist Palliative Care Services 1997c Ethical decision-making in palliative care: cardiopulmonary resuscitation (CPR) for people who are terminally ill. NCHSPCS, London

National Council for Palliative Care 2005a Guidance on the Mental Capacity Act 2005. NCPC, London

National Council for Palliative Care 2005b Artificial hydration for people who are terminally ill. NCPC, London

National Council for Palliative Care 2006 Response to The Assisted Dying for the Terminally Ill Bill 2005. NCPC, London

National Institute for Clinical Excellence 2004 Guidance on cancer services: improving supportive and palliative care for adults with cancer. NICE, London

NHS Modernisation Agency 2004 Preferred place of care. Department of Health, London

Nursing and Midwifery Council 2004 The Professional Code of Conduct for Nurses, Midwives and Health Visitors. NMC, London

Oregon Department of Human Services 2006 Eighth annual report on Oregon's Death with Dignity Act. Department of Human Services, Oregon

Rachels J 1975 Active and passive euthanasia. In: Singer P (ed.) 1986 Applied ethics. Oxford University Press, Oxford, p 29–36

Randall F, Downie R S 1996 Palliative care ethics: a good companion. Oxford University Press, Oxford

Roberts A L 1997 Dehydration and the dying patient. International Journal of Palliative Nursing 3(3):156–160

Stone C 1993 Prescribed hydration in palliative care. British Journal of Nursing 2(7):353–357

The Mental Capacity Act 2005 HMSO, London

Thomas K 2003 Caring for the dying at home: companions on the journey. Radcliffe Medical Press, Abingdon

Twycross R 1999 Introducing palliative care, 2nd edn. Radcliffe Medical Press, Oxford

Chapter **12**

The Liverpool Care Pathway (LCP) for the dying patient

Anita Roberts and Maureen Gambles

INTRODUCTION

Despite all of the advances in medicine, the fact remains that each and every one of us will die at some point in time. Death and dying are often regarded as taboo subjects but recently have started to gain more prominence. End-of-life care is being recognised as a discrete and important aspect of healthcare delivery. It requires specialist management and is the responsibility of all professionals caring for dying patients. The importance of this issue is reflected not only in prestigious medical journals such as the *British Medical Journal,* which devoted an entire issue to these topics in 2003, but also through mainstream media such as the recently televised BBC production 'How to have a good death' (March 2006) and current government policy (Department of Health [DoH] 2006).

Medical technological advances in the 20th century resulted in healthcare that was focused towards the medical model of disease, diagnosis and cure. This resulted in the marginalisation of care for patients who were dying from advanced disease. These patients were often not even told that they had incurable illness, and symptom control was relatively poor. The importance of psychological, social and spiritual care was often not recognised and, therefore, not adequately addressed.

In the 1960s the pioneering work of Dame Cicely Saunders was the catalyst for the development of the modern hospice movement. This hospice movement recognised the tension between the need for appropriate and effective care for patients dying from advanced disease and the increasingly prevalent 'cure focused' model of healthcare in the National Health Service (NHS). The palliative care approach, pioneered by the hospice movement, promoted the quality of life of patients and their families via the prevention and relief of suffering through early identification and impeccable assessment and treatment of physical, psychological and spiritual concerns and problems.

The hospice movement continued to develop this model of best practice in the provision of care at the end of life. However, this was accomplished largely in the voluntary sector and evolved separately from mainstream healthcare. Despite the increasing expertise and the proliferation of hospices (and to some extent, specialist palliative care services), the majority of people continued to die in the acute setting (Higginson 2003) where the medical model prevailed and the focus remained firmly on cure.

In recent years the imperative to provide quality care to *all* dying patients and their families has become a feature of UK government policy. In 2000, the Cancer Plan (DoH 2000) highlighted a lack of resources in mainstream healthcare that was undermining the provision of high-quality end-of-life care for patients dying from cancer. In 2004, the End of Life Care Initiative (EOLI) extended the focus to encompass the care of all dying patients regardless of diagnosis. In particular, the EOLI focused on the implementation of three frameworks aimed at promoting best practice in end-of-life care: the Liverpool Care Pathway for the dying patient (LCP); the Gold Standards Framework (GSF) and the Preferred Place of Care document (PPC). In the same year, the LCP framework was identified as recommended practice within the National Institute for Clinical Excellence guidance on supportive and palliative care (NICE 2004), and more recently the government White Paper 'Our health, our choice, our say: a new direction for community services' (DoH 2006) prioritised the need for training and recommended roll-out of the LCP across the UK.

WHAT ARE INTEGRATED CARE PATHWAYS?

Integrated care pathways (ICPs) gained prominence within the British healthcare system in the 1990s. However, the original concept developed within the USA as a model for assessing quality in engineering by defining processes and auditing variances and outcomes (Overill 2003). Karen Zander, a nurse educator from Massachusetts, is credited with recognising the salience of such principles for the effective and consistent delivery of healthcare in the USA in the 1980s. Clinicians saw the need to redefine care delivery and identify outcomes in a measurable way as a means of demonstrating high-quality yet cost-effective care (Overill 2003).

Development of these pathways requires consensus by multidisciplinary teams to agree a comprehensive and holistic process for a specific episode of care that is anchored in available evidence-based practice. The function of care pathways is to map the required care for a specific clinical condition and attempt to describe all of the tasks that should be undertaken together with the timing and sequence of those tasks. The resultant multidisciplinary documentation, which generally replaces all existing documentation, then acts as a template that guides practitioners to deliver appropriate care and enables the recording of outcomes. The ability to record essential clinical information in a way that is easy to complete results in a more comprehensive and concise clinical record that can be easily interrogated for audit purposes (Baker 1996).

However, use of an ICP is in no way meant to replace clinical judgement and decision-making. Whenever clinicians feel that the prescribed course of action is not the most appropriate one for a given individual, or it is not possible to undertake a particular action in a given circumstance, it is perfectly acceptable to deviate from the ICP by recording the variation in practice ('variance') on the documentation. A clear indication of the rationale underpinning the decision or reason for deviation is then also documented, along with subsequent actions taken. The combination of the provision of guidance and the ongoing recording of progress and 'variance' is what differentiates an ICP from a clinical guideline.

Campbell et al (1998) suggested that well constructed ICPs have the potential to:

- facilitate the introduction of guidelines and systematic and continuing audit into clinical practice
- improve multidisciplinary communication and care planning
- reach or exceed existing quality standards
- decrease unwanted variation in practice
- improve clinician–patient communication
- identify research and development questions.

Non-randomised studies examining a variety of clinical areas have reported a number of benefits, including a reduction in the length of stay in hospital (e.g. Weingarten et al 1993), a reduction in the costs of patient care (e.g. Trubo 1993), improved patient outcomes (such as quality of life and reduced complications – e.g. Mosher et al 1992, Ogilvie-Harris et al 1993), increased patient satisfaction with the service (e.g. Stead et al 1995), improved communication between doctors and nurses (e.g. Hoyle et al 1994), increased participation of patient or carer(s) in patient care (e.g. Williams et al 1993) and reduction in the time spent by health staff in carrying out paperwork (e.g. Trubo 1993).

Some randomised controlled trials examining the effectiveness of ICPs for patient and organisational outcomes in acute and rehabilitative stroke care have been reported in a systematic review (Kwan & Sandercock 2005). Although no evidence was found that the use of a care pathway provided significant additional benefit over conventional multidisciplinary care in terms of death or discharge destination, there was some evidence that use of an ICP may be associated with fewer urinary tract infections and readmissions, and more comprehensive use of computed tomography brain scans. They concluded that the impact of care pathways on length of stay and hospitalization was still unclear and that more detailed research was required. It could be argued that it is not surprising that the studies did not detect any discernible differences as stroke units, like hospices, already offer a model of best practice for a specific cohort of patients. The real benefits of a pathway could be to transfer this high standard of care into the generalist arena, and this became the imperative for the development of an ICP for care of the dying patient.

DEVELOPMENT OF THE LCP

Developing an ICP to guide the delivery of palliative care in its entirety is fraught with challenge because of the inherent complexity and wide-ranging nature of this specialty. Increasingly, the principles of good palliative care are seen as being important from the point of initial diagnosis of advancing disease to death. It would have been unrealistic to attempt to establish a pathway of care that could meet the needs of all patients throughout such a complex and protracted care trajectory. It was, therefore, vital to identify an important, yet discrete and time-bound, element of palliative care that could be mapped successfully. To this end, in the late 1990s the Hospital Specialist Palliative Care Team (HSPCT) at the Royal Liverpool and Broadgreen University Hospitals NHS Trust, together with staff from the Marie Curie Hospice in Liverpool, identified ICPs as a way to improve care for dying patients and their families.

Although the hospice and hospital environments were clearly very different, it was felt that the development of an ICP to translate the hospice model of best practice in care for the dying into a template of care for use by ward staff in the acute setting would empower generalist workers and improve care for patients and families. By enabling ward staff to manage the majority of expected deaths appropriately, it would also allow the HSPCT to concentrate its efforts into supporting patients and families with more complex specialist need.

Defining the scope of the document

A multidisciplinary working party made up of those professionals representing elements of care felt to be important in the dying phase was set up. Included were representatives from nursing, palliative medicine, social work, pastoral care, pharmacy, members of the pilot wards teams and an ICP coordinator. It was important that the group also included representation from senior management within the Trust to ensure executive endorsement of the project.

The next step was to identify examples of best practice in care of the dying. Appropriate outcomes in palliative care are often difficult to define and measure owing to the complexity of the specialty, and the literature provides many examples of the challenges inherent in conducting research in this area (Rinck et al 1997, Westcombe et al 2003). However, literature searches were undertaken to identify any existing evidence regarding end-of-life care on which to base the document. Although the evidence base was limited, this search identified a number of symptoms that were commonly experienced in the dying phase. These are illustrated in Box 12.1.

Alongside these sources of 'external' evidence it was also important to identify current practice at the university hospital. Data were gathered to identify the number of 'expected' deaths per annum across the hospital and the wards on which they occurred. From this information, it was possible to identify wards that frequently cared for dying patients. Two of these wards were selected as pilot wards for the implementation phase at the hospital.

Box 12.1 Symptoms commonly experienced in the dying phase

Main symptoms	Other symptoms
Excessive respiratory tract secretions	Inability to swallow
Pain	Constipation
Restlessness	Bleeding
Dyspnoea	Seizures
Nausea and vomiting	

A retrospective audit of a subset of the case notes of patients who had died recently on the two identified 'pilot' wards was then undertaken in order to establish how care was routinely being delivered and recorded. This audit revealed that the standard of documentation of the care of the dying patient was relatively poor. This exercise provided useful information regarding the potential role of the pathway in improving documentation and care.

Medical and nursing staff are often exposed to death and its aftermath, and when things don't go to plan they can be left feeling extremely demoralised. They can experience feelings of helplessness and failure when their knowledge and understanding of symptom management and appropriate care in the dying phase is lacking. In order to establish the level of knowledge and understanding of medical and nursing staff prior to implementation of the pathway, questionnaires were distributed to all staff on the pilot wards. These questionnaires sought information about symptom control and other elements of appropriate care. There was also space for staff to provide examples of how care of the dying could be improved on their ward. It was clear from the results of the questionnaires that knowledge and understanding of palliative care drugs and control of end-of-life symptoms varied enormously. Organisational and environmental issues such as the lack of private space and an inability to provide such things as hot drinks for families were also very apparent. It was interesting that there was a view that improvement in the quality of care for dying patients and their families could be achieved only by employing more specialist palliative care nurses. This suggested that care of the dying was perceived to be a specialist area of care rather than integral to the role of ward-based staff.

A focus group involving nurses from the pilot wards was set up to explore their perceptions of caring for dying patients. They were asked to talk about their experiences of 'good' and 'bad' deaths in an attempt to understand better the environment in which the new pathway would function. The nurses were able to identify many factors that influenced their experiences. Poor symptom management, poor communication between staff and families, and lack of facilities were often associated with the perception of a 'bad death'. Conversely, good symptom management, minimal invasive procedures or treatments, and relatives being present at the time of death were more often associated with the perception of a 'good death'.

The working group considered all of the 'evidence' and information gathered during this process with the aim of developing a draft pathway that could be piloted and refined via a continuous and cyclical process. It became clear that, to influence the culture of death and dying in the acute sector in a positive way, the pathway would need not only to guide the delivery of appropriate holistic care in the dying phase, but also to take into account those organisational and environmental issues that impact on the experiences of patients and families. Four major stages of care emerged as essential elements of the pathway:

1. Recognition that the patient has entered the dying phase
2. Assessment of the needs of the patient (and family) and initiation of appropriate care
3. Ongoing assessment and care delivery
4. Care after death.

In addition, it was apparent that the pathway would need to address the physical, social, psychological and spiritual aspects of care for patients and families. Developing a pathway that embraced all of these issues would result in a relevant and useful document that could be used to structure appropriate care for patients dying in the acute setting (Fig. 12.1).

Developing the document

The steering group used the evidence gathered to identify key outcomes and goals. There was also further consultation and development of the initial

Framework of LCP document

1 Aim
- To improve care of the dying in the last hours/days of life

2 Key themes
- Knowledge and process
- Quality

3 Key sections in LCP
- Initial assessment
- Ongoing care
- Care after death

4 Key domain in LCP
- Physical
- Psychological
- Social
- Spiritual

Figure 12.1   Framework of the LCP document.

ideas with the community palliative care nurses and hospice specialists. The LCP is structured into three main sections: initial assessment, ongoing assessment and care after death (Table 12.1). However, before the development of these main sections it was important that attention be paid to how and when the decision to commence a pathway should be made. To avoid the pathway from being used inappropriately, consideration was given to how clinicians make the diagnosis that a patient has entered the dying phase.

Recognising that the patient has entered the dying phase

It is essential that clinicians are able to 'diagnose dying', yet this is an extremely complex process. Clinicians may be reluctant to make such a diagnosis if there is hope that the patient's condition may improve. This is particularly so in the acute setting as the prevailing culture is aimed at cure with an associated pressure to continue investigations, invasive procedures and treatments rather than focus on maintaining the comfort of the patient.

It is crucial that staff are able to recognise the key signs and symptoms seen in the dying phase. However, the predictability of the dying phase may vary depending on which disease the patient has. For example, with cancer patients death may sometimes be unanticipated (e.g. fatal haemorrhage), but more commonly is preceded by gradual deterioration in the patient's general condition. The patient will often become:

- bedbound
- semicomatose
- able to take only sips of fluid
- unable to take oral medication.

With other incurable illnesses the dying trajectory may differ. In heart failure, for example, it is particularly difficult to predict when death is imminent as worsening heart failure is not always due to an irreversible underlying pathology and corrective action may bring about a worthwhile remission (Ellershaw & Ward 2003). However, even here there are some indicators that may suggest the prognosis is very poor and alert staff to the fact that the patient may be entering the last few days of life. Such patients often (Ellershaw & Ward 2003):

- have repeated admissions with worsening heart failure
- have no identifiable reversible cause
- are receiving optimal tolerated medication

- have deteriorating renal function
- fail to respond to changes in medication (e.g. diuretics or vasodilators) within 2–3 days.

Other diseases will have slightly different trajectories and challenges, but the most important elements in diagnosing dying are that:

- all reversible causes have been considered
- the patient fails to improve despite receiving optimal care
- the multidisciplinary team members caring for the patient have discussed and agreed that the patient is dying.

Once the team is in agreement that the patient is likely to be in the last days of their life, care can be revised appropriately. The criteria for starting to use the LCP for a particular patient (Fig. 12.2) were developed as a general guide to assist decision-making.

It is also very important to remember that the LCP is a document that is put in place because it represents the most appropriate care for a patient who is deemed to be in the dying phase. If the patient's condition does improve at any time and it is considered that the patient is no longer dying, the LCP should be discontinued and management refocused appropriately.

The initial assessment – assessing the needs of the patient (and family) and initiating appropriate care

Section 1 begins with the initial physical assessment of the patient that provides a snapshot of their

---

Criteria for use of the LCP

• All possible reversible causes for current condition have been considered

• The multiprofessional team has agreed that the patient is dying, and two of the following may apply:–

The patient is bedbound ☐

Only able to take sips of fluids ☐

Semi-comatose ☐

No longer able to take tablets ☐

Figure 12.2 Criteria for use of the LCP.

condition at the time the decision was made to commence the pathway. This can act as a useful comparator for evaluating continued use of the pathway.

The initial assessment section consists of 11 goals (see Table 12.1) focusing on:

- maintaining patient comfort through anticipatory prescribing of medications for the most common symptoms in the dying phase and ensuring that consideration is given to the need for medical and nursing interventions
- promoting appropriate communication and information giving for patients, families and other relevant healthcare colleagues
- assessing insight and psychosocial and spiritual needs of both patient and family.

Ongoing assessment and care delivery

The second section of the pathway facilitates the ongoing recording of the condition of the patient and the family at 4- or 12-hourly intervals in inpatient units (hospital, hospice and care home sectors), and per visit in the community. The patients are assessed for discomfort arising from any of the following:

- uncontrolled symptoms including pain, agitation, nausea and vomiting, respiratory tract secretions, dyspnoea
- micturition, mouthcare or bowel care issues
- psychological or spiritual issues.

In addition, family members are assessed for ongoing insight and psychological and spiritual well-being.

Table 12.1   Goals of care for patients in the dying phase

Stage of care	Goal	Description
Initial assessment	1	Current medication assessed and non-essentials discontinued
	2	As required, subcutaneous drugs written up according to protocol (pain, agitation, respiratory tract secretions, nausea and vomiting, dyspnoea)
	3	Discontinue inappropriate interventions (blood tests, antibiotics, intravenous fluid or drugs, document 'not for CPR', deactivate cardiac defibrillators)
	3a	Discontinue inappropriate nursing interventions
	3b	Syringe driver set up within 4 hours of doctor's order
	4	Ability to communicate in English assessed as adequate (patient/carer)
	5	Insight into condition assessed in patient and/or carer:
	5a1	Diagnosis patient
	5a2	Diagnosis carer
	5b1	Recognition of dying – patient
	5b2	Recognition of dying – carer
	6	Religious and spiritual needs assessed patient/carer
	7	How family/other to be informed of patient's impending death
	8	Family or other people involved given relevant hospital information (accommodation, car parking, dining room facilities, etc.)
	9	General practitioner is aware of patient's condition
	10	Plan of care explained and discussed with patient/carer
	11	Family/other express understanding of plan of care
Ongoing assessment	4-hourly[a]	Pain, agitation, respiratory tract secretions, nausea and vomiting, dyspnoea, mouth care, micturition, medication given safely and accurately, syringe driver checked (where appropriate)
	12-hourly[a]	Mobility, bowels, psychological, religious/spiritual, care of the family
Care after death	12	General practitioner informed of patient's death
	13	Procedure for laying out followed
	14	Procedure following death discussed or carried out
	15	Family/other given information on procedures
	16	Policy followed re collection of valuables
	17	Documentation and advice given to the appropriate person
	18	Bereavement leaflet/information given

[a]Frequency.

Care after death

The third section of the LCP is concerned with care delivered immediately after the death of the patient. Communication of the death to the primary care team is highlighted as well as policy and procedures around laying out and the collection of valuables. Prompts are also included to ensure that information and supporting leaflets are given to family members to advise them of local and national procedures and where they can access support in the immediate post-bereavement phase.

Variance

Variance reporting is an extremely important element of the LCP that has a vital role in all three sections of the pathway. This recording ensures that care can be individualised to the specific needs of the patient, that healthcare professionals are alerted to the need for action in support of patient comfort and that information is readily available to audit the care that has been delivered. In essence, it provides a mechanism through which any deviation from the goals on the pathway can be recorded and monitored.

In the initial assessment and care after death sections, deviation from the suggested template of care can occur for various reasons, such as:

- Clinicians decide that following the template of care would not be in the patient's best interest; for example, taking the decision to continue using antibiotics for a patient who may be experiencing distressing symptoms due to infection.
- A lack of resources or other organisational barriers prevent the delivery of that care; for example, a syringe driver is not available owing to a shortage within a given Trust, or there are no bereavement leaflets available to give to relatives.

Recording a tick in the 'no' box on the pathway against those specific goals and detailing on the variance sheet the rationale for the decision not to follow the pathway or the reason why it has not been possible to achieve a particular goal provides important information about care delivery.

In the ongoing assessment section, where the goals relate to the patient's condition at a given moment in time, variance reporting allows the healthcare professional to record when a patient was not 'comfortable' against particular aspects of their condition and to detail any action taken to right this situation. In addition, the variance sheet includes a section where the outcome of any action should be detailed.

Regular analysis and feedback of entries on the variance sheets then allows healthcare professionals to evaluate their practice. This evaluation can focus on the care delivered to an individual patient over time, or can involve scrutiny of a cohort of patients with the aim of identifying any recurrent themes that could lead to a change in practice.

Any ICP needs to be continually responsive to emerging evidence relating to best practice in order to remain relevant and valid. Thus, the LCP document is subject to regular review by a multidisciplinary LCP central steering group that includes representation from medical, nursing and allied health professionals such as social workers, as well as bereaved carers. Some 10 years on from its inception, the document now exists as the current version 11 of the 'Liverpool Care Pathway for the dying patient'.

IMPLEMENTING THE LCP INTO THE CLINICAL ENVIRONMENT

With any major change within an organisation, the time required to establish the new way of working must not be underestimated. In a generic setting such as a hospital or in the community, this process may take up to 1–2 years. In smaller specialist units such as hospices, the implementation process is likely to take less time. Implementing the LCP in the care home setting has specific challenges that may influence the time required. Despite the fact that deaths frequently occur in care homes, death and dying may not be central to care home policy which may result in a lack of end-of-life care education for staff. Changing practice can also be further hampered by the practicalities of working with multiple general practices (Hockley et al 2005).

Since 2004, a more formal process for involvement with the LCP framework (both nationally and internationally) has been in place that provides tangible central support to participating organisations at various important phases of the implementation process (Fig. 12.3):

- registration
- base review analysis
- education
- post-implementation analysis
- benchmarking.

In this way, the LCP framework is an exemplar of continuous quality improvement (CQI). CQI applies scientific methodology to everyday work with the aim of improving outcomes for patients. Graham

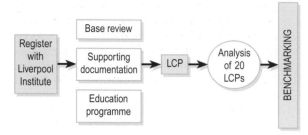

Figure 12.3 Continuous quality improvement (CQI) programme. (Reproduced with kind permission of the Marie Curie Palliative Care Institute liverpool.)

(1995) suggests that CQI involves a focus on systems and processes requiring the analysis of objective data to promote quality management.

A 10-step CQI programme (Table 12.2) was developed to support the introduction of the LCP into any specific clinical area.

Step 1: Establishing the project

In order to start this process it is vital to gain executive endorsement from within the organisation. This endorsement will allow the LCP to become embedded within the culture and process of the organisation. However, to ensure success, the project needs to

Table 12.2   The 10-step continuous quality improvement programme

Step	Details
1: Establishing the project	Obtain executive support and multidisciplinary team endorsement for LCP programme and establish steering group
	Nominate a lead for the project and appoint a LCP facilitator
	Identify pilot site(s)
	Register with LCP central team
	Provide appropriate education for key staff, including attendance at LCP foundation study day
2: Development of documentation	Multidisciplinary team discuss LCP and revise prompts according to local need
	Identify or write all supporting documentation, such as clinical guidelines, information leaflets, etc.
3: Retrospective audit of documentation	Undertake a base review (20 sets of notes)
	Feedback results of base review to staff
4: Induction education programme	Key staff undertake further appropriate education, including attendance at LCP advanced study day
	Establish an intensive education programme for clinical staff
	Ensure that resource folders are available to clinical areas
5: Implementation programme	LCP implemented as a pilot project over an agreed timeframe
	LCP facilitator(s) provide ongoing education and support to staff whenever LCP is used
6: Reflective practice	LCP documents are reviewed whenever they are completed
	LCP facilitator works closely with staff to reflect on care given, outcomes achieved and the process of completing the documentation
7: Evaluation and further training needs	Data from the first 20 pathways used are analysed and results fed back to staff
	LCP facilitator reviews the specific resource/educational needs of the clinical teams with support from the specialist palliative care team
8: Maintenance education programme (development of competencies)	Regular update/teaching sessions provided by LCP facilitator with the support of specialist palliative care team
9: Development of ongoing educational strategy within the organisation	Key staff trained to take on ongoing education and training in their own area with support of specialist palliative care team
	Key staff attend training events (e.g. annual national LCP conference)
10: Programme of ongoing feedback from analysis of the LCP	Establish links with local audit/clinical governance systems
	Develop system of ongoing analysis for LCP data
	Participate in local or national benchmarking programmes (e.g. National Hospital Audit)

be planned carefully, key players identified and relevant clinical staff involved. It is essential to identify a key member of staff to provide leadership and a local steering group to oversee the project. The appointment of LCP facilitators to provide this leadership and direction can be extremely beneficial in achieving successful implementation (Mellor et al 2004).

Registering the project with the LCP central team brings a number of benefits. This team can offer much support and advice on implementing and sustaining the use of the pathway at various milestones throughout the implementation process. For example, data from the recommended retrospective audit of practice (base review – see step 3) can be analysed by the central team and fed back to implementing teams, not only in the form of a database but also as part of a powerpoint presentation that can be used to provide feedback locally to staff. The central team will also undertake analysis of the first 20 pathways used (see step 6). Registration provides the opportunity for organisations to receive up-to-date information regarding the pathway, including updated versions of the document and news of developments.

The central team also provides an education programme in the form of foundation and advanced study days, and an annual conference. This programme aims to support key staff in implementing and sustaining the use of the LCP within the clinical environment.

The foundation study day focuses on techniques for priming the environment for change. It is helpful if key staff can attend this day prior to the commencement of the implementation phase. It discusses the concept of pathways, the development of the LCP, and also enables staff to understand the purpose and process of base review. In addition staff are encouraged to identify issues relating to implementing the pathway in their own clinical areas.

Step 2: Development of the documentation

The local steering group should review the LCP document and amend it according to local need. However, it is vital that the goals on the pathway should not be altered as this would mean that the document would become fundamentally different from the LCP and might not be suitable to be included in any future benchmarking or national audit programmes. Nevertheless, the prompts that support the goals can be adapted to reflect local practice better, provided that they do not alter the meaning of the stated goals. Extra goals may also be added to the document, should the need arise locally.

Another essential task for the local steering group is to agree the symptom control guidelines that support the pathway. It is crucial that the guidelines are agreed by the multidisciplinary team and have executive endorsement. Example guidelines are included in the document and may be adapted to meet local requirements.

Consideration must also be given to supporting literature such as information leaflets for patients and carers relating to the LCP, facilities within the organisation (parking, dining facilities, etc.), what needs to be done following a death and bereavement support. Some of this information is available nationally, such as:

- Information from the Department for Work and Pensions including
  — bereavement benefits (BB1)
  — what to do after a death in England and Wales (D49).
- Information from the LCP central team including
  — information on the LCP for relatives/carers
  — guidelines for use of the LCP for healthcare professionals
  — coping with dying leaflet.

Some leaflets will be available locally, such as information regarding facilities or bereavement provision, but it may become obvious that some information leaflets still need to be written or revised.

Step 3: Retrospective audit of documentation

Participating organisations are encouraged to undertake a retrospective audit (base review) of the routine documentation of care given to dying patients in their organisation. The main purpose of this exercise is to highlight and reinforce the need for change. The base review involves organisations identifying a set of 20 recent consecutive notes from within the proposed pilot area. The information contained within the notes is then scrutinised for evidence that appropriate care has been delivered in the dying phase against the goals of care identified on the LCP. A set of guidance notes is available from the LCP central team to assist organisations in systematically coding the information on to scannable pro formas. Patient demographic information regarding primary diagnosis, sex and age is also collected. The information is then returned to the LCP central team, which analyses the data descriptively and reports back the results to participants within 4–6 weeks. In the main, the feedback consists of simple charts that illustrate, at a glance, where the documentation of care is good

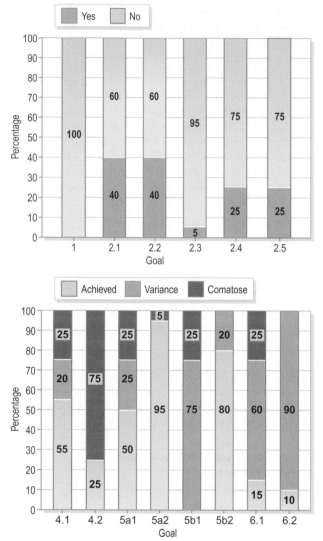

Figure 12.4   Examples of base review feedback.

areas, including LCP facilitators, to attend the LCP advanced study day. This day brings together colleagues from different organisations who are facing similar issues during the implementation phase, facilitates discussion of shared challenges and provides opportunities for subsequent networking.

It is important at this stage that the LCP facilitators/identified project leads work closely with their palliative care colleagues to devise a locally relevant induction programme for staff in the chosen pilot sites. Successful implementation of the programme requires wide-ranging education to be delivered to staff involved in the pilot, and steps should be taken to ensure that all relevant members of the multidisciplinary team have received appropriate education.

Education at this stage is primarily focused into making sure that staff understand the document fully and are able to complete it accurately. They may, in addition, require education related to the wider issues involved in using the pathway, such as communication skills, pain and symptom control, cultural and spiritual issues. The provision of a resource folder containing relevant evidence-based documentation and guidance is recommended to support the implementation process.

Increasingly, a package of educational and information resources is being sought to support the endeavours of LCP facilitators in providing timely educational input at an appropriate level. A project has recently begun within the Marie Curie Palliative Care Institute Liverpool to develop and evaluate an 'educational toolkit' for use with the LCP. The planned 'action research' based project will develop a variety of learning resources, both lecture format and more informal teaching approaches, to support medical and nursing colleagues in their use of the LCP.

and where it might be improved; see Figure 12.4 for examples.

An important method to gain support for the implementation of the LCP into any environment is to invite various members of the multidisciplinary team in the pilot site to be involved in the base review process. In this way, healthcare professionals responsible for the delivery of the care under scrutiny can experience first hand the frustration that occurs when the documentation is not as consistent or comprehensive as it could or should be.

Step 4: Induction education programme

At this point it is helpful for key staff responsible for or involved in providing education to the clinical

Step 5: Implementation programme

Once the relevant group of staff has received their educational input, the implementation phase can begin. This is likely to be the most 'hands on' phase of the project, where LCP facilitators/project leads will need to ensure that they are available within the pilot sites to offer ongoing support each time the document is used. Maintaining a 'high profile' during this period is imperative for success, as is ensuring strong links between staff in the pilot areas and the specialist palliative care team. Liaison between staff and the LCP facilitator/specialist team each time an LCP is used is a good way to increase specific knowledge and confidence in caring for dying patients and their families.

Step 6: Reflective practice

This process of ongoing review each time a pathway is used provides the opportunity for staff to engage actively in reflective practice. Schön (1983) suggested that the capacity to reflect on action in order to engage in a process of continuous learning was one of the defining characteristics of professional practice. This practice should continue at least for the first few months after the introduction of the document. Taking the opportunity to reflect formally on and discuss the specific elements of the care delivered allows the transfer and cementing of knowledge and helps to build confidence in the use of the document. Such ongoing reflection not only has the potential to highlight any inherent barriers to the delivery of optimal care, but also provides an opportunity to acknowledge and celebrate success whenever appropriate.

Although ongoing reflection with the staff directly involved in the delivery of care using the LCP is of paramount importance, it is also useful to take the opportunity to reflect in a more formal, quantitative way once a sizeable number of pathways have been used within the pilot sites. The LCP central team offers assistance to participating organisations to audit the first 20 LCPs used in the pilot site(s) in order to provide tangible feedback that can be disseminated more widely to key staff and to highlight any improvements in the environment since the implementation of the LCP. The information gained from the audit can point to areas where further education or training would be useful and can lead to appropriate amendments to the ongoing education programme. It can also provide useful information about organisational issues, such as the availability (or otherwise) of resources – something that may need to be addressed in order to facilitate the delivery of high-quality care.

The feedback report is of a similar format to that of the base review, and is returned to organisations within 4–6 weeks. The reports are designed to provide useful information in an accessible and easily interpretable format, using bar charts to illustrate the proportion of 'achieved' (goal met), 'variance' (goal not met) and 'not applicable' coded on the pathway at the time of delivery of care, along with the proportion of missing data (i.e. nothing coded on the pathway against that particular goal).

Step 7: Evaluation and further training needs

The ongoing evaluation and review of current status to inform future education and training continues.

Step 8: Maintenance – education programme (development of competencies)

Maintaining ongoing education around the LCP and more generally around palliative care has proven to be pivotal to the continued success of the LCP framework. An example of how this can be achieved is the Palliative Care Team Network Nurse Programme that has been running for some years within the Royal Liverpool and Broadgreen University Hospitals NHS Trust. The aim of this programme is to enhance the knowledge and skills of generic nurses interested in the palliative care approach (via regular liaison with the HSPCT) to enable them to take a lead role in the management of patients with palliative needs, including those in the dying phase. The programme specifically addresses issues such as the management of pain and other symptoms, communication and psychological support, care of the dying, and dealing with complex placement issues. Network nurses are encouraged to share their knowledge and skills (including how and when to use a LCP) with others in their immediate environment. The programme was subjected to a recent questionnaire evaluation (Jack et al 2004), in which respondents reported that it had been beneficial, particularly in providing them with increased palliative care knowledge, support and important networking opportunities.

Step 9: Development of ongoing educational strategy within the organisation

Passing on specialist skills and knowledge to generic healthcare workers for further dissemination directly into the clinical environment is a valuable mechanism in the spread and sustainability of the LCP programme. It is vital, however, that such clinicians are able to develop skills that will allow them to facilitate the work of others. This means that they will need to be updated regularly in all aspects of palliative care, but most importantly in current developments relating to the LCP. There is a national LCP conference held annually which provides an effective forum not only for clinicians to keep up to date with developments, but also to disseminate work that they may be undertaking locally themselves.

Step 10: Programme of ongoing feedback from analysis of the LCP

One of the major challenges to organisations using the framework is to find ways to spread and sustain the use of the LCP beyond the initial implementation phase. The development of the toolkit and the Network Nurse Programme will undoubtedly be important elements in this regard, but equally vital is the timely feedback of data on progress to clinical staff working with the document, to staff responsible for the delivery of education and to organisational managers who have responsibility for the allocation of scarce resources. The structure of the LCP makes it relatively easy to audit and, through the establishment of links with local clinical audit departments, it should be possible to provide ongoing relevant and up-to-date information concerning aspects of the delivery of care in the dying phase. This type of information is also likely to be useful in performance management within an organisation.

In addition, using the LCP to deliver and track care in the dying phase facilitates comparative audit with other organisations who are using the document. Data can be brought together to illustrate care in a wider context and to allow organisations to understand their own level of comparative performance in relation to that of similar settings. A national audit of care delivered in the dying phase using the LCP in acute hospital Trusts in England is currently under way, and around 118 individual hospitals from 94 Trusts have successfully registered to participate. The results from this audit are due in the summer of 2007. Prior to this national audit, two pilot collaborative audit exercises were undertaken in neighbouring strategic health authorities in the north west of England. Sixteen organisations (five hospitals, five community samples and six hospices) took part in phase 1A, and 24 organisations (12 hospitals, six community samples and six hospices) took part in phase 1B of the project. Data from 315 and 394 patients were included in each phase respectively. Each goal on the pathway was analysed descriptively to ascertain the proportion of 'achieved' or 'yes' coded (i.e. goal met), 'variance' or 'no' coded (i.e. goal not met), 'not applicable' and 'missing' (nothing coded on the pathway). Each organisation was given feedback to illustrate its own performance on each of the goals compared with the sector as a whole. In general, the results indicated high levels of achievment across the board for many of the goals on the pathway, but also highlighted those areas where further education would be useful to underpin improvements in practice. Participants came together in a workshop environment to share and discuss results and to future action plan – something they reported as a useful and informative undertaking.

LCP – THE CURRENT POSITION

Originally, the LCP programme represented a local development that was designed to improve the care of patients dying from cancer in one university hospital. However, over the years the programme has been increasingly recognised nationally as a model of best practice for use in all care settings and for dying patients irrespective of their diagnosis. To date, across England alone, more than 200 acute hospitals, 103 hospices, 384 community teams and 272 care homes have registered their involvement with the project. Furthermore, interest is spreading outside of the UK, and the LCP is increasingly being adopted internationally. A series of collaborating centres are now working with the LCP in countries in Europe, Australasia and Asia. Of these, the Dutch healthcare system has the longest association with the framework; the first formal process for translation of the pathway into another language was successfully undertaken using the method established by the European Organisation for Research and Treatment of Cancer (Cull et al 1998).

Over the past decade, teams working with the LCP have spontaneously used the document to guide care for patients dying from conditions other than cancer. However, in recognition of the particular challenges in certain areas of healthcare, the imperative to develop the pathway more formally has also been identified. This has led to a systematic approach using action research methodology, firstly to revise the pathway for use with a specific cohort patients, then to undertake local and national piloting, and finally to refine the document prior to wider dissemination. Currently, pilots are under way to develop and test pathways for use in paediatric and intensive care settings. In addition, two national pilots have taken place in collaboration with colleagues working with patients with heart failure and renal failure.

THE MARIE CURIE PALLIATIVE CARE INSTITUTE LIVERPOOL

The expanding LCP programme is now firmly established within the Marie Curie Palliative Care Institute Liverpool, which was launched in November 2004.

The Institute is a partnership between Marie Curie Cancer Care, the University of Liverpool and the Royal Liverpool and Broadgreen University Hospitals NHS Trust. This is an exciting collaboration between the voluntary sector, university and NHS, and has a multiprofessional profile. Part of the Division of Neurosciences in the University of Liverpool, the Institute is based at the Marie Curie Hospice in Liverpool with a satellite unit at the Royal Liverpool and Broadgreen University Hospitals Trust.

The key aims of the Institute are:

- to promote best practice in the care of the dying
- to be a leading institute in palliative care research, development and education, with a programme directed to making a difference to patient care
- to promote effective collaboration and spread of best practice between the voluntary and NHS sectors at local, national and international levels.

The key research theme of the Institute is 'care of the dying'. The subthemes are:

- Direct patient care
  — physical
  — psychosocial
  — ethical
  — spiritual
- Frameworks of care (e.g. LCP, rapid discharge pathway)
- Service organisation and delivery
- Education and training
- Policy.

The structure and stated aims of the Institute provide a context for the further development of the LCP programme to incorporate more formal research and audit of care of the dying. The difficulties involved in identifying appropriate outcomes and outcome measures for palliative care patients and undertaking robust research have been widely documented (Rinck et al 1997, Westcombe et al 2003). Obtaining views directly from patients and, to some extent their carers, is fraught with practical, moral and ethical dilemmas that are further exacerbated for patients in the dying phase. We have already seen that retrospective audit using the LCP can provide a useful alternative form of assessment. Evidence regarding the use of the LCP to provide information about the delivery of care in the dying phase is now emerging. For example, the LCP has been used to audit symptom control in the last days and hours of life (e.g. Ellershaw et al 2001, Hugel et al 2006, Kaas & Ellershaw 2003), and a study is currently under way within the Institute to evaluate the views of bereaved carers regarding care provided to patients in the last days and hours of life.

SUMMARY

End-of-life care is now firmly established as an important aspect of healthcare delivery. The LCP has developed from its humble beginnings to be nationally and internationally recognised as an effective means of improving end-of-life care. The framework incorporates change management techniques, education programmes, audit and research of demonstrable outcomes of care, but Dame Cicely Saunders provides a timely reminder of perhaps the most important aspect of all:

... the careful details of the pathway ... are a salute to the enduring worth of an individual life. Such an ending can help those left behind to pick up the threads of memory and begin to move forward

(Saunders 2003, p vi)

References

Baker J 1996 Shared record keeping in the multidisciplinary team. Nursing Standard 10:39–41

Campbell H, Hotchkiss R, Bradshaw N, Porteous M 1998 Integrated care pathways. British Medical Journal 316:133–137

Cull A S M, Bjordal K, Aaronson N 1998 EORTC Quality of Life Study Group translation procedure. EORTC Quality of Life Study Group, Brussels

Department of Health 2000 The NHS Cancer Plan: a plan for investment, a plan for reform. DoH, London

Department of Health 2006 Our health, our care, our say: a new direction for community services. DoH, London

Ellershaw J, Ward C 2003 Care of the dying patient: the last hours or days of life. British Medical Journal 326:30–34

Ellershaw J, Smith C, Overill S, Walker S E, Aldridge J 2001 Care of the dying: setting standards for symptom control in the last 48 hours of life. Journal of Pain and Symptom Management 21(1):12–17

Graham N O 1995 Quality in health care: theory, application, and evolution. Aspen Publications, New York

Higginson I 2003 Priorities for end of life care in England, Wales and Scotland. National Council for Palliative Care, London

Hockley J, Dewer B, Watson J 2005 Promoting end of life care in nursing homes using an integrated care pathway for the last days of life. Journal of Research in Nursing 10(2):135–152

Hoyle R M, Jenkins J M, Edwards W H, Edwards W H, Martin R S, Mulherin J L 1994 Case management in cerebral revascularization. Journal of Vascular Surgery 20:396–401

Hugel H, Ellershaw J, Gambles M 2006 Respiratory tract secretions in the dying patient: a comparison between glycopyrronium and hysocine hydrobromide. Journal of Palliative Medicine 9(2):279–284

Jack B, Gambles M, Saltmarsh P, Murphy D, Hutchinson T, Ellershaw J E 2004 Enhancing hospital nurses' knowledge of palliative care: a network nurse programme. International Journal of Palliative Nursing 10(10):502–506

Kaas R M, Ellershaw J E 2003 Respiratory tract secretions in the dying patient: a retrospective study. Journal of Pain and Symptom Management 26(4):258–264

Kwan J, Sandercock D M 2005 In-hospital care pathways for stroke. An updated systematic review. Stroke 36:1348

Mellor F, Foley T, Connolly M, Mercer V, Spanswick M 2004 Role of a clinical facilitator in introducing an integrated care pathway for the care of the dying. International Journal of Palliative Nursing 10(10):497–501

Mosher C, Cronk P, Kidd A, McCormick P, Stockton A, Sulla C 1992 Upgrading practice with critical pathways. American Journal of Nursing 1:41–44

National Institute for Clinical Excellence 2004 Guidance on cancer services: improving supportive and palliative care for adults with cancer. NICE, London

Ogilvie-Harris D J, Botsford D J, Hawker R W 1993 Elderly patients with hip fractures: improved outcome with the use of care maps with high quality medical and nursing protocols. Journal of Orthopaedic Trauma 7:428–437

Overill S 2003 The development, role and integration of integrated care pathways in modern day healthcare. In:

Ellershaw J, Wilkinson S (eds) Care of the dying: a pathway to excellence. Oxford University Press, Oxford, p 1–10

Rinck G C, van den Bos G A, Kleijnen J, de Haes H J, Schade E, Veenhof C H 1997 Methodologic issues in effectiveness research on palliative cancer care: a systematic review. Journal of Clinical Oncology 15(4):1697–1707

Saunders C 2003 Foreword. In: Ellershaw J, Wilkinson S (eds) Care of the dying: a pathway to excellence. Oxford University Press, Oxford, p vi

Schön D A 1983 The reflective practitioner: how professionals think in action. Temple Smith, London

Stead L, Arthur C, Cleary A 1995 Do multidisciplinary pathways of care affect patient satisfaction? Health Care Risk Report Nov:13–15

Trubo R 1993 If this is cookbook medicine, you may like it. Medical Economics 69:69–82

Weingarten S, Agocs L, Tankel N, Sheng A, Ellrodt A G 1993 Reducing lengths of stay for patients hospitalized with chest pain using medical practice guidelines and opinion leaders. American Journal of Cardiology 71:259–262

Westcombe A M, Gambles M A, Wilkinson S M et al 2003 Learning the hard way! Setting up an RCT of aromatherapy massage for patients with advanced cancer. Palliative Medicine 17(4):300–307

Williams J G, Roberts R, Rigby M J 1993 Integrated patient records: another move towards quality for patients? Quality in Health Care 2:73–74

Chapter **13**

Sexuality in palliative care: the problems and prospects

Valerie Forster

CHAPTER CONTENTS

INTRODUCTION

Sexuality is part of living, yet current practice portrays that diagnosis of a life-limiting illness terminates this aspect of being human from the outset.

Palliative care specialists enthuse about quality of life and provision of patient-centred holistic care, with Dom (1999) acknowledging holistic care to be governed by a social, psychological, physical and spiritual influence. Despite this, sexuality, which touches all of these domains, remains an obvious omission in clinical practice.

It may seem uncomfortable, low priority and indeed inappropriate to consider the sexuality of patients who are in the palliative stages of illness and often burdened with multiple and complex problems that render them physically and emotionally dependent. Nevertheless, sexuality is a universal phenomenon, unique to each individual, and holds a much deeper meaning than sexual intercourse. Sexuality can affirm love, relieve stress and anxiety, and distract one from the emotional and physical sequelae of an eventually terminal chronic illness (Lamb 2001).

The multifaceted nature of sexuality does make it difficult to prioritise and separate this chapter into a coherent form; therefore, a broad approach will be taken, trying not to disentangle an integrated concept.

The aim of this chapter is to:

- explore the nature of sexuality and the impact of advanced illness and treatment modalities
- consider patients' psychosexual support needs and the barriers that prevent sexuality from being addressed in clinical practice
- clarify the nurse's role and ability to provide psychosexual support and the appropriateness of its application to palliative care

- contemplate the operational, educational and research agenda required to inform and change practice.

It must be acknowledged that, although the focus is largely disease-specific (cancer), many issues addressed also apply to caring for people with non-malignant disorders requiring palliative care.

THE NATURE OF ALTERED SEXUALITY IN PALLIATIVE CARE

It is important to have an appreciation of sexuality in health to be able to consider its meaning in illness. Sexuality is a complex and broad phenomenon yet a basic human need; its thread runs through the physical, psychosocial and spiritual domains. It exceeds the physical act of sexual intercourse and varies in its meaning, importance, expression, gender and sexual orientation. Although no universal definition is agreed, Rice (2000a) references the World Health Organisation (1975), which translates sexual health as the somatic, emotional, intellectual and social aspects of sexual being, in ways that are positively enriching and that enhance personality, communication and love. This would fit the 'socially accepted norm', yet not all sexual encounters are based on enhancing personality and love, and may be predominantly physical and casual in nature.

The Royal College of Nursing (RCN 2000) provides a modern interpretation and describes sexuality as an individual self-concept, shaped by the personality and expressed as sexual feelings, attitudes, beliefs and behaviours expressed through a heterosexual, homosexual, bisexual and transsexual orientation. This reflects today's society and considers its multidimensional nature. Arguably a universal definition should not be sought as it could be considered too restrictive and fail to capture the uniqueness of sexuality, but on the other hand it may be purposeful to communicate its core meaning.

Sexual intercourse and the need to reproduce is a fundamental component of one's sexuality. Gallo-Silver (2000) describes Masters and Johnson's (1970) sexual response cycle which consists of four phases:

1. Desire – interest in sex (emotional and physical)
2. Arousal – sense of sexual pleasure with physiological changes of pelvic vasocongestion, vaginal lubrication and penile erection
3. Orgasm – period of peak sexual pleasure
4. Resolution – sense of relaxation.

The ability to complete this cycle is influenced not only by physical health but also by emotional well-being. Sexuality is communicated through behaviour as well as physical appearance, which is demonstrated at both a conscious and an unconscious level, through efforts to exaggerate one's femininity or masculinity. This is achieved by the way we dress, wear our hair, right down to adopted mannerisms which are emphasised or suppressed when interacting with others. It interlinks with the psychosocial domain whereby religion, culture, law, education, life experience and our peers influence sexual beliefs, values and expression. However, as discussed by Rafferty (1995) and the RCN (2000), sexuality remains a concept unique to each individual and constantly changes throughout our life, with variable levels of importance.

Historically sexuality was portrayed as a personal, private and taboo subject, whereas the sexual revolution of the 1960s and improved contraception encouraged acceptance of sexual relations outside marriage, varied sexual preferences and liberal sexual expression. This is portrayed by the media in an idealistic manner whereby sex is synonymous with youth, beauty and health. Nevertheless sexuality can be an important part of life for all people, male and female, young and old, healthy and ill (Jefferies 2002, Ooijen 1996).

The impact of advanced cancer on human sexuality

Following a diagnosis of advanced cancer, initial concerns are likely to be that of prognosis, yet through time other aspects of daily living will come into question. Nishimoto (1995) refers to Schwartz et al (1994), who suggest that the primary goal of someone diagnosed and treated for cancer is survival followed by normalisation, which is not static as what is perceived as normal will change in a patient's life. Although cancer may have a negative and sustained impact on sexuality, the extent to which it alters the concept of normal will be variable.

Altered sexuality is considered by Anderson (1990) and cited by Hughes (1996), who state that cancer, its treatment, or treatment side-effects interfere with sexual functioning and that the sexual response cycle changes, resulting in dysfunction and inability to express one's sexuality in a manner that is consistent with personal needs and preferences. This is illustrated by Ramage (2005), who refers to the sexual arousal circuit (Fig. 13.1) which represents the positive and negative factors that influence sexuality; these are not restricted to the genitals, but involve links between mind, body and emotions. Negative factors such as pain, poor body image, lowered self-

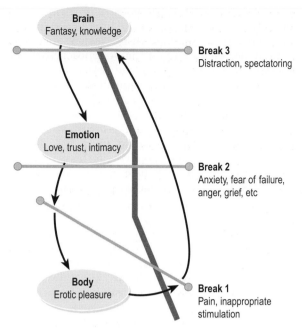

Figure 13.1 The sexual arousal circuit. (Redrawn from Ramage 2005, with kind permission of John Tomlinson and Blackwell Publishing Ltd.)

Case Study 13.1   The impact of advanced cancer on sexuality

Mary is 53 and has lived with her boyfriend, Jim, aged 44 for 3 years. She was diagnosed with lung cancer and widespread bone metastases 6 months ago and has been admitted to the hospice with symptoms of breathlessness, fatigue, pain, weight loss, dry mouth, anxiety, depression and insomnia.

Jim is very supportive and remains affectionate towards Mary, but now sleeps in the spare room as Mary has wakeful nights. When asked by a nurse which symptoms were most problematic she replied:

'All of them really, as they are preventing me from making love to Jim and it has always been so important to us. We don't talk about it but I know it must bother him; it's not that I don't want to but I just don't have the energy. I don't know why he stays with me really, especially looking like this.'

Mary explained to the nurse that anxiety was not about prognosis but about being separated from Jim and worried that they would never be intimate and engage in sexual intercourse again.

Thinking about the sexual arousal circuit, what factors may link or break the circuit and affect Mary's sexuality?

esteem, pressure to perform, anxiety, anger, irritability, loss of control, fear, grief or depression may break the circuit and alter one's sexuality.

Improved treatment means that cancer may now lie under the umbrella of chronic illness, thereby augmenting the importance of quality of living that is fundamental to palliative care. Altered sexuality threatens this quality.

As mentioned above, sexuality touches all life domains, yet it seems difficult to comprehend its place in life-limiting illness when contemplating the complex and debilitating nature of cancer. Case Study 13.1 demonstrates the impact of advanced cancer on sexuality.

Case Study 13.1 supports Thaler-DeMers' (2001) opinion that altered sexuality occurs in all patients with cancer at all stages, not just those of sexual origin, yet research appears to be predominantly site-specific, namely prostate, breast and gynaecological cancers. Kurtz et al (2000) identified the most problematic symptoms of lung cancer to be fatigue (82.2%), cough (67.4%), difficulty breathing (61.2%), pain (58.9%) and weakness (55%), all of which potentially alter sexuality. This list is not exhaustive, yet Sutherland & Gamlin (1999) argue that physical and mental fatigue itself prevents sexual activity, particularly penetrative intercourse, from taking place.

Despite this it would seem that sexuality remains important, with Rice (2000a) stating that sexual contact may have special meaning for the cancer patient as sexuality and sexual expression convey being alive.

Altered body image and an altered sexual self

Factors that threaten one or more phases of the sexual response cycle or cause a break in the sexual arousal circuit are multifaceted and have fundamental affiliations with body image. This is supported by Heath & McCormack (2002, p 66), who emphasise the correlation between altered body image and sexuality by stating:

We live in our bodies, yet are more than our bodies. The body is the medium through which we experience our lives and the showcase of our inner being.

Body image consists of three components (Price 1990, cited by Price 1998):

1. Body reality – the body as it really is
2. Body ideal – beliefs and ideas about how the body should be

3. Body presentation – efforts to maintain an attractive social appearance.

Cancer and its treatment challenge the equilibrium of these components, compromising self-esteem and emotional well-being. All the same, Price (1998) states that body image is influenced by the circumstances of the patient, by his or her personal make-up and the level of support that he or she receives from professionals or carers. The extent to which appearance is altered may also influence adaptation to an altered sexual self, with examples of mastectomy scars, cachexia, lymphoedema and alopecia being visual reminders. Case Study 13.2 considers the correlation between body image and sexuality.

In Case Study 13.2, Kim appeared to avoid Dave's wound, suggesting that she struggled with his disfigurement or simply saw her husband and not the wound. Price (2000) explains that avoidance is not to be confused with denial as the lay carer accepts the illness but chooses to focus on the parts of the patient's body function or personality that still seems whole. Conversely, nurses focused on the wound to improve presentation, perception and adaptation, yet the impact this had on the couple's sexuality was unknown as neither was ever asked because the nurses considered it inconsequential due to severe disfigurement and associated symptoms. Monga et al (1997), who studied sexual function in 54 men with head and neck cancer, refute such assumptions. Data collection using the validated Derogatis inventory of sexual functioning identified that 85% showed

---

Case Study 13.2   Body image and sexuality

Dave is 57 years old and has basal cell carcinoma of the face with an extensive fungating wound that obstructs his nasal airway, causing communication difficulties and pain. Dave has worked in the media for many years and is always immaculate in his hygiene and dress. He has a close relationship with his wife, Kim, and demonstrates affection through holding hands and writing loving notes. One pertinent observation is that Kim never makes reference or demonstrated unease at his disfigurement.

The district nurse visits Dave at home each day to provide education and support in caring for his tracheostomy and gastrostomy, as well as changing the dressing to his facial wound. At one visit Dave wrote on his notepad that he felt worthless, unsightly and extremely anxious about Kim seeing him without his dressing and desperately wished he could look normal and be the man he was.

How may changes to Dave's body influence body reality, ideal and presentation, and affect his sexuality and marital relationship?

---

interest in sex despite existing sexual problems. Interestingly there was no significant difference in interest between men with severe disfigurement and those with none, confirming its importance across the disease trajectory. This study did not consider sexual function prior to illness or treatment, rendering it difficult to quantify its true impact. Rafferty (1995) proposed that awareness of factors affecting body meaning can improve the care of those with altered body image. However, in Case Study 13.2, despite nurses being able to address changing body issues by improving presentation, they failed to recognise sexual problems consequential of such change.

Changing relationships

The impact of life-shortening illness should never be underestimated (Webster & Heath 2002) and patients who have a sexual partner will find that the quality of their relationship will significantly influence their sexuality, body image and self-esteem, especially when its foundations are fundamentally based on strong sexual attraction. Vulnerability, fear of rejection, feeling undesirable, emotionally overwhelmed and miscommunication between couples are common compounding factors that may not be fully appreciated by healthcare professionals.

Trauma caused by disability may reverse normal roles and polarities within a relationship (Webb 1994), with the couple's adaptive response to illness potentially being diverse and influencing ability to be intimate with one another. Altered relationship dynamics where the roles of lover and carer become blurred have been illuminated by Roe & May (1999, p 575), who quoted Parkes (1993) recalling a partner's words:

'It takes the edge off it, it isn't as though desire is not there but it's like I said, when you stop being a nurse and become a husband'

Searle (2002) looks more closely and considers the transactional analysis framework by Berne (1964), which describes changing dynamics in ill-health whereby adult, child and parent roles are adopted, with the carer forced into a parent role and the patient towards a child role, causing negative sexual relations. Kiss & Meryn (2001) also remind us that supporting and caring for others is a core feature of female but not male identity, so being mindful of this is important when offering support to couples.

Ooijen (1995) postulates that partnerships and marriages fail when either partner cannot cope with the illness. Northouse et al (1991), cited by Hordern (2000), challenge this by revealing no increase in marital breakdown in a study of breast cancer patients. Conversely, a negative impact on sexual relationships was found by Kralik et al (2001) when studying 81 middle-aged American women with chronic illness, including cancer. Wilmoth & Ross (1997), on the other hand, report varied experiences through a triangulation study of 105 American breast cancer survivors. Quantitative data using the Wilmoth Sexual Behavior Questionnaire contained 49 statements measured on a Likert scale with seven subscales. Qualitative methodology involved an open questionnaire asking about changes in sexuality since diagnosis, and responses ranged from feeling trapped and unworthy to one woman writing:

'I feel more in touch with my body and more connected to life, generating more intense sexuality.'

Data presented in this manner are powerful and real, complementing the structured questionnaire, and although they identified sexual problems it is reassuring that some people report positive outcomes through re-evaluation of life. Thaler-DeMers (2001) acknowledges this response, stating that the cancer experience is one that encourages more intimate and intense interpersonal relationships.

Although sexuality in gay, lesbian and single people is referenced, it is less recognised in research; this may also reflect practice where assumptions of healthcare professionals wrongly render patients either heterosexual or asexual, as well as putting less value on their relationships.

REFLECTION POINT

- Do you assume that all patients in your care are heterosexual?
- How do you feel about caring for people who have different sexual orientations, such as homosexual and bisexual?
- How does your view influence the care you give?

Treatment modalities: are we making matters worse?

Surgery, radiotherapy, chemotherapy and hormone treatments are increasingly employed to control symptoms and delay the disease process; however, short-term and irreversible sexual dysfunction, consequential of curative and palliative treatment, may jeopardise quality of living. It is therefore paramount that both inherited and current treatment side-effects are recognised in order to give appropriate care. Examples are presented in Table 13.1.

Surgery such as an amputation due to cancer has sexual implications, with Shell & Miller (1999) stating that men may equate loss of a limb to loss of manhood. In addition, the formation of a stoma for bowel cancer is known to affect sexuality (Bond 1997).

Radiotherapy generally results in localised side-effects, with Anderson & Van der Does (1994), cited by Rice (2000b), identifying pelvic radiotherapy as having the most serious effect on sexual function for both sexes.

Schover et al (1995) found chemotherapy to be most debilitating in 218 breast cancer patients, who experienced more sexual dysfunction, poorer body image and long-term impairment. Data collection involved standardised questionnaires and, although the sample group was not palliative, findings may be transferable to those with advanced disease. Lamb (2001) also considered long-term chemotherapy side-effects such as paraesthesia, making the simple act of touch no longer pleasurable, and creating potential dangers of neutropenia and thrombocytopenia when receiving chemotherapy, whereby intercourse may increase risk of infection or haemorrhage. Lack of knowledge and awareness means that such information is not communicated to couples by health professionals. As the side-effects of chemotherapy are numerous, careful consideration is warranted in order to minimise dysfunction; however, this may be true of all modalities, as Hughes (2000) identifies fatigue as the most frequent and distressing side-effect, with Rice (2000b) suggesting that it can persist long after treatment has ended, impacting negatively on sexuality.

Pharmacological management of symptoms such as pain, nausea, vomiting, agitation and depression is multifarious. In palliative care polypharmacy is common, with side-effects of sexual dysfunction remaining unrecognised by clinicians. Tomlinson (2005) identifies commonly prescribed drugs that potentially alter sexual function (Fig. 13.2). For example, antidepressants, which cause erectile and ejaculatory dysfunction, and some antiemetics, which reduce libido and cause erectile problems, are both widely used in palliative care, yet their side-effects are rarely discussed. Centrally acting depressant drugs, particularly antispasmodics, benzodiazepines and opiates, may also impair sexual function (Glass

Table 13.1   Possible effects of cancer treatment on sexual function

Cancer site	Surgery	Radiotherapy	Chemotherapy	Information source
Brain metastases		Alopecia causing body image problems		Hoskin 1999
Head and neck	*Removal of part of facial structure* – reduced libido, difficulty maintaining erection due to body image and psychological changes	Nausea, vomiting, drooling, altered taste and smell. Malaise, stomatitis, xerostomia		Wilmoth & Botchway 1999 Lamb 1995 Hordern 2000 Rydholm & Strang 2002
Breast	*Mastectomy* – loss of sensation in the breast and also after reconstructive surgery; lymphoedema. Limited physiological impact but major psychological and body image issues	Lymphoedema, fatigue, nausea, erythema	Stomatitis, weakness, nausea, vomiting, fatigue, infertility, premature menopause causing mood changes, reduced libido, vaginal dryness and thickening, urinary problems, diarrhoea, alopecia, emotional distress/depression	Wilmoth & Ross 1997 Hordern 2000 Wilmoth & Botchway 1999 Rice 2000b Fenlon 2001
Lung		Used in symptomatic non-small cell lung cancer. Symptoms include fatigue, nausea, erythema	Weakness, nausea, vomiting, as above; alopecia, fatigue, depression, altered body image and sexual dysfunction	Schwartz & Plawecki 2002
Colorectal cancer	Abdominoperineal resection *Men* – damage to the pelvic nerve, affecting all stages of sexual arousal *Women* – dyspareunia *Both* – body image/ psychological issues due to formation of an ostomy	Faecal incontinence, rectal bleeding, anal pain, fistula, ulceration, nausea, diarrhoea, cramps	As above	Bond 1997 Rice 2000b Faithfull 2001

Table 13.1 Possible effects of cancer treatment on sexual function – cont'd

Cancer site	Surgery	Radiotherapy	Chemotherapy	Information source
Bladder	Cystectomy – retrograde ejaculation problems. Body image issues due to formation of ileal conduit		Inhibited desire, painful intercourse	Ofman 1995 Rice 2000b
Prostate	Radical prostatectomy – autonomic nerve damage causing erectile dysfunction/urinary incontinence	Decreased secretion of testosterone and fibrosis in the pelvis – diminished blood supply and nerve damage	Hormonal manipulation – oestrogens, antiandrogens, gonadatropin releasing agents cause loss of libido, erectile dysfunction and changes in hair distribution	Waxman 1993
	Bilateral orchidectomy – diminished libido, erectile dysfunction, dry orgasm			Rice 2000b
Gynaecological (cervical, endometrial, ovarian)	Radical hysterectomy/bilateral oophorectomy – vaginal shortening, reduced lubrication, decreased desire or orgasmic ability, menopause, dyspareunia	Pelvic irradiation for endometrial cancer causes vaginal dryness, thinning and stenosis resulting in chronic problems including vaginal bleeding, bowel changes, cystitis, postcoital bleeding	Alopecia, anorexia, weight loss, lethargy, fatigue, bone marrow suppression. Hormone therapy may be contraindicated in hormone-dependent tumours	Lamb 1995
	Pelvic nerve damage causing altered response to G-spot stimulation. Infertility, depression/anxiety. Lymph node involvement causing lymphoedema in legs			Wilmoth & Botchway 1999 Rice 2000b Dennison 2001

Commonly prescribed drugs associated with sexual dysfunction (list not fully comprehensive)

Drug	Erectile dysfunction	Loss of desire	Ejaculatory disorder	Orgasmic disorder	Priapism
Anticonvulsants		Also gynaecomastia			
Carbamazepine	✓		✓	✓	
Phenytoin	✓	✓			
Primidone	✓	✓			
Valproate	✓	✓			
Antidepressants*					
Tricyclics					
Amitriptyline	✓	✓	✓	✓	
Amoxapine	✓	✓	✓		
Clomipramine	✓	✓	✓	✓	
Imipramine	✓	✓	✓	✓	
Maprotiline	✓	✓			
Nortriptyline	✓	✓			
Trimipramine	✓	✓	✓	✓	
Monoamine oxidase inhibitors					
Phenelzine	✓	✓	✓	✓	
Selective serotonin reuptake inhibitors					
Fluoxetine	✓		✓		
Fluovoxamine	✓		✓		
Paroxetine	✓		✓		
Sertraline	✓		✓		
Venlafaxine	✓	✓			
Lithium		✓			
Antipsychotics					
Chlorpromazine	✓	✓	✓		✓
Fluphenazine	✓	✓	✓		
Haloperidol	✓		✓		
Amisulphide	✓	✓			
Risperidone	✓	✓			
Zotepine	✓	✓			
Benzodiazepines	✓	✓	✓	✓	
Antihypertensives					
Atenolol	✓				
Bisprolol	✓	✓	✓	✓	
Carvedilol	✓	✓	✓	✓	
Clonidine	✓		✓	✓	
Enalapril	✓				
Felodipine					
Guanethidine	✓	✓	✓		
Hydralazine	✓				✓
Labetalol	✓	✓	✓		✓

Drug	Erectile dysfunction	Loss of desire	Ejaculatory disorder	Orgasmic disorder	Priapism
Lisinopril	✓				
Methyldopa	✓	✓	✓	✓	
Metoprolol	✓	✓			
Pindolol	✓	✓	✓	✓	
Prazosin					✓
Propranolol	✓	✓	✓	✓	
Quinapril	✓				
Ramipril	✓				
Reserpine	✓	✓	✓		
Terazosin					✓
Timolol	✓	✓			
Verapamil	✓				
Lipid regulators					
Bezafibrate	✓				
Fenofibrate	✓				
Gemfibrozil	✓				
H$_2$ antagonists					
Cimetidine	✓				
Famotidine	✓				
Nizatidine	✓				
Ranitidine	✓				
Diuretics					
Amiloride	✓	✓			
Chlorthalidone	✓	✓			
Indapamide	✓	✓			
Spironolactone	✓	✓			
Thiazides	✓				
Antiemetics					
Metoclopramide	✓	✓			
Non-steroidal anti-inflammatory drugs					
Naproxen	✓		✓		
Anticholinergics					
Atropine	✓				
Diphenhydramine	✓	✓	✓	✓	
Hydroxyzine	✓	✓			
Propantheline	✓				
Scopolamine	✓				
Antispasmodics					
Baclofen	✓		✓		
Hypnotics		✓			
Barbiturates	✓	✓	✓		

* The following antidepressants have little or no sexual side-effects: mitrazapine, trazodone, reboxetine, moclobemide and nefazodone available only on a named patient basis. Clozapine seems to be without sexual side-effects.

Figure 13.2 Commonly prescribed drugs associated with sexual dysfunction (list not fully comprehensive). (From Tomlinson 2005, with kind permission of Blackwell Publishing Ltd.)

& Soni 2005, Parkinson & Bateman 1994). Steroids, commonly used to treat many symptoms of cancer, have numerous side-effects yet Cushing's syndrome alone may compromise body image and self-esteem, and thus feelings of attractiveness. Failure to address such issues with patients when making treatment decisions creates not only ethical dilemmas but potentially unnecessary distress for patients.

Literature suggests that symptoms of cancer and its treatment leave palliative care patients with inevitable dysfunction, advocating greater recognition of drug side-effects and consideration of non-pharmacological approaches.

It is difficult to verify the prevalence and severity of sexual dysfunction amongst this patient group, yet Ananth et al (2003) conducted a controlled study of 50 cancer care, palliative care and healthy patients from general practitioners to explore the impact of treatment on sexuality at different stages of illness. There was a 75% response rate to the questionnaire, which measured status of sexual frequency, activity, strength and emotional status of relationships, and sexual satisfaction using visual analogue and Likert scales. It was tested against the validated Derogatis subscale, with data mirroring changes in response. Both cancer groups reported more sexual difficulties than the healthy controls, with palliative patients being most impaired. The fundamental importance of this study is that it specifically included palliative care patients through controlled sample selection. Findings suggest that serious sexual dissatisfaction does not occur until advanced stages of illness, as echoed by Lamb (2001), who states that the trajectory of palliative care may force celibacy on an otherwise sexually active couple.

This section looked at the broad meaning of sexuality in Western society and considered its place in palliative care. Prevalence and severity of sexual dysfunction is difficult to confirm owing to the many influencing factors and lack of clinical inquiry. Nonetheless, the literature suggests that patients experience serious problems that have a close affiliation with disease progression, altering body image, altered relationship dynamics and treatment modalities.

PITFALLS IN PRACTICE: ADDRESSING SEXUALITY

Although discomfort in talking about death is dissolving, it is rarely discussed synonymously with sexuality, with Wells (2002) stressing that trying to address the sexual needs of palliative care patients seems one of the great last taboos across health professions. Why is it that it remains an omission of care in a Western society that boasts sexual liberation? Reasons seem multiple, with pitfalls fundamentally being patient and professional communication difficulties whereby an unspoken agreement exists that sexual issues, which are considered private and personal, should remain so. Such silence leaves many uncertainties, including the disparity between patients' psychosexual support needs and actual care given.

What are the psychosexual support needs of patients?

Because patients' psychosexual support needs are not enquired about, nurses work on the basis of assumptions that to some extent reflect those in the literature. Evidence appears fragmented regarding patients' needs and is largely embedded in research of oncology treatments, with partners' views and experience unexplored. However, more recently Ananth et al (2003) identified in their study that significantly more cancer patients wanted the opportunity to discuss sexual concerns with professionals than did the healthy controls ($P < 0.001$). Level of need appears variable, as demonstrated by Sanson-Fisher et al (2000), who studied the response of 888 Australian surgical and oncology patients across nine cancer centres to a psychological needs survey. Those receiving chemotherapy or hormone therapy were significantly more likely to report sexual support needs than other treatment groups.

Contrasting findings were reported by McIllmurray et al (2001), who explored unmet psychological needs of 380 patients from four hospitals in the west of England. A cross-sectional quantitative approach using the psychological needs inventory assessing breast, colorectal, lymphoma and lung cancer patients generated comprehensive data, demonstrating changing needs at crucial stages of the cancer journey (diagnosis, end of treatment, first recurrence, and from active to palliative care). Interestingly, 59% considered sexual support not applicable, with the 14% who identified it as important being healthier. Clinician bias excluded those from the study considered too poorly, accounting for the low percentage of palliative care patients. A more balanced representation may have altered results, as would looking at less crucial stages of illness, as demonstrated in a Canadian study by Lemieux et al (2004). This research examined the importance of sexuality for 10 cancer patients in a tertiary palliative care unit, hospice or home care through face-to-face interviews. Those in the sample group were all married, and consisted of six men and four women aged 44–81 years. They had been diagnosed from 6 months to 10 years previously, with one person dying 4 days after the interview. Findings demonstrated that the importance of sexuality had changed minimally since becoming ill, with one interviewee stating: 'Intimacy is more important to me than basically anything in life'.

Most interviewees identified that progressive disease decreased the frequency of sexual contact as a consequence of becoming ill, and that emotional connection to others was an integral component of sexuality, taking precedence over physical expression. One interviewee considered sexuality and their illness, and stated: 'It doesn't necessarily have to be lovemaking every night kind of thing. But just to be close or caressing each other'.

Patients unanimously believed that a holistic approach to palliative care would include opportunities to discuss the impact of illness on their sexuality, yet only one subject had previously been asked about it. Limitations of the study included a small sample size which was not selected at random and those who refused to participate were uncomfortable speaking about the subject and concerned about being physically able to tolerate the interview. Partners were not included, but in three interviews they were present and two participated in discussion, which may have affected the results. Even so, the worth of this study must be noted as it provides qualitative data emphasising the fact that sexuality and psychosexual support is a real issue in palliative care.

Patient barriers contribute to unmet needs with the very factors that determine one's sexuality influencing disclosure of sexual concerns. This is illustrated in Case Study 13.3.

McIllmurray et al (2001) identified that women have more information and support needs than men, which is representational of gender differences in our society. Bond (1997) and Kiss & Meryn (2001) implied that women want to talk and share feelings, whereas men make light of illness, joke and block purposeful conversation, as mirrored in Case Study 13.3. Yet following the doctor's direct approach, John's support needs involved ongoing dialogue which helped him grieve his sexual loss. Such variance affirms the importance of an individualised approach to addressing psychosexual support needs, yet at the same time avoiding gender generalisation.

Rice (2000a) claims that patients may make assumptions about cancer and sexuality, with Schover & Jensen (1988) identifying myths such as:

Case Study 13.3   Expression of sexual loss

John is 36 and has multiple sclerosis causing limited movement and muscle spasms in his arms and legs, and difficulty with eating and talking. John is bisexual but has not had a sexual partner since diagnosis 4 years ago. He lives with his mother, who is his main carer, and has been attending day hospice for 4 months. John obstructs dialogue regarding psychological issues through jokes, laughter and sexual innuendo, as well as making inappropriate comments of a sexual nature to the nurses about their appearance. The care team was concerned that John may have issues regarding his sexuality and was uncertain about how best to support him and handle the unwelcome comments. Following discussion, a male doctor approached the issue directly by saying to John:

'It is not unusual for people with your condition to experience sexual problems. In what ways has this been a concern for you since becoming ill?'

John cried and expressed feelings of loneliness and isolation. He also expressed shame regarding his conduct with the nurses, as well as sadness about not having or ever likely to have a loving sexual relationship.

What do you think John's psychosexual support needs are?

- Cancer is contagious through sexual activity.
- Resuming sex will prompt a recurrence.
- A sexual partner is exposed to radiation during radiotherapy treatment.
- Cancer is a punishment for past sexual misdeeds.

Such misconceptions may evoke feelings of fear, guilt or shame, reducing intimacy between couples and inhibiting discussion. It is also not uncommon for patients to adopt a passive role, with Jenkins (1988), cited by Rice (2000a), stating that patients fail to ask questions, assuming that if it were important the nurse or doctor would have told them. There are also social and cultural barriers, such as it being important to speak to someone of the same age group, religion or sex, the latter proving difficult for male patients in a female-dominated profession. Sexual orientation also creates barriers, with Matthews (1998) stating that lesbians hold fears of self-disclosure and negative consequences of homophobia and compromised care. Regardless of orientation, patients may be all too worried about staff opinions to voice concerns, believing it inappropriate to ask.

The nurse's role: responsibility versus capability

Nursing practice is influenced by internal, external, professional and personal factors. In 2002 the Nursing and Midwifery Council (NMC) stated that nurses are personally accountable for their practice. This renders them answerable for their omissions as well as actions. Despite the National Institute for Clinical Excellence (2003) failing to reference sexuality within their draft of supportive palliative care guidelines, the RCN (2000) clearly stated that sexuality and sexual health was an appropriate, legitimate area of nursing activity, and that nurses have a professional and clinical responsibility to address it.

The literature indicates that patients want to talk about sexual problems (Ananth et al 2003, Lemieux et al 2004, Rubin 2005, Steinke 1994), with Waterhouse (1996) voicing patient preference to be that health professionals initiate discussion. In addition, research by Stead et al (2001) revealed that 15 women with ovarian cancer identified that the benefits of talking about sexual issues outweighed any embarrassment. On the other hand, this study, which also explored attitudes of 43 clinicians and nurses through interviews using grounded theory, found that nurses wait for patients to raise the issue. Grounded theory involves developing a theory from methodically obtained data from real life; Benton (2000) considers this approach suitable for investigating topics of which little is known. Omission of methodology regarding interviews renders it difficult to quantify this study's validity. Cort (1998) explored the perspective of 50 hospice nurses through a questionnaire and interviews; this revealed liberal views, yet it is noteworthy that only 10 nurses volunteered for interview, signifying discomfort with the subject.

Wells (2002), a hospice reverend, took a wider view and explored attitudes of the multidisciplinary team in relation to sexuality through interviews. This is important as palliative care is strongly based on effective team working. Themes that emerged from the study included a need to identify a team member who could talk to patients or alternatively look for help, and for the team as a whole to work together to find a solution. It is, however, a contentious issue, as sexuality would seem too big a task to be left to the skilled few. Although Wells (2002) advocates a multidisciplinary team approach, the literature suggests that nurses are best placed as they have the most sustained contact with patients and their partners (Hughes 1996, Lewis & Bor 1994). Ideally patients should be able to choose the person to whom they talk and share experiences, rather than having someone imposed upon them; however, working on an *ad hoc* basis has failed, with the very same barriers to practice being echoed in dated literature (Bor & Watts 1993, Fisher & Levin 1983, Waterhouse & Metcalfe 1991, Webb 1988). Gamel et al (1993) reinforced this in a literature review; they identified knowledge, attitude, comfort levels, views about professional responsibility, and education as key issues. Literature across specialties was included, yet may still be applicable to palliative care, and although methodology was not referenced the concerning issue is that the same problems remain, rendering practice static. Logic suggests that a greater number of healthcare professionals with the necessary attitudes, knowledge and interpersonal skills would allow patients greater choice of whom they discuss their concerns with.

REFLECTION POINT

- Discuss with your colleagues the extent to which sexuality should be part of your role.
- Consider the practical and professional barriers in your clinical area that prevent you from addressing the issue.

Attitudes and knowledge: do nurses have what it takes?

No literature to date disputes the role of the nurse, who is in an influential position, yet assumptions and attitudes may prove detrimental to patient care, as considered by Schwartz & Plawecki (2002), who state that patients are generally hesitant to initiate discussion about sexuality with nurses because they fear being rebuffed, embarrassed or labelled as sexually aggressive. A qualitative study of surgical nurses by Guthrie (1999) recognised that the upbringing of some nurses, where beliefs are deep-rooted, makes discussing sexuality difficult. Nevertheless nurses must be more self-aware of personal values in order to give non-judgemental care and support patients effectively (Herson et al 1999, Ooijen 1996). It may be questioned whether this means asking nurses to compromise their own beliefs. Goldsborough (1970), cited by Hayter (1996), argues that being non-judgemental does not mean giving up beliefs or challenging them to fit in with what others believe to be morally right.

Health professionals should not make assumptions about the level of interest or capacity a couple have for physical intimacy (Lamb 2001). Such assumptions lead to omission of care, such as unfounded beliefs that older people are asexual despite increased recognition in the literature that they consider sexuality an important aspect of daily living (Gregoire 1999, Russell 1998, Shell & Smith 1994). Many receive palliative care, yet Jones (1994) states that carers accept a liberal attitude towards themselves while still considering their elders as holding more Victorian values. Steinke (1994) studied 308 healthy elders and found that the majority were sexually active up to four times per month with some degree of sexual satisfaction and no divergence of attitude between sexes. Conversely, Johnson (1996) reported men to have greater interest and satisfaction than women. Women were more interested in hearing loving words, yet both sexes had similar interest in holding hands, sexual conversations, kissing and hugging. Other assumptions include patients being too unwell with more important things to worry about, thinking that someone else has addressed the issue, or that initiating discussion about their sexuality would offend or embarrass patients (Nishimoto 1995, Ooijen 1995).

REFLECTION POINT

- What are your views of young, middle-aged and elderly people?
- How do your beliefs and values affect how you care for people?

Assumptions and attitudes are closely related to knowledge and nursing practice. Lewis & Bor (1994) studied 160 qualified nurses (mean age 27 years) using questionnaires including the sex, knowledge and attitude test (SKAT) to assess nursing practice and sexual attitudes and knowledge. Findings identified that nurses practising religion had lower knowledge levels and attitude scores, male nurses were more likely to discuss sexuality with patients than female nurses (11.9% were male), and 64.8% rarely or never assessed patients despite 68.1% receiving pre-registration training. Variables of lack of time and privacy were considered, but only a small significant correlation between receiving teaching about taking a sexual history and questioning patients was found. Although informative, these results should be used with caution as the validity of SKAT is untested and limited to physical aspects of sexuality rather than its broader meaning.

The literature appears conflicting, as Matocha & Waterhouse (1993), cited by Waterhouse (1996), found that continuing education programmes significantly influenced the likelihood of addressing sexual issues with clients. Gamlin (1999), in fact, argues that little knowledge is required to initiate conversation, with Clifford (1998) endorsing the value of careful listening. On the other hand, Risen (1995) understands core qualities to be empathy, warmth and positive regard to encourage patients to talk and to undertake accurate assessment of underlying problems and their cause. Sears et al (1988), cited by White (2002), takes a global view, believing that the relationship between cognitive (knowledge) and affect (feelings and emotions) is predictive of behaviour (practice), rather than the influence of either component in isolation. The literature does, however, consider that nurses must feel comfortable to address sexuality effectively (Guthrie 1999, Lamb 2001, Nishimoto 1995, Waxman 1993), with Ooijen (1996) and Crouch (1999a) postulating that nurses must first come to terms with their own sexuality.

REFLECTION POINT

- What does sexuality mean to you?
- What and who has influenced your beliefs and values?
- How important is it and how do you express your sexuality?

Nurse–patient communication: a collaborative effort?

Being comfortable, non-judgemental and knowledgeable about sexuality is fruitless without good interpersonal skills. Palliative care functions on the ethos of effective communication with patients, family and colleagues, which the National Council for Hospice and Specialist Palliative Care Services (NCHSPCS 1995) believes is an essential component and the focus and drive of palliative care teams. The NCHSPCS (1997) also produced a discussion paper relating to psychosocial care, promoting the provision of holistic care, but interestingly little attention was given to sexuality other than to reference the term 'family' and the importance of acknowledging unmarried, gay or heterosexual patients.

Guidelines are based largely on expert opinion and the principles of basic counselling skills, yet the literature concerning nurse–patient communication across the healthcare spectrum proves largely critical of nurses. The opinion of Heaven & Maguire (1996) is that hospice nurses lack the therapeutic skills to assess patients' individual needs. Despite 44 nurses completing 10 weeks of communication skills training, they failed to elicit 40% of patients' concerns, with a significant rise in blocking behaviour that coincided with increased emotional disclosure, bringing into question the benefit and quality of training. In addition, standardised questionnaires that identified patient concerns may have restricted and guided responses, so reducing their worth. Researchers recognised that patients may wish to share concerns with specific multidisciplinary team members; this included sexual difficulties, which patients may not consider part of the nurse's remit.

Bailey & Wilkinson (1998) used semi-structured questionnaires, which were more personalised and less leading, to study the views of 36 advanced cancer patients to nurses' communication skills. They believed that good communicators possess good verbal and non-verbal skills, demonstrate approachable personal attributes, and have knowledge of their subject. Nurse–patient interviews elicited at least one concern in 81% of patients, yet 19% had not discussed any. Some patients who failed to discuss concerns were happy to write emotional issues down, suggesting that patients themselves purposefully block communication; this presents a dilemma for nurses in knowing when to encourage dialogue and when to use it as a cue that sexuality is not up for discussion. This begs the question as to what the patient's contribution is in nurse–patient communication. Jarrett & Payne (1995) argue that research has overemphasised the nurse's role, with the patient's contribution being largely ignored. Illness may restrict patients' ability to communicate due to pain, fatigue, cognitive impairment or depression, for example; even so, Jarrett & Payne (1995) propose that although patients have less power than nurses they are not completely passive, and play a part in nurse–patient communication.

Professionals can use their expertise to exercise power over patients or to empower them (Lugton 1999). Penman (1998) found this when exploring the therapeutic nurse–patient relationship in addressing sexual problems using action research. As a psychosexual nurse–counsellor, she led seminars for nurses from various specialties, including terminal care, to consider their own and their patients' responses, which were used to inform future encounters. Seminars were documented in a reflective manner, gradually building on knowledge. Results demonstrated development of interpersonal skills and changing

dynamics in nurse–patient relationships which initially prevented therapeutic interaction, progressed to the expert nurse and the vulnerable patient, ending in the nurse and patient working effectively to address psychosexual difficulties. This not only created therapeutic space for patients to be aware of their own protective barriers but empowered them to take control of the pace and depth of discussion. This study is difficult to quantify as the sample size, prior knowledge, frequency and format of seminars, and researcher involvement, are unknown. However, according to Clark (2000) action research is about professionals carrying out research in their own practice, for and with people rather than on people, and checking theory against practice in a continuum of care. Despite reliability and validity being weak, and limited control over the form the research takes, advantages include facilitating the application of a difficult concept in a systematic and supportive manner, encouraging its success, and narrowing the theory–practice gap.

Wallace (2001) believes that the development of interpersonal skills cannot be left to chance, and suggests that palliative care nurses are conversant with communication theories and models. Although it is unrealistic to expect all patients and their partners to disclose sexual concerns on the basis of excellent communication skills, it would seem an essential prerequisite for health professionals attempting to help those requesting psychosexual support.

Considerations in this section included professional barriers to addressing sexuality (Box 13.1). Despite support needs of patients being varied and indistinct what is obvious is that several of their concerns and difficulties run parallel with those of health care professionals. Regardless, the key message is that palliative care patients wish to talk about sexual difficulties

---

Box 13.1   Common barriers to addressing sexuality in practice

- Lack of time
- Lack of privacy
- Little or no training
- Lack of awareness
- Comfort levels
- Assumptions that it is not important
- Assumptions that patients will bring the subject up
- Personal beliefs and values
- Communication difficulties
- Ambiguity regarding professional responsibilities

with nurses being considered key players. To do this effectively it would seem that a diversity of skills presently beyond the capabilities of many nurses is required.

THE POTENTIAL: ASSESSMENT AND MANAGEMENT OF SEXUALITY

Strategies for supporting patients with sexual loss and adaptation to a new sexual self require careful consideration, with essential questions of how, when and by whom remaining. Selected assessment and management issues related to psychosexual care will be explored using Annon's (1976) PLISSIT framework (cited by White 2002). This considers need for:

- Permission
- Limited Information
- Specific Suggestion
- Intensive Therapy.

This framework is widely referenced and considered helpful in education and clinical practice across specialties, with few employed alternatives. White (2002) believes its strength to be its capacity to clearly identify the key contribution that can be made by nurses and healthcare practitioners, depending on role and expertise, with Gamlin (1999) considering it a useful basis for discussion.

Permission

Giving permission to discuss sexual concerns legitimises the topic (Hughes 1996, Lamb 2001), and may in fact be sufficient to resolve many problems (Herson et al 1999, Risen 1995). This is because mechanical difficulties result in psychological responses, and vice versa, so that talking may help to reverse the problem or facilitate acceptance of loss and adjustment to a new sexual self.

Primarily it is important that a private and confidential forum is ensured (Howlett et al 1997, Lamb 2001) and that patients and their partners know that sexuality is on the agenda. This may be done verbally and through patient information booklets.

Roper et al (1996) state that if patients' expectations are to be understood and problems addressed then assessment must be undertaken. Risen (1995) recognises a need for individual time spent with both patient and partner, with Wilmoth (1998) advocating that partners should be included in discussion with the patient. The ability of nurses to do this is, however, questionable as relationships and comfort levels with each may vary considerably. Extramarital relation-

ships also make joint discussions both inappropriate and uncomfortable, highlighting need for discretion. Assessment should include past and present sexual issues and their meaning to the individual, although approaches may differ, with Gregory (2000) stating that the extent to which sexual issues should be considered depends on the setting, role and skill of the nurse and patient need.

LeMone & Jones (1997) suggest that nurses would be more likely to include sexuality in initial and ongoing assessment and interventions using objective measures, and reference two instruments specific to cancer care – the Cancer Inventory of Problem Situations (Heinrich et al 1984) and the Sexual Adjustment Questionnaire (Waterhouse & Metcalfe 1986) – yet only the latter shows validity and reliability. As palliative care includes the care of people without malignancy, an instrument for general use may be more appropriate, such as the Derogatis Sexual Functioning Inventory (Derogatis & Melisaratos 1979), cited by LeMone & Jones (1997). This is a 245-item self-report questionnaire that examines multiple dimensions of sexuality, but, like many instruments, it would seem to be too time consuming for use in clinical practice; thus a tool designed specifically for palliative care that is short, holistic, sensitive, easy to complete and practicable for daily use would help guide health professionals. It may, however, be argued that standard assessments generally separate the physical from the psychosocial and are restrictive, so compromising the subjective and unique nature of sexuality. Dennison (2001) proposes that asking patients to tell their story is most effective.

The initiation of discussion is considered by many authors (Dennison 2001, Howlett et al 1997, Wells 2002, Wilmoth 1998), yet knowing the correct time to do this is uncertain. Risen (1995) states that the ideal time is when gathering psychosocial and developmental information, with Dittemar (1989), cited by Howlett et al (1997), highlighting that nurses first need to create an atmosphere of trust. McKee & Schover (2001) dispute this, advocating a brief assessment as part of initial information-gathering for all new patients. Nurses carry out assessment of multiple problems on admission, some of a sensitive nature, and can be instrumental in prioritising patients' problems. Allowing patients themselves to identify the priority of sexuality in their life would help determine if and when a more detailed assessment should be conducted.

Once the existence of a sexual problem has been established, its severity and importance to the patient need to be understood before the most appropriate management can be offered (Ramage 2005). Roper et al (1996) employ a problem-solving approach in their model of care, but the opinion of Williams (1999) is that it is not always necessary or indeed possible for a solution to be found, which may be very true in palliative care where reversible causes of sexual dysfunction decrease as illness progresses.

Limited information

Limited information is when nurses provide non-expert information related to sexuality or sexual health (RCN 2000), and actual and potential problems are addressed following assessment (Lamb 2001). The Calman–Hine report (1995) states that patients, families and carers should be given clear information and assistance in a form they can understand about treatment options and outcomes available to them at all stages of treatment from diagnosis onwards. This should include verbal and written information to help patients accept and adapt to altered sexuality, and, for couples, relationship changes. Waxman (1993) endorses the provision of educational materials, yet Payne (2002) states that information leaflets give medical aspects of care rather than experiential, which may be known only by fellow patients. Cancerlink (1998) and Cancer-BACUP (Openshaw et al 2001) booklets do in fact provide clear information regarding cancer, treatment and its impact on sexuality, based on service-user feedback. Educating patients in the use of the sexual arousal circuit mentioned above may also help to explain problems that result from psychosocial stresses and physical changes experienced.

The literature portrays other specialties as no better at providing information (Guthrie 1999, Stead et al 2001), and that is why identifying a patient's level of knowledge and information needs is vital, as they may never have talked about sexuality since diagnosis. To do this, nurses surely require significant insight and, as highlighted by Herson et al (1999), need to know their limitations, where to access information, and where to refer on to if necessary. A multidisciplinary approach, working collaboratively with associated specialties, is crucial to dispel myths and misconceptions, and facilitate informed decision-making regarding treatment modalities and quality of living.

Specific suggestion

Dennison (2001) understands specific suggestions to include giving information about strategies to help overcome problems related to disease and treatment, with Gregory (2000) stressing that it would be unethi-

cal to encourage a patient to disclose highly emotional information without trying to resolve the issues revealed. This imposes huge expectations on the nurse and prompts us to question to what extent sexuality is a nursing concern. The RCN (2000) propose the need for specialist training, with White (2002) identifying the clinical nurse specialist (CNS) as appropriate to work at this level. This is supported by Dennison (1997), who states that the emergence of the CNS in cancer care and site-specific specialties such as gynaecology and breast care has gone some way to addressing sexuality. Maughan & Clarke (2001) conducted a randomised controlled trial of women recovering from gynaecological cancer. Women who received counselling from a CNS trained in psychosexual medicine were found to have improved quality of life and sexual function. The control group of seven patients received standard care and 19 patients in the intervention group were seen by the CNS prior to surgery and on three occasions at home. Data obtained using the European Organisation for Research and Treatment of Cancer (EORTC) Quality of Life Questionnaire C30 (QLQC30) and the Lasry Sexual Function Scale showed that the intervention group resumed intercourse within 12 weeks, whereas two of the control group did not and experienced lower libido. The difference, however, was not statistically significant, and criticism of the Lasry scale and the small sample size limits the worth of this study.

Some aspects of care are clearly outside the nurse's remit, yet it is not practical to rely on the CNS to make suggestions regarding all sexual concerns in daily practice, such as indwelling urinary catheters (White 2002), altered body image (Howlett et al 1997) or relationships. Appointment of a link nurse in each clinical area, trained to a recognised level, may help guide and support members of the multidisciplinary team accordingly.

It may be argued that sexual rehabilitation is an unrealistic option in palliative care and that emphasis on adapting to changing sexuality is more appropriate. Literature does, though, provide suggestions for cancer care ranging from vaginal lubricants, sexual positions, importance of touch, sexual expression, communication, reading materials, videos, symptom control, relaxation techniques, assisting with improving self-image (Gallo-Silver 2000, Hordern 2000, Hughes 1996, Shell & Smith 1994) to facilitating sex (Earle 2001). This was demonstrated by Francis (1998), who along with care workers assisted a disabled couple to consummate their marriage. Although uncomfortable, she felt proud that she cared enough to act on their behalf. Such examples illuminate the diversity and uncertainty of the nurse's role which is fraught with legal, ethical, practical, professional and personal dilemmas.

Intensive therapy

Before the patient is exposed to the emotional stress of discussing sex and relationship issues it is important to know what help is available (Gregory 2000). Intensive therapy may mean referral to a clinical psychologist, sex therapist, social worker or nurse specialist (RCN 2000, Sutherland & Gamlin 1999, Waxman 1993).

White (2002) states that psychosexual therapists frequently use physical devices or pharmacological interventions in conjunction with education and psychotherapeutic strategies. Conversely Wilmoth (1998) reminds us that treating the sexual consequences of cancer therapies is more problematic than addressing the problems of healthy individuals. Treatments such as vaginal dilators, oestrogen creams, penile injections, vacuum devices or intraurethral medications considered in cancer care have poor compliance (McKee & Schover 2001, Thaler-DeMers 2001). McKee & Schover (2001) report on the benefits and limitations of drug therapy such as Sildenafil and bupropion in the treatment of erectile problems in men who are prescribed antidepressants or opioids. Other pharmacological approaches include testosterone replacement therapy to treat reduced libido following anticancer treatment in some men and women.

Psychosexual work, which White (2002) states involves behavioural, cognitive and psychodynamic approaches, may help patients to grieve their sexual loss, cope with changing relationships and facilitate sexual expression throughout the cancer journey. Palliative care is committed to caring for the bereaved, yet Elliott (1997) identifies their sexual difficulties as largely unexplored. Cognitive therapy and bereavement support is available in some areas of palliative care, as is counselling from a trained marriage guidance counsellor. Some team members may consider working at this level after additional training; Lamb (2001), on the other hand, recognises that intensive therapy is not usually suggested in end-of-life care. The likelihood of accessing specialist services is also uncertain, with patchy commitment from neighbouring specialties. Nonetheless Payne & Haines (2002) encourage palliative care practitioners to be mindful of the skills that psychologists may bring when negotiating boundaries, referrals and contracts. It is unclear whether lack of referral is a consequence of limited resources, unrecognised patient need, or the fact that intensive therapy requires emotional energy and conscious effort from patients who are often fatigued, weak and living with poor prognosis.

This section has highlighted the need for an individualised and sensitive approach in the assessment and management of sexual problems, yet advice on how, when and by whom this is carried out is conflicting. The PLISSIT framework, although widely referenced and favoured when exploring professional boundaries, is of limited value to the novice nurse and difficult to use in isolation to guide practice. In addition, intensive therapy is arguably incongruous for the majority of patients, for whom prognosis, well-being and available resources dictate the potential for providing comprehensive care.

IMPLICATIONS FOR PRACTICE

Although evidence indicates that sexual problems are synonymous with advanced cancer and that nurses are instrumental in providing support, the reality is that nurses are already overstretched by the physical and emotional demands of palliative care, and, despite specialties such as coronary care and genitourinary medicine demonstrating its feasibility, introducing sexuality into daily practice is likely to be met with resistance. How can managers enthuse and empower nurses to address this complex and sensitive issue? Strategies demand careful engineering and, although many aspects are worthy of discussion, focus will be on organisational issues, educational and research, which are key themes in addressing sexuality and fundamental to initiating change.

Organisational issues: what needs to change?

Changing practice can be a slow and uncomfortable process that necessitates management support, economical use of resources and essential commitment. The literature considers giving 'permission' as paramount; this means embracing new ways of working to encourage a cultural shift that runs parallel with our liberated society. However, first and foremost the level of psychosexual support that can be offered needs to be established to determine change.

Barriers identified by patients include room-sharing, no privacy, staff intrusion, and single beds in hospice and hospital settings (Lemieux et al 2004). Practical changes such as private rooms with locked doors, double beds, privacy signs and information booklets should prove conducive to creating an environment that accepts and encourages intimacy. More conscious use of resources such as aromatherapy massage, therapeutic touch, hypnosis and counselling could also be employed to help improve self-esteem and coping strategies, and reduce pharmacological interventions associated with sexual dysfunction.

Nursing care plans are central to the implementation of high-quality care (Mallet & Bailey 1996, cited by Gregory 2000), with literature identifying the need for sexuality assessment. This requires careful consideration in the light of conflicting data, yet it may be appropriately linked with spiritual care, which includes the meaning of life – sexuality seems to be very much part of that meaning. Nurses may consider assessment impractical due to time constraints, but arguably long-term benefits may reduce patient distress and so demands on time. Confidentiality is essential in developing trusting relationships, and patients may not wish sexual disclosure to be documented or shared with the multidisciplinary team. This may restrict care provision as documentation facilitates awareness plus systematic assessment, planning, implementation and evaluation of care. In addition, measurement of care outcomes in clinical practice is absent in the literature yet crucial to evaluate quality and efficacy of care and identify need for change.

A policy is mandatory to establish a standard, identify professional, legal and ethical boundaries, and guide practice. Surprisingly one area that has received little attention is the vulnerability associated with addressing sexuality. Fears of misinterpretation and abuse are real, so comprehensive guidelines are needed to protect the patient, partner and professional. Assessment should begin at diagnosis and continue throughout the disease trajectory, so liaison with neighbouring CNSs as well as hospital and community palliative care teams, and the use of shared policies and guidelines, may augment collaborative working and continuity of care. Finally, the Department of Health's clinical governance paper (DoH 1998) and the NHS Cancer Plan (DoH 2000), both committed to quality care, advocate the involvement of service users, whose views could be identified through audit.

The educational challenge

Post-registration education on sexuality and nurses' knowledge base are unknown. All the same, nurses have a responsibility to enhance practice within their clinical area (UK Central Council 1996), ensuring a safe, supportive environment to manage debilitating side-effects and address psychosexual needs. Crouch (1999b) considers it crucial in pre- and post-

registration training, yet Dennison (1997), reporting on 33 professionals (doctors, nurses, CNSs, radiographers) working in cancer care who attended a sexuality study day, found that 66% had received no sex education during training and 45% had none post-registration.

Bearing in mind the professional barriers identified, education should aim to (Crouch 1999b, Grigg 1997, Irwin 1997, Muir 2000, Ooijen 1996):

- heighten awareness of self and others
- increase knowledge base
- recognise sexual orientation and cultural differences
- dispel myths and misconceptions
- change attitudes
- improve interpersonal skills
- augment comfort levels
- provide a safe forum for reflection and discussion.

Duldt & Pokorny (1999) advocate a holistic approach using strategies involving body, mind and spirit that not only correlates with the sexual arousal circuit but also reflects palliative care philosophy. A series of workshops dedicated to sexuality should encourage participation across professions and specialties. In addition, in response to the literature, core elements pertinent to palliative care, namely treatment modalities, body image issues, relationship dynamics and their correlation with sexual dysfunction, should be included.

Success relies largely on the ability to identify suitably trained professionals to commit to the challenge. Morrissey & Rivers (1998) state that nurse tutors need advanced training and relevant experience with the English National Board (1994), cited by Rafferty (1995), stating that those uncomfortable with the topic should not be expected to teach. Arguably an expectation exists for nurses to address sexuality in clinical practice; therefore tutors also need to step out of the comfort zone and develop their knowledge at varied levels if progress is ever to be made.

Payne & Haines (2002) contemplate the contribution of psychologists in palliative care and identify their teaching role. Such external support, as well as facilitating interested staff to study and practise at a recognised level, could influence practice through educating colleagues and acting as a role model. Alderman (2000) cites Jamieson (2000), who envisages satellite modules at diploma and degree level as the way forward. Such commitment demands careful consideration from all concerned, as Penman (1998) rightly states that short bursts of training are not sufficient to influence practice, but need to be ongoing.

Additionally Hayter (1996) advocates clinical supervision as a means of support and learning by reflecting on practice.

Sexuality and research

The NMC (2002) states that nurses have a responsibility to deliver care based on best practice and, where applicable, validated research. Unfortunately evidence is limited in volume and value, with the few palliative care studies restricted to small sample size, exploring staff knowledge and attitudes, and occasionally the patient's perspective. Neglecting patients' contribution results in bias and misrepresentation of nursing skills, so more equitable research is necessary to provide a true picture at the palliative stage of the disease trajectory.

Available literature exploring sexuality in palliative care ranks low in the hierarchy of evidence despite some studies using quantitative methodology with validated questionnaires. Perhaps this approach may hold less value as structured questionnaires attempt to fit this broad and unique concept into a rigid framework and therefore risk losing sensitivity. All the same, Wilkes (1998) advocates quantitative research in palliative care, with Seymour & Ingleton (1999) questioning the ethical implications of qualitative methodologies. Although considered burdensome to involve palliative care patients in research, its importance in guiding practice and the therapeutic benefit of allowing patients to tell their story is increasingly being recognised.

Evidence predominantly refers to site-specific studies conducted early in the disease trajectory. Longitudinal studies (from diagnosis onwards) involving both sexes, varied cancers and non-malignancies are required to identify common themes in sexual dysfunction consequential of treatment and disease progression, to assist informed treatment decision-making and provision of appropriate support. Triangulation studies (quantitative and qualitative approaches), where Porter (2000) identifies conclusions drawn to be all the stronger, are required to provide strong evidence that determines the prevalence and severity of sexual problems, and their impact on quality of life.

The probabilities of such recommendations being employed are uncertain; however, the NHS Cancer Plan (2000) has finally acknowledged the government's financial responsibility to palliative care services, which should include research and education.

CONCLUSION

Sexuality is a legitimate concern in palliative care and, although this chapter may have provoked thinking, many unanswered questions remain. The small pool of palliative care research indicates that advanced disease and treatment modalities clearly impact on patients' sexuality, but the extent to which their quality of life is affected needs further enquiry. It would, however, seem that the inherent factor determining psychosexual support needs is the significance of dysfunction to the individual and ability to adjust and cope with their sexual loss. Nevertheless, until palliative care research augments exploration of service users' perspective, care provision will leave a question mark regarding efficacy of care.

Overall, palliative care literature is based predominantly on expert opinion and guidelines, of which its evidence base is dubious, yet it may be argued that just because it has not yet been proven it is not rendered invalid. Further longitudinal and triangulation studies exploring the impact of cancer and its treatment are essential to inform practice.

Patient and professional barriers are widely referenced yet fail to correlate with anecdotal evidence that nurses are considered best placed to take a leading role. The PLISSIT framework identifies varied levels of practice, yet Gamlin (1999) suggests that nurses never get past the 'P' stage. It would, however, seem that this level is in fact most relevant to palliative care, followed by 'limited information' to promote informed treatment decision-making. Unfortunately the reality is that nurses are not adequately equipped to work at either level; nonetheless, Yaniv (1995) states that we have a crucial role in encouraging our patients not to give up the effort to gain a better quality of life, whatever it means to them.

The healthcare culture needs to change to be in line with our liberated society so that sexuality is legitimised and patients have permission to talk. How realistic it is for psychosexual care to be part of daily practice, considering the many problems identified, is difficult to forecast. One certainty does remain though: unless educators commit to the challenge and health professionals develop their knowledge, change their outlook and become more self-aware, practice will stand still and patients will remain asexual while receiving 'holistic' palliative care.

References

Ananth H, Jones L, King M, Tookman A 2003 The impact of cancer on sexual function: a controlled study. Palliative Medicine 17:202–205

Anderson B L 1990 Cited by Hughes M 2000 Sexuality and the cancer survivor: a silent coexistence. Cancer Nursing 23(6):477–482

Anderson B L, Van der Does J 1994 Cited by Rice A 2000b Sexuality in cancer and palliative care 1: effects of disease and treatment. International Journal of Palliative Nursing 6(8):392–397

Annon J 1976 Cited by White I 2002 In: Heath H, White I (eds) The challenge of sexuality in health care. Blackwell Science, Oxford, p 249

Bailey K, Wilkinson S 1998 Patients' views on nurses' communication skills: a pilot study. International Journal of Palliative Nursing 4(6):300–305

Benton D 2000 Grounded theory. In: Cormack D (ed.) The research process in nursing, 4th edn. Blackwell Science, Oxford, p 153–164

Berne E 1964 Cited by Searle E 2002 In: Heath H, White I (eds) The challenge of sexuality in health care. Blackwell Science, Oxford, p 164

Bond C F 1997 Men and sexuality in stoma care. British Journal of Community Health Nursing 2(5):260–263

Bor R, Watts M 1993 Talking to patients about sexual matters. British Journal of Nursing 2(13):657–661

Calman K, Hine D 1995 A policy framework for commissioning cancer services. The Stationery Office, London

Cancerlink 1998 Close relationships and cancer. Cancerlink, London

Clark J 2000 Action research. In: Cormack D (ed.) The research process in nursing, 4th edn. Blackwell Science, Oxford, p 183–197

Clifford D 1998 Psychosexual awareness in everyday nursing. Nursing Standard 12(39):42–45

Cort E 1998 Nurses' attitudes to sexuality in caring for cancer patients. Nursing Times 94(42):54–56

Crouch S 1999a Sexual health 1: sexuality and nurses' role in sexual health. British Journal of Nursing 8(9):601–606

Crouch S 1999b Sexual health 2: an overt approach to sexual health education. British Journal of Nursing 8(10):669–675

Dennison S 1997 Psycho-sexual care for patients with cancer and their partners: a service development. Journal of Cancer Nursing 1(3):141–143

Dennison S 2001 Sexuality and cancer. In: Corner J, Bailey C (eds) Cancer nursing. Care in context. Blackwell Science, London, p 420–427

Department of Health 1998 A first class service: quality in the new NHS. DoH, London

Department of Health 2000 Implementing the NHS Cancer Plan. Online. Available: http://www.dh.gov.uk/ PolicyAndGuidance/HealthAndSocialCareTopics/ Cancer/CancerArticle/fs/en?CONTENT_ ID=4068463&chk=hvKSOI March 2006

Derogatis L, Melisaratos N 1979 Cited by LeMone P, Jones D 1997 Nursing assessment of altered sexuality: a review of salient factors and objective measures. Nursing Diagnosis 8(3):120–128

Dittemar S 1989 Cited by Howlett C, Swain M, Fitzmaurice N, Mountford K, Love P 1997 Sexuality: the neglected component in palliative care. International Journal of Palliative Nursing 3(4):218–221

Dom H 1999 Spiritual care, need, and pain – recognition and response. European Journal of Palliative Care 6(3):87–90

Duldt B, Pokorny M 1999 Teaching communication about human sexuality to nurses and other healthcare providers. Nurse Educator 24(5):27–32

Earle S 2001 Disability, facilitating sex and the role of the nurse. Journal of Advanced Nursing 36(3):433–440

Elliott B 1997 Sexual needs of those whose partner has died. Bereavement Care 16(1):2–5

English National Board 1994 Cited by Rafferty D 1995 Putting sexuality on the agenda. Nursing Times 91(17):28–31

Faithfull S 2001 Radiotherapy. In: Corner J, Bailey C (eds) Cancer nursing. Care in context. Blackwell Science, London, p 222–261

Fenlon D 2001 Endocrine therapies. In: Corner J, Bailey C (eds) Cancer nursing. Care in context. Blackwell Science, London, p 262–278

Fisher S, Levin D 1983 The sexual knowledge and attitudes of professional nurses caring for oncology patients. Cancer Nursing February:55–61

Francis H 1998 The agony and the ecstasy. Nursing Times 94(24):34–35

Gallo-Silver L 2000 The sexual rehabilitation of persons with cancer. Cancer Practice 8(1):10–15

Gamel C, Davis B, Hengeveld M 1993 Nurses' provision of teaching and counselling on sexuality: a review of the literature. Journal of Advanced Nursing 18:1219–1227

Gamlin R 1999 Sexuality: a challenge for nursing practice. Nursing Times 95(7):48–50

Glass C, Soni B 2005 Sexual problems of disabled patients. In: Tomlinson J (ed.) ABC of sexual health, 2nd edn. Blackwell Publishing, London, p 53–56

Goldsborough J D 1970 Cited by Hayter M 1996 Is non-judgmental care possible in the context of nurses' attitudes to patient sexuality? Journal of Advanced Nursing 24:662–666

Gregoire A 1999 ABC of sexual health. Male sexual problems. British Medical Journal 318:245–247

Gregory P 2000 Patient assessment and care planning: sexuality. Nursing Standard 15(9):38–41

Grigg E 1997 Guidelines for teaching about sexuality. Nurse Education Today 17:62–66

Guthrie C 1999 Nurses' perceptions of sexuality related to patient care. Journal of Clinical Nursing 8(3):313–321

Hayter M 1996 Is non-judgmental care possible in the context of nurses' attitudes to patients' sexuality? Journal of Advanced Nursing 24:662–666

Heath H, McCormack B 2002 Nurses, the body and the body work. In: Heath H, White I (eds) The challenge of sexuality in health care. Blackwell Science, Oxford, p 66–86

Heaven C, Maguire P 1996 Training hospice nurses to elicit patient concerns. Journal of Advanced Nursing 23:280–286

Heinrich R, Schag C, Ganz P 1984 Cited by LeMone P, Jones D 1997 Nursing assessment of altered sexuality: a review of salient factors and objective measures. Nursing Diagnosis 8(3):120–128

Herson L, Hart K, Gordon J, Rintala D 1999 Identifying and overcoming barriers to providing sexuality information in the clinical setting. Rehabilitation Nursing 24(4):148–151

Hordern A 2000 Intimacy and sexuality for the woman with breast cancer. Cancer Nursing 23(3):230–236

Hoskin P 1999 Radiotherapy fractionation in palliative care. European Journal of Palliative Care 6(4):111–115

Howlett C, Swan M, Fitzmaurice N, Mountford K, Love P 1997 Sexuality: the neglected component in palliative care. International Journal of Palliative Nursing 3(4):218–221

Hughes M 1996 Sexuality issues: keeping your cool. Oncology Nursing Forum 23(10):1597–1600

Hughes M 2000 Sexuality and the cancer survivor: a silent coexistence. Cancer Nursing 23(6):477–482

Irwin R 1997 Sexual health promotion and nursing. Journal of Advanced Nursing 25:170–177

Jamieson S 2000 Cited by Alderman C 2000 On a sex drive. Nursing Standard 14(38):18

Jarrett N, Payne S 1995 A selective review of the literature on nurse–patient communication: has the patient's contribution been neglected? Journal of Advanced Nursing 22:72–78

Jefferies H 2002 The psychosocial care of a patient with cervical cancer. Cancer Nursing Practice 1(5):19–25

Jenkins B 1988 Cited by Rice A 2000a Sexuality in cancer and palliative care 2: exploring the issues. International Journal of Palliative Nursing 6(9):448–453

Johnson B 1996 Older adults and sexuality: a multidimensional perspective. Journal of Gerontological Nursing February:7–15

Jones H 1994 Mores and morals. Nursing Times 90(47):55–59

Kiss A, Meryn S 2001 Effect of sex and gender on psychosocial aspects of prostate and breast cancer. British Medical Journal 323:1055–1058

Kralik D, Koch T, Telford K 2001 Constructions of sexuality for midlife women living with chronic illness. Journal of Advanced Nursing 35(2):180–187

Kurtz M, Kurtz J, Stommel M, Given C, Given B 2000 Symptomology and loss of physical functioning among geriatric patients with lung cancer. Journal of Pain and Symptom Management 19(4):249–256

Lamb M A 1995 Effects of cancer on the sexuality and fertility of women. Seminars in Oncology Nursing 11(2):120–127

Lamb M A 2001 Sexuality. In: Ferrell B, Coyle N (eds) Textbook of palliative nursing. Oxford University Press, Oxford, p 306–315

Lemieux L, Kaiser S, Pereira J, Meadows L 2004 Sexuality in palliative care: patient perspectives. Palliative Medicine 18:630–637

LeMone P, Jones D 1997 Nursing assessment of altered sexuality: a review of salient factors and objective measures. Nursing Diagnosis 8(3):120–128

Lewis S, Bor R 1994 Nurses' knowledge of and attitudes towards sexuality and the relationship of these with nursing practice. Journal of Advanced Nursing 20:251–259

Lugton J 1999 Support processes in palliative care. In: Lugton J, Kindlen M (eds) Palliative care. The nursing role. Churchill Livingstone, Edinburgh, p 93–95

Mallet J, Bailey C 1996 Cited by Gregory P 2000 Patient assessment and care planning: sexuality. Nursing Standard 15(9):38–41

Masters W H, Johnson V E 1970 Cited by Gallo-Silver L 2000 The sexual rehabilitation of persons with cancer. Cancer Practice 8(1):10–15

Matocha L, Waterhouse J 1993 Cited by Waterhouse J 1996 Nursing practice related to sexuality: a review and recommendations. Nursing Times Research 1(6):412–417

Matthews A 1998 Lesbians and cancer support: clinical issues for cancer patients. Health Care for Women International 19:193–203

Maughan K, Clarke C 2001 The effect of a clinical nurse specialist in gynaecological oncology on quality of life and sexuality. Journal of Clinical Nursing 10(2):221–229

McIllmurray M B, Thomas C, Francis B, Morris S, Soothill K, Al-Hamad A 2001 The psychosocial needs of cancer patients: findings from an observational study. European Journal of Cancer Care 10:261–269

McKee A, Schover L 2001 Sexuality rehabilitation. Cancer 92(suppl 4):1008–1012

Monga U, Tan G, Ostermann H, Monga T 1997 Sexuality in head and neck cancer patients. Archives of Physical Medicine and Rehabilitation 78:298–304

Morrissey M, Rivers I 1998 Applying the Mims–Swenson sexual health model to nurse education: offering an alternative focus on sexuality and health care. Nurse Education Today 18:488–495

Muir A 2000 Counselling patients who have sexual difficulties. Professional Nurse 15(11):723–726

National Council for Hospice and Specialist Palliative Care Services 1995 A statement of definitions. Occasional Paper 8. NCHSPCS, London

National Council for Hospice and Specialist Palliative Care Services 1997 Feeling better: psychosocial care in specialist palliative care. Occasional Paper 13. NCHSPCS, London

National Institute for Clinical Excellence 2003 Clinical guidelines: supportive and palliative care. Online. Available: http://www.nice.org.uk/ March 2006

Nishimoto P 1995 Sex and sexuality in the cancer patient. Nurse Practitioner Forum 6(4):221–227

Northouse L, Cracchiolo-Caraway A, Pappas A 1991 Cited by Hordern A 2000 Intimacy and sexuality for the woman with breast cancer. Cancer Nursing 23(3):230–236

Nursing and Midwifery Council 2002 Code of professional conduct. NMC, London

Ofman U S 1995 Preservation of function in genitourinary cancers: psychosexual and psychological issues. Cancer Investigation 13(1):125–131

Ooijen E 1995 How illness may affect patients' sexuality. Nursing Times 91(23):36–37

Ooijen E 1996 Learning to approach patients' sexuality as part of holistic care. Nursing Times 92(36):44–45

Openshaw S, Elworthy R, Coats D (eds) 2001 Sexuality and cancer. A guide for people with cancer and their partners. CancerBACUP, London

Parkes G 1993 Cited by Roe B, May C 1999 Incontinence and sexuality: findings from a qualitative perspective. Journal of Advanced Nursing 30(3):573–579

Parkinson M, Bateman N 1994 Disorders of sexual function caused by drugs. Prescribers' Journal 34(5):183–190

Payne S 2002 Information needs of patients and families. European Journal of Palliative Care 9(3):112–114

Payne S, Haines R 2002 The contribution of psychologists in specialist palliative care. International Journal of Palliative Nursing 8(8):401–406

Penman J 1998 Action research in the care of patients with sexual anxieties. Nursing Standard 13(13–15):47–50

Porter S 2000 Qualitative analysis. In: Cormack D (ed.) The research process in nursing, 4th edn. Blackwell Science, Oxford, p 399–410

Price B 1990 Cited by Price B 1998 Cancer: altered body image. Nursing Standard 12(21):49–55

Price B 1998 Cancer: altered body image. Nursing Standard 12(21):49–55

Price B 2000 Altered body image: managing social encounters. International Journal of Palliative Nursing 6(4):179–185

Rafferty D 1995 Putting sexuality on the agenda. Nursing Times 91(17):28–31

Ramage M 2005 Management of sexual problems. In: Tomlinson J (ed.) ABC of sexual health, 2nd edn. Blackwell Publishing, London, p 1–4

Rice A 2000a Sexuality in cancer and palliative care 2: exploring the issues. International Journal of Palliative Nursing 6(9):448–453

Rice A 2000b Sexuality in cancer and palliative care 1: effects of disease and treatment. International Journal of Palliative Nursing 6(8):392–397

Risen B 1995 A guide to taking a sexual history. Psychiatric Clinics of North America 18(1):39–53

Roper N, Logan W, Tierney A 1996 The elements of nursing: a model for nurses based on a model of living, 4th edn. Churchill Livingstone, New York

Royal College of Nursing 2000 Sexuality and sexual health in nursing practice. RCN, London

Rubin R 2005 Communication about sexual problems in male patients with multiple sclerosis. Nursing Standard 19(24):33–37

Russell P 1998 Sexuality in the lives of older people. Nursing Standard 13(8):49–56

Rydholm M, Strang P 2002 Physical and psychosocial impact of xerostomia in palliative cancer care: a qualitative interview study. International Journal of Palliative Nursing 8(7):318–323

Sanson-Fisher R, Girgis A, Boyes A, Bonevski B, Burton L, Cook P 2000 The unmet supportive care needs of patients with cancer. Cancer 88:225–236

Schover L R, Jensen S B 1988 Sexuality and chronic illness. A comprehensive approach. Guilford Press, New York

Schover L, Yetman R, Tuason L et al 1995 Partial mastectomy and breast reconstruction. A comparison of their effects on psychosocial adjustment, body image, and sexuality. Cancer 75(1):54–64

Schwartz C L, Hobbie W L, Constine L S 1994 Cited by Nishimoto P 1995 Sex and sexuality in the cancer patient. Nurse Practitioner Forum 6(4):221–227

Schwartz S, Plawecki H M 2002 Consequences of chemotherapy on the sexuality of patients with lung cancer. Clinical Journal of Oncology Nursing 6(4):212–216

Searle E 2002 Sexuality and people who are dying. In: Heath H, White I (eds) The challenge of sexuality in health care. Blackwell Science, Oxford, p 163–164

Sears D et al 1988 Cited by White I 2002 In: Heath H, White I (eds) The challenge of sexuality in health care. Blackwell Science, Oxford, p 246

Seymour J, Ingleton C 1999 Ethical issues in qualitative research at the end of life. International Journal of Palliative Nursing 5(2):65–73

Shell A, Smith C 1994 Sexuality and the older person with cancer. Oncology Nursing Forum 21(3):553–558

Shell J, Miller M 1999 The cancer amputee and sexuality. Orthopaedic Nursing 18(5):53–57

Stead M, Fallowfield L, Brown J, Selby P 2001 Communication about sexual concerns in ovarian cancer: qualitative study. British Medical Journal 323:836–837

Steinke E E 1994 Knowledge and attitudes of older adults about sexuality and aging: a comparison of two studies. Journal of Advanced Nursing 19:477–485

Sutherland N, Gamlin R 1999 Body image and sexuality: implications for palliative care. In: Lugton J, Kindlen M (eds) Palliative care. The nursing role. Churchill Livingstone, Edinburgh, p 141–162

Thaler-DeMers D 2001 Intimacy issues: sexuality, fertility, and relationships. Seminars in Oncology Nursing 17(4):255–262

Tomlinson J 2005 Taking a sexual history. In: Tomlinson J (ed.) ABC of sexual health, 2nd edn. Blackwell Publishing, London, p 13–16

UK Central Council for Nursing, Midwifery and Health Visiting 1996 Guidelines for professional practice. UKCC, London

Wallace P 2001 Improving palliative care through effective communication. International Journal of Palliative Nursing 7(2):86–90

Waterhouse J 1996 Nursing practice related to sexuality: a review and recommendations. Nursing Times Research 1(6):412–418

Waterhouse J, Metcalfe M 1986 Cited by LeMone P, Jones D 1997 Nursing assessment of altered sexuality: a review of salient factors and objective measures. Nursing Diagnosis 8(3):120–128

Waterhouse J, Metcalfe M 1991 Attitudes towards nurses discussing sexual concerns with patients. Journal of Advanced Nursing 16:1048–1054

Waxman E S 1993 Sexual dysfunction following treatment for prostate cancer: nursing assessment and interventions. Oncology Nursing Forum 20(10):1567–1571

Webb C 1988 A study of nurses' knowledge and attitudes about sexuality in health care. International Journal of Nursing Studies 25(3):235–244

Webb C 1994 Living sexuality. Issues for nursing and health. Scutari Press, London

Webster C, Heath H 2002 Sexuality and people with disability and chronic illness. In: Heath H, White I (eds) The challenge of sexuality in health care. Blackwell Science, Oxford, p 211–225

Wells P 2002 No sex please, I'm dying. A common myth explored. European Journal of Palliative Care 9(3):119–122

White I 2002 Facilitating sexual expression: challenges for contemporary practice. In: Heath H, White I (eds) The challenge of sexuality in health care. Blackwell Science, Oxford, p 243–263

Wilkes L 1998 Palliative care nursing research: trends from 1987 to 1996. International Journal of Palliative Nursing 4(3):128–133

Williams S 1999 In search for the skills to talk about sexual issues. Nursing Times 95(26):50–51

Wilmoth M C 1998 Sexuality resources for cancer professionals and their patients. Cancer Practice 6(6):346–348

Wilmoth M C, Botchway P 1999 Psychosexual implications of breast and gynecologic cancer. Cancer Investigation 17(8):631–636

Wilmoth M, Ross J 1997 Women's perception. Breast cancer treatment and sexuality. Cancer Practice 5(6):353–359

World Health Organisation 1975 Cited by Rice A 2000a Sexuality in cancer and palliative care 2: exploring the issues. International Journal of Palliative Nursing 6(9):448–453

Yaniv H 1995 Sexuality of cancer patients – a palliative approach. European Journal of Palliative Care 2(2):69–72

Chapter **14**

Complementary therapies

Pippa Lovell, April Joslin, Linden Tansley, Kathy Roberts, Helen Richardson, Karen Merkin–Eyre and Sharon Macnish

INTRODUCTION

Without my journey
And without the Spring,
I would have missed this dawn

                                    SHIKI

Complementary therapies are becoming an increasingly acceptable adjunct to palliative care. There is considerable pressure to make complementary interventions more available within the National Health Service (NHS) cancer services (Walker 2006). More than 30% of people with cancer use complementary therapies (Rees et al 2000), and nearly 50% of those not receiving complementary therapies would like to do so (Lewith et al 2002, cited by Kohn 2003). Most provision is in hospices (36%) and hospitals (31%) (Kohn 2003). Patients are known to prefer to receive complementary therapies from therapists employed by a specialist unit because they are reassured that the therapist would have a knowledge of cancer, its treatment and the side-effects (Watson & Watson 1997). Coss et al (1998) found that 75% of patients would like to be referred by a doctor and 85% would like complementary therapies to be offered as part of the service at the cancer centre.

A study by Morris et al (2000), cited by Hann et al (2005), showed that breast cancer sufferers were more likely to use complementary therapies than other cancer patients. This may be changing, and a Europe-wide survey carried out by Molassiotis et al (2005) found that the patient groups most likely to access complementary therapies included those with pancreatic, liver, bone and brain cancers. The latter three may be evidence of metastases; however, owing to communication difficulties in the survey it was not always possible to clarify the diagnosis. Patients with these cancers are often deteriorating rapidly, have a poor prognosis, and may have run out of conventional medical options. They may turn to complementary therapies to improve the quality of their life. This survey, carried out across 33 countries with responses from 956 patients, showed that patients were satisfied with the use of complementary therapies even when they did not see an obvious benefit (Molassiotis et al 2005). The authors suggest that complementary therapies such as aromatherapy, massage, relaxation and reflexology may not need to be proved to be effective before allowing their use, because they are low risk and patients feel good after their use. In palliative care, where the goal is an improvement in quality of life rather than cure, patient satisfaction is a suitable measure for evaluation rather than hard clinical data.

INTEGRATION INTO CONVENTIONAL CARE

There are many obstacles to the integration of complementary therapies into mainstream cancer care and the attitudes of doctors are an important factor (Barnett 2001). It may be difficult to change the attitudes of those already in practice. However, the British Medical Association (2005) has recommended in a document entitled 'Medicine in the 21st century – standards for the delivery of undergraduate medical education' that medical students should have a basic understanding of the principles and side-effects of evidence-based complementary therapies, and of their interactions with conventional medicine, and that this should be integrated into the core curriculum in response to greater NHS involvement and increasing public popularity. Students at our local medical school are now offered an optional module during their fourth year, in which they can spend 6 weeks learning about and experiencing complementary therapies from qualified therapists. It is most encouraging to see how experiential learning can change attitudes.

Nurses, on the other hand, have readily responded to public demand for complementary types of treatment and applied them in practice, particularly in palliative care (Rankin-Box 1997). Palliative care nurses are ideally placed to deliver complementary therapies because of their wealth of knowledge and experience in cancer care. The use of complementary therapies involves a more hands-on approach and promotes a more caring philosophy. This is becoming increasingly important as palliative care becomes more technical with emphasis on physical symptoms at the expense of psychosocial and spiritual concerns (Clark 2002). Touch, in particular, enhances verbal communication and conveys empathy (Watson &

Watson 1997). The development of the therapeutic relationship through touch reduces fear, induces peace of mind, and promotes trust and hope in cancer patients (McNamara 1999).

COMPLEMENTARY THERAPIES

The term 'complementary therapies' or 'complementary medicine' encompasses many distinct therapies. Some authors have suggested that there may be as many as 58 or more different types, so this chapter will employ the following collective definition:

> Diagnosis, treatment and or prevention which complements mainstream medicine by contributing to a common whole, by satisfying a demand not met by orthodoxy or by diversifying the conceptual framework of medicine.
> (Ernst et al 1995, p 506)

Complementary therapies in the palliative care setting do not aim to cure, but to alleviate symptoms and reduce adverse effects of conventional treatment (McNamara 1999). They aim to improve quality of life and well-being by helping people to cope with being ill in a holistic way. They help patients to use their inner resources, to make a healthy adaptation to facing their death. Illich (2003) defined health as a process of adaptation through which one is empowered to control one's own destiny. By improving quality of life it may become possible to improve the quality of death.

Once patients have been diagnosed with cancer they often feel that they lose their identity and are viewed in terms of their disease and the treatment plans designed to fight the cancer. Loss of control in decision-making may inhibit normal coping strategies (Burke & Sikora 1992). Complementary therapies redress the balance, empowering the patient, encouraging self-responsibility and enhancing personal autonomy. Patients are able to regain control by becoming partners with the therapist in the decision-making about their therapy – they can choose the therapy, and influence the choice of oils if used, etc., depending on their mood and symptoms. Therapists see patients as 'people with cancer' rather than 'cancer patients', and the person's choice is honoured and respected in this area of care. The most popular therapies chosen by patients are aromatherapy, acupuncture, relaxation, massage and nutrition (Lewith et al 2002).

The term 'alternative medicine' may be used interchangeably with 'complementary therapy' or 'complementary medicine', or reserved to describe unconventional treatments and therapies intended to cure cancer. In this chapter, 'complementary therapy' refers to those therapies that are used alongside conventional treatment. Alternative therapies – some examples include Traditional Chinese Medicine and Ayurvedic medicine – may be used by patients for the treatment of cancer as well as for symptom control. Therapies that intend to cure are not covered in this chapter.

It is estimated that conventional medicine is in fact used by only 30% of the world's population – the rest use alternative methods. Most people seeking an alternative treatment for cancer do so when conventional approaches have failed or the effects of treatment are considered detrimental.

Therapies, including herbalism, cross both complementary and alternative camps. Herbal compounds such as ESSIAC (burdock root, sheep sorrel, slippery elm bark and turkey rhubarb) and Iscador (a mistletoe extract) are promoted as treatments aimed at supporting the patient and enhancing the effects of conventional treatment. Homoeopathy also offers remedies that can be used alongside conventional treatment to treat symptoms ranging from radiation fatigue to nausea and vomiting. Hahnemann, in the 18th century, developed the principles of homoeopathy when he felt there was little to offer patients apart from a bedside manner. It is interesting to consider that nowadays there is so much to offer patients in conventional medicine that perhaps the bedside manner has become of secondary importance. Complementary therapies have been able to elevate this most important aspect of treatment, offering perhaps a charismatic and empathic attitude in contrast to the often cool and professional approach of the conventional medicine practitioners (Furnham 2001).

RESEARCH

The 'gold standard' of research in the biomedical field is the randomised controlled trial. This technique is reductionist and seeks to standardise as many variables as possible in human attributes – removing our individuality. Clinical trials aim to measure the effect of a single treatment technique on the human body. Complementary therapies, however, are holistic in their methods, individualised for each patient, and offer multifaceted treatment packages. Attempts to study a single aspect of these multifaceted packages lead to a negative outcome in a trial. The multifaceted treatment package encompasses the personalities of the patient and therapist as well as the therapy; clinical trials are designed to evaluate the latter and neglect the former (Ernst et al 2003). This package is an example of the original meaning

of 'holism' – that the whole is greater than the sum of its parts. In some respects palliative care is similarly holistic and individualised, and presents similar problems to research.

The effects of complementary therapy are subtle and require clinical trials designed appropriately for symptoms and treatment as well as the research question under consideration. With certain complementary therapies, for example acupuncture or magnetic therapy, it can be difficult to find adequate control groups or to 'blind' the trial. Research can be achieved through qualitative methods more readily than quantitative ones using validated measures of quality of life, well-being and patient-directed symptoms. Ernst et al (2003) suggest that a debate exists between proof of effectiveness through randomised control trials versus accepting it is enough that patients adopt complementary therapies with satisfaction, and that neither stance is entirely right or wrong. However, at the end of the day, in such a strongly biomedical environment the absence of vigorous science will critically hinder progress to the detriment of future patients (Ernst et al 2003).

COMPLEMENTARY MEDICINE IN PALLIATIVE CARE

Although an examination of the wide range of therapeutic applications is outside the scope of this chapter, it is useful to consider several therapies that are most popularly used by nurses in palliative care (Rankin-Box 1997). These are the physical therapies concerned with touch and the senses, as well as the mental therapies concerned with emotions and empowerment.

The following section is written by complementary therapists who are involved in providing complementary therapies and acupuncture for cancer patients and their carers. They work in a variety of settings, including hospital and patients' homes. Linden Tansley and Kathy Roberts now work with a newly formed charity (Lifespan, Minsteracres Monastery, County Durham), which enables therapies to be offered free of charge to the patients who are terminally ill in the community. The use of massage, aromatherapy, Reiki, reflexology, relaxation, meditation and acupuncture with people who have cancer will be considered.

Massage and other touch–based therapies

Skilled touch is beneficial at nearly every stage of the cancer experience . . . not only are physical needs addressed, but emotional, social, and spiritual ones as well. Receiving comforting, attentive bodywork reminds the patient that the body can still be a source of pleasure.

(MacDonald 1999, p vi)

Therapists always carry out a full consultation with a patient or carer wishing to receive a complementary therapy, to identify any contraindications or precautions that need to be considered in relation to choice of treatment, necessary adaptations and, in the case of aromatherapy, selection of essential oils. Unfortunately, it is outside the scope of this chapter to discuss such contraindications and our guidelines for safe practice end here. Whilst reference to the research literature has been made, we have also been concerned to describe our own experience with our patients.

The majority of people we see with cancer are shocked and frightened by their diagnosis and further traumatised by medical treatments whose side-effects leave them feeling ill and exhausted. The patients who come to our centre often find that complementary therapies can help provide emotional as well as physical support. In addition to helping with the control of specific side-effects and symptoms, such as digestive problems, breathlessness and fatigue, the therapies can also aid in reducing anxiety and depression, and promoting relaxation, which in turn can help the patient to cope better with the effects of their orthodox treatment. Tavares (2003, p 39) lists the 'best available evidence' for the usefulness of massage, aromatherapy and reflexology in providing such support.

Massage

Massage is the giving and receiving of touch for therapeutic purposes. A variety of techniques can be used to encourage the muscles to release tension and the body to feel toned and relaxed. When used with cancer patients, however, the emphasis is on a treatment that feels gentle, safe and comforting.

Historically, there has been concern that even gentle massage could encourage the spread of cancer through the lymphatic and circulatory systems. As more becomes known about the way in which cancer cells metastasise, the more these fears are seen to be unfounded (MacDonald 1999, McNamara 1994). This is made evident by the fact that massage and other therapies are now available to cancer patients in a growing number of medical settings, including the regional cancer treatment centre, which offers massage to chemotherapy patients. Even though the massage treatments are quite short (usually 15–20 minutes), they are nevertheless perceived as valuable by the patients, who are often feeling stressed and tense prior to their chemotherapy.

An Australian study (Grealish et al 2000, p 237) which examined the impact of brief foot massage on cancer patients reported that 'a 10-minute foot massage (5 minutes per foot) was found to have a significant immediate effect on the perceptions of pain, nausea, and relaxation'.

Feedback from our hospital chemotherapy patients has included comments such as:

'The therapy is very beneficial in reducing the tension caused by both the chemotherapy and by the presence of the Hickman line which causes stiffness in the neck area' (male patient, evaluation form 2004)

'Totally relaxing and immediately beneficial' (male patient, evaluation form 2005).

As well as helping to alleviate physical discomfort and anxiety levels, massage can also affect the way in which patients see themselves. Cancer patients can easily feel that they are defined by their illness. Their orthodox treatment is often perceived as invasive and unpleasant. Massage, however, can be experienced 'as an antidote to the rigours of cancer treatments by addressing the whole person rather than the diseased part' (McNamara 1994, p 25). Gentle, soothing touch can help reconnect a patient with the body that they may feel has let them down and which may also have been changed by surgery or drug treatments. As MacDonald (1999, p vi) says: 'Touch reminds them they are still lovable and worthwhile. For a moment, this person, who may be disfigured, lonely, or without hope, feels whole again'.

One of the writers remembers working with John:

He asked for an Indian head massage because his shoulders were quite stiff. At the end of his treatment, I asked if the massage had helped. He moved his shoulders tentatively and said that, yes, they felt easier. 'But,' he said, 'that's not all. The massage took me back – back to the person I used to be, before I was ill – the person I'd completely lost sight of.'

As McNamara (1994, p 25) says: 'When the vast majority of time and attention is directed towards the cancer, it can be easy to lose sight of the self, the person who was before, and will be during and after the cancer treatments'. The power of touch can help remedy this.

Aromatherapy

Aromatherapy involves the use of essential oils to promote physical and emotional well-being. These aromatic oils, extracted from a wide range of plants, are believed to have certain healing properties, affecting the body and mind in different ways. For example, some oils are understood to be analgesic, anti-inflammatory or antiseptic, whereas others are thought to have antidepressant, calming and relaxing properties, and can be used to influence mood.

There are a number of ways in which the oils can be administered, including through massage, inhalation, baths and compresses. At our centre the most common aromatherapy treatment is in the form of massage, where the beneficial effects of gentle touch, outlined above, combine with the healing properties of the oils. Research studies cited in Tavares (2003, p 44) suggest that 'aromatherapy massage confers some additional benefit when compared with non-aromatherapy massage'. In addition, patients receiving other complementary therapies may also be given a tissue to smell, impregnated with drops of an appropriately calming or uplifting oil.

Full body massage would not usually be appropriate if the patient was very ill or undergoing active treatment. Instead, a part body massage could be offered using a low concentration of essential oil, as both massage and certain oils can have a detoxifying effect. Price & Price (1995, p 196) support this, saying: 'For people undergoing chemotherapy, it may be preferable to administer only specific area massage. This releases fewer toxins at a time and at a slower rate'. Therapist and patient together decide upon which areas of the body are massaged.

The choice of oils will reflect the patient's needs and concerns. Thus, oils such as ginger or Roman chamomile may be selected for a patient suffering from nausea, and lavender, frankincense and ylang ylang may be among the oils of choice for someone who is anxious. However, our selection of essential oils is also very much guided by the patient's preference, because as Price & Price (1995, p 192) affirm: 'An important consideration when selecting essential oils holistically is that the patient should like the aroma . . . The psychological effect of a welcomed aroma can do much to begin the healing process'.

Two examples of anecdotal evidence given by our patients for the efficacy of their massage with essential oils are as follows:

- One gentleman, who suffered with painful scarring on his back following cancer surgery, was given a single aromatherapy back massage using analgesic oils. He reported an unprecedented total reduction in pain for a number of days afterwards.
- Another patient found that regular aromatherapy massage with uplifting oils has helped her to reduce her antidepressant medication, saying: 'Aromatherapy really helps me relax' (personal conversation).

Reiki

Reiki is a form of healing, originating in Japan. It is based on the understanding that energy (*ki*) flows through us and within us, and that this energy can be directed from its universal source by the practitioner to the patient to help maintain and restore balance and well-being, as it supports the body's own healing system. The word *Reiki* means *universal life energy*.

During a treatment, the patient usually sits or lies down fully clothed while the practitioner places his or her hands either gently on or above different areas of the body. There are no physical contraindications, although Tavares (2003, p 47) lists certain other precautions to be taken into account, such as ascertaining that the patient does not assume that the word *healing* is synonymous with *cure*. Reiki is, therefore, a safe, non-invasive therapy that can be carried out in almost any setting and with patients at all stages of their cancer. It can be used as a stand-alone therapy, or in some cases combined with another therapy, such as massage.

There is at present very little scientific evidence on the effects of Reiki, although one recent study (Mackay et al 2004) concluded that 'Reiki has some effect on the autonomic nervous system' as 'heart rate and blood pressure decreased significantly in the Reiki group'. We can, however, provide a wealth of anecdotal evidence from our own work. Patients report a range of physical and mental, emotional and spiritual benefits. These include pain relief, alleviation of breathing difficulties and, in one case – much to the surprise of the practitioner – a reduction in lymphoedema. Another surprise came when two of us witnessed an extraordinary effect, albeit temporary. A female patient, who had entered our centre in pain and using sticks because of her extensive cancer, found she could walk normally and comfortably for the whole day following her Reiki treatment.

Patients often inform us that their Reiki treatment has helped calm persistent, anxious thoughts, and also that it has given them a better night's sleep. It may give a needed boost of energy, improve mental clarity or perhaps bring about a turning point after which the patient can cope more easily with their illness. Reiki can provide valuable support for patients who are close to the end of their life, alleviating certain symptoms and also bringing a sense of calm and quiet. We have worked with patients near the time of their death, and family members often tell us that they believe Reiki to have helped their relative towards an easier and more peaceful death. For an example, see Case Study 14.1, an account by one of the writers of her work with a patient, Rick. This is included to illustrate the place and benefit of complementary therapies within holistic cancer care.

Reflexology

For patients who are terminally ill, quality of life takes priority and the focus of care is to keep them as comfortable as possible. This may include the use of complementary therapies, including reflexology, to provide comfort and relaxation (Federation of Holistic Therapists 2005).

Reflexology works on the principle that there are reflex areas on the feet and hands that correspond to all the glands, organs and parts of the body (Byres 1983). In short, the feet contain a mini-map of the body (Booth 2000).

The linkage of the body parts to the hands and feet is known as zone theory. There are ten zones or lines, five on each side, right and left (Byers 1983), that run longitudinally through the body terminating in each toe and finger. Organs contained in zone 1 in the centre of the body are represented in the reflexes of the hands and feet in zone 1.

Reflexology involves working these reflex areas in a systematic way using finger and thumb pressure (Pinder et al 2005). A cream, lotion or talc is used for lubrication purposes during the treatment. A reflexology treatment usually lasts about 45 minutes to 1 hour, with a case history being taken at the first visit and any changes noted at subsequent visits. The aim of the treatment is to bring balance or homeostasis to the body. Any reflex area that feels congested or gritty to the touch is thought to indicate an area of imbalance (Botting 1997).

Reflexology is a useful therapy to offer in the palliative care setting as it can be given when the client is seated or reclining in bed, on a couch or recliner. The feet are usually easily accessible with minimal disturbance, and if there is a contraindication to using the feet then the hands can be treated. It also gives the client the opportunity to talk to the therapist if they wish, or to switch off and relax completely.

Botting (1997) and Milligan et al (2002) point out that there is little research into the underlying physiology of reflexology, or the reported effects of its use.

Case Study 14.1   My work with Rick

Rick first started coming to our centre after his bowel cancer had returned. His prognosis was poor, and he wanted to do whatever he could to help himself and his family.

He came for complementary therapies, and also attended a group to learn relaxation and self-healing techniques. To begin with he would come with other members of his family for several hours on a Thursday; they would attend the relaxation group, stay for lunch, and then Rick would have an individual therapy. Initially, Rick was interested in trying all the therapies on offer: aromatherapy, massage, Indian head massage, reflexology and Reiki.

Rick could only lie on his back on a massage couch or sit upright in a chair. The therapies he chose initially were reflexology, which helped with the nausea caused by chemotherapy at that time, and Indian head massage to help ease muscle tension in his neck and shoulders, and soothe headaches resulting from anxiety.

As his cancer progressed, Rick became too ill to manage more than his individual therapy session, maintaining how important it was for him to come. Eventually, Rick would only leave the house to come to the centre as he said: 'There are only two places I feel safe: home and the centre'. At this time, his therapy preference was for a very gentle aromatherapy foot massage, using his favourite oils of lavender and bergamot, followed by Reiki, both of which relaxed him and soothed his spirits.

It was important to Rick and his family that he should die at home. During the last few weeks of his life, I worked closely with him and his family, visiting their home on a weekly basis and giving treatments to both him and his wife. Rick still chose to have his foot massage and Reiki combination, on a reclining chair in the living room or, as he became increasingly frail, in his bed. Towards the end of his life, when the family felt the need to restrict visitors, as a therapist from our centre, I was always warmly welcomed. By this time, the treatment of choice was Reiki, which helped bring calmness and comfort.

My last visit to Rick was in September, 6 months after I had first met him. He was asleep, heavily medicated. I gave him a Reiki treatment as he slept, and then gave a relaxing Indian head massage to his wife as she watched over him. Rick died peacefully in his sleep about an hour and a half after I left.

Rick's wife firmly believes that Rick had an easier death, a longer life and a better last few months because of the complementary care he had received.

Tavares (2003) found that the touch therapies (including reflexology) were helpful in the following areas:

- *By promoting relaxation, alleviating anxiety, reducing stress and tension* (Dobbs 1985, Gambles et al 2002, Hodgson 2000, Milligan et al 2002, Stephenson

2000). Relaxation seems to be one of the most common benefits of reflexology, and may be the key to many of the other benefits listed below. When someone experiences a therapy that involves caring touch, the body usually exhibits a relaxation response, which also involves the production of endorphins, the body's natural painkiller and 'feel good' hormone. It is no real surprise that this can have a positive impact upon factors such as quality of life, sleep, pain and nausea. Reflexology gave:

'A feeling of peace and relaxation.'
'It had the most calming effect.'
'I am less anxious and it is helping me to come to terms with my illness.'
(Source of comments: Gambles et al 2002)

- *By improving well-being and quality of life* (Dobbs 1985, Gambles et al 2002, Hodgson 2000, Milligan et al 2002).

- *By reducing depression and psychological distress* (Milligan et al 2002). As reflexology can promote relaxation, alleviate anxiety and provide the opportunity to talk to a therapist, it can provide a coping mechanism for those experiencing depression and psychological distress (Mackereth & Tiran 2002).

'Sometimes when I go for treatments I feel so weak that I am sure I will dissolve into tears, when in fact each time the reverse happens. I leave the session feeling strong and calm. My brain feels empty of all worry and I feel positive about the future.'
(Milligan et al 2002, p 489)

- *By providing emotional support* (Gambles et al 2002). Mackereth & Tiran (2002) suggest that reflexology is a powerful form of non-verbal communication that fulfils the human need to be touched in a caring and comforting way; this can be very soothing for people experiencing palliative care. The following comment was made by a client attending a chemotherapy unit at a general hospital where reflexology is offered:

'I look forward to the small space in time just for me. Talking to the therapist is also very soothing and makes you feel special.'

- *By improving sleep patterns* (Gambles et al 2002, Hodgson 2000, Hodkinson 2001a, Milligan et al 2002). It is quite common for a client to be so relaxed that they fall asleep during a reflexology treatment. The fact that someone has relaxed during a reflexology treatment seems to benefit their overall sleep patterns.

'I have found that I have been able to have a deep sleep – a good sleep for a couple of hours after each session, which is not something I get at any other time.'
(Gambles et al 2002, p 40)

- *By alleviating chemotherapy side-effects of nausea, fatigue and poor appetite* (Federation of Holistic Therapists 2005, Gambles et al 2002, Yang 2005). For many people, having chemotherapy can be a stressful experience in itself. They may, for example, have anxiety about cannula insertion or whether their blood count will be adequate for chemotherapy, and be fearful of the possible side-effects. Reflexology has the potential to change the patient's perspective.

- *By reducing pain* (Hodgson 2000, Hodkinson 2001a, Milligan et al 2002, Stephenson et al 2000).

'It helped to ease my backache and helped me to relax so much so that I fell asleep.'
(Gambles et al 2002, p 40)

- *By reducing constipation* (Eriksen 1995, Hodgson 2000, Hodkinson 2001a). One client who had a stoma was convinced that having reflexology resolved any problems she had with constipation.

- *By providing spiritual support* (Hodkinson 2001b). A reflexology session provides the individual attention of a therapist, giving the client the chance to talk about their innermost feelings and fears – subjects that they may be unable to talk about with family and friends (Hodkinson 2001b).

- *By providing support for carers* (Mackereth & Tiran 2002). Reflexology can offer valuable support for the carers and family of those receiving palliative care, offering relaxation and time for themselves at a challenging time in their lives (Mackereth & Tiran 2002).

The increased understanding of the mind–body connection in psychoneuroimmunology, and the greater understanding of the effects of relaxation on the body, with the production of endorphins and their effect on the immune system, help to explain the positive impact that reflexology, or any other relaxing therapy, can have in the palliative care setting.

The 'National guidelines for the use of complementary therapies in supportive and palliative care' (Tavares 2003) has been a valuable document both in evaluating the literature for evidence of the effectiveness of complementary therapies and in producing guidelines for their use in the cancer care setting. It is suggested that they could be accessed for further reading.

Acupuncture

Acupuncture is an ancient form of healing, dating back more than 2000 years in China (Ma 1992). The practice is based on the theory that energy – 'Qi' or 'Chi' – flows through the body along specific pathways called 'channels' or 'meridians'. The purpose of Qi is to circulate throughout the body, maintaining its physiological functions (Tavares 2003). Most of the meridians correspond to an organ system of the body (Cohen et al 2005). There is considerable evidence supporting the claim that opioid peptides are released during acupuncture and may be antagonised by naloxone (National Institutes of Health [NIH] 1997). There are several types of acupuncture in existence, including Traditional Chinese Medicine and auricular acupuncture, and other forms of intervention based on the acupuncture model include trigger point acupuncture, acupressure, electroacupuncture and transcutaneous electrical nerve stimulation (Cohen et al 2005).

In diagnosis, in traditional Chinese medicine, equal importance is given to physical, emotional and psychological symptoms and causes of disease, which together identify what are called 'pattern(s) of disharmony'. These patterns of disharmony indicate the exact ways in which the flow of the vital lifeforce is disrupted and how this imbalance of energy is affecting and has affected the patient.

The appearance of the tongue and the nature of the radial pulse are also taken into account, together with the patient's voice, demeanour and appearance. The radial pulse is palpated in three positions on the wrist. The pulse variance indicates an excess or deficiency in the 'yin' and 'yang' energies which is used to help make the diagnoses (Helms 1995, cited by Cohen et al 2005).

Treatment usually involves up to 12 fine needles being inserted at specific points along the channels to restore balance and the smooth flow of energy, easing symptoms and distress. The needles may be left in place for up to 40 minutes, whilst the patient relaxes or sleeps. Heat may also be used over certain areas or points, as well as 'cupping' and massage. Ideally, the patient should receive regular treatments, although this is not always possible. Dietary advice might also be offered.

Not everybody responds to acupuncture. The rate of responders to non-responders is not currently known as results from trials give conflicting patterns (NIH 1997).

The patient with cancer is subjected to an onslaught of physical, emotional and psychological shocks which can overwhelm the body's natural restorative capabilities. Many patients use traditional Chinese acupuncture effectively, to help them manage these; for example:

- *Treatment side-effects*
    — nausea and vomiting (NIH 1997)
    — xerostomia (Blom et al 1996)
    — fatigue (Vickers et al 2004) – this initial study suggests that further research in this area would be of benefit
    — low white cell count – there is evidence that acupuncture produces alterations in immune functions (NIH 1997). Petti et al (1998, cited by Cohen et al 2005) showed changes in B- and T-cell populations that would favour antibody production after acupuncture
    — loss of appetite
    — sweats and hot flushes (Towlerton et al 1999).

- *Psychological and emotional effects* – these include stress, depression, anger, frustration, guilt, loss of control, anxiety and panic attacks, fearfulness, altered body image and loss of confidence and self-esteem. Patients attending for physical complaints have often experienced marked changes to their emotional and mental states (Gould & Macpherson 2001).

- *General* – insomnia, pain and loss of sense of well-being. Filshie & Redman (1985, cited by Cohen et al 2005) were amongst the first to investigate outcomes for efficacy of acupuncture for malignant cancer pain. They studied 183 patients with malignant pain and found an overall amelioration rate of 82%.

The author advises patients seeking help with the direct side-effects of chemotherapy to have an acupuncture treatment shortly before their orthodox treatment, preferably the day before. This may not always be possible, but it does seem to maximise the benefits. Patients frequently report having more energy, increased appetite, fewer mouth ulcers, reduced nausea and vomiting, and less reliance on antiemetic medication – in some cases no longer needing it at all. Some patients who are particularly badly affected choose to have acupuncture every week while they are undergoing chemotherapy, and the regularity of treatments assists in supporting them through their orthodox treatment regimen.

Leng (1999) found that the response to acupuncture seemed to reflect the stage of the disease. Any tolerance to treatment may be an indication of tumour recurrence, requiring reassessment of the cancer status of the patient (Tavares 2003).

Auricular acupuncture

Auricular acupuncture (using points found on the ears) is proving, in the author's experience, to be an extremely effective and efficient treatment for many patients, including those with widespread metastases for whom the use of body points to help control pain are often contraindicated (Tavares 2003). Alimi et al (2003, cited by Cohen et al 2005) have shown a statistically significant reduction in pain intensity in patients treated with auricular acupuncture compared with controls. For patients suffering from night sweats and hot flushes, for example women on oestrogen depressants such as tamoxifen and anastrozole (Arimidex), and men with similar symptoms from hormone manipulation for prostate cancer, the National Acupuncture Detoxification Association (NADA) protocol of five ear points is of particular benefit. This calming treatment also appears to help with stress, insomnia and raised blood pressure, and patients report improved energy levels and a greater sense of well-being. This treatment is offered to both patients and carers on a weekly basis in a group setting, thereby enabling a greater number of people to be treated as well as affording patients the many benefits of group support.

Meditation

Mind–body therapies are becoming more popular within cancer populations as methods to treat physical and psychiatric symptoms in conjunction with conventional allopathic care (Ott et al 2006). Meditation is a mind–body therapy that tries to engage the mind in the present moment, letting go of past experiences and the anticipated future. Meditation can help direct attention and develop the skill of controlling one's responses to stressful situations. As cancer patients experience loss of control over their lives, mindfulness meditation helps by providing an internal focus of attention, empowering them to take a proactive stance by consciously directing their attention (Ott et al 2006).

Mindfulness meditation uses the physical experience of breathing or other body sensations. Focusing on the process of breathing helps to quieten the mind and takes the attention away from the outer world of action, demands and distractions. Meditation involves achieving a state of 'thoughtless awareness' in which the excessive stress producing activity of the mind is neutralised without reducing alertness and effectiveness (Manocha 2000). In this state, people often develop a different perception of their problems; the things that normally agitate us become less important when they are addressed from a point of balance and alignment within.

Unlike certain other therapies, such as cognitive behavioural therapy, mindfulness encourages non-striving and makes no attempt to distract or reframe (Ott et al 2006). Relaxation may occur as a side-effect rather than an aim. In America 'mindfulness based stress reduction' (MBSR) has been developed by Jon Kabat-Zinn as a patient-focused intervention with formal training in mindfulness meditation. It has been used to treat a wide range of stress and pain disorders, and chronic diseases (Grossman et al 2004). It is useful not only for physical pain but also for emotional pain.

A pilot study carried out by Bauer-Wu et al (2004) using mindfulness meditation with cancer patients undergoing stem cell transplant showed a statistically significant decrease in pain and increases in levels of relaxation, happiness and comfort. Meditation has also been found to affect immune markers in some patients with prostate and breast cancer. Carlson et al (2003, cited by Ott et al 2006) measured the immune parameters as well as quality of life, mood and symptoms of stress of patients attending outpatients with these cancers, and found statistically significant changes in T-cell production of cytokines in those following a MBSR programme over 8 weeks. The change in cytokines suggested a shift towards an anti-inflammatory response from a pro-inflammatory state.

Relaxation and guided imagery

The physiological mechanisms that connect mind and body lie at the heart of relaxation and guided imagery. A central belief is that what a person believes, thinks and feels affects every cell in the body. This is the basis of psychoneuroimmunology – the connections of the mind, neurological system and immunity. Imagery (thoughts, pictures, sounds, memories, feelings, sensations) forms the basis of how we experience ourselves – our bodies, our relationships, our work, our environment, and our emotional and spiritual lives. Guided imagery makes conscious and creative use of this faculty, to create a psychophysiological change to reduce stress, adjust to change, and promote health and healing. Patients develop ways of tapping into the powerful resources of the mind to effect physical, psychological or spiritual change according to their needs.

Walker et al (1999) carried out a prospective randomized controlled trial looking at the effects of relaxation training and guided imagery during primary chemotherapy in 96 women with newly diagnosed large or locally advanced breast cancer. The effects included improved quality of life, less emotional suppression, and a clinical response correlating to imagery ratings. Molassiotis et al (2002) studied 71 patients in Hong Kong who took part in a randomized controlled trial to assess the effectiveness of progressive muscle relaxation training in clinical management of chemotherapy-related nausea and vomiting. There was a significant decrease in the duration of nausea and vomiting, a trend towards less frequent episodes of nausea and vomiting, but no reduction in intensity between the two groups. Sloman (1995) suggests that relaxation with guided imagery may reduce cancer pain by breaking the pain–muscle–tension–anxiety cycle and thereby improving pain relief through a calming effect.

Many studies to date have looked at the effectiveness of relaxation and guided imagery in patients with breast cancer. Professor Walker at Hull University has proposed a research project to study the psychoneuroimmunological effects of relaxation therapy and guided imagery in a group of 180 people with operable colorectal cancer suitable for adjuvant chemotherapy (Walker 2006). It is only through continuing high-quality research that widens the evidence base that those who work in conventional medicine will begin to accept the importance of integrating these therapies into routine cancer care.

In the author's experience, many patients quickly respond to relaxation and guided imagery, enjoying the fact that they have some control over events in their life and the part that they are able to contribute to the healing process. As with any other therapeutic intervention, there are pitfalls, dangers and contraindications for the use of guided imagery. These dangers include leaving patients unsupported when they are most vulnerable, and being left with a sense of guilt for having caused their cancer (or failed to cure it) because of perceived faults and psychological or spiritual blocks in their lives. Guilt and remorse are ordinary human emotions that can be sympathetically addressed without reinforcement. This was expressed by Moore (1992), who argued for the reintegration of science and art in healing. He wrote:

A poetic reading of the body as it expresses itself in illness calls for a new interpretation for the laws of imagination . . . In recent years some have spoken against a metaphoric view of disease because they don't want us blaming patients for their physical problems . . . Rather than blame, we should respond. Listening to the messages of the body is not the same as blaming patients.

(Moore 1992, p 159)

Many patients actively seek to understand and resolve their emotional and spiritual pain by using interventions such as counselling, relaxation and guided imagery. The issue for nurses is how best to offer advice or how to train in these therapies and avoid the simplistic 'solutions' of popular self-help books.

ADVANTAGES OF COMPLEMENTARY MEDICINE FOR THE PATIENT

- The therapies provide an opportunity to learn new skills that can help a person gain control. Such skills may reduce the sense of helplessness that frequently accompanies a cancer diagnosis (e.g. guided imagery for pain control).

- The therapies require the active participation of the patient, who is expected to work towards recovery or improvement and to achieve something for her or himself. The power base is shifted toward the patient, who is usually kept fairly passive and disempowered by the technological interventions of conventional medicine.

- Time spent on these interventions is greater than with conventional ones. This allows sharing and exchange of information and provides an opportunity for patients to be heard and recount their own unique story.

- Complementary medicine offers non-pharmacological options for symptom control and reduces the drug risk for patients (e.g. acupuncture for pain, relaxation for anxiety, aromatherapy for sleeplessness).

- Complementary medicine may provide physical contact and intimacy (e.g. therapeutic massage from a therapist or family member). Touch therapies provide an opportunity to return to the innate skill of meaningful touch, which has its own non-verbal language and allows the body to speak and communicate.

- Complementary medicine can reconnect the individual to her or his emotional and spiritual self.

- Complementary medicine frequently augments and strengthens the effects of other treatments.

- Patients often experience immediate results, although these may be short term.

It is important to view these benefits with objectivity and to consider some possible disadvantages of using complementary medicine.

DISADVANTAGES OF COMPLEMENTARY MEDICINE FOR THE PATIENT

- There is no such thing as a completely safe therapy. Any intervention has potential hazards and this must be assessed by all parties involved.

- Some people prefer passivity in their treatment and would not welcome decision-making, empowerment and change when they are only just coping.

- Complementary medicine remains too expensive in most circumstances for the majority to afford.

- Each doctor and nurse has a duty of care and is, therefore, vicariously liable for any referral made to a complementary practitioner. Most doctors know very little about complementary medicine (NHS Confederation 1997). Subsequently, they remain reluctant to make a professional referral without a greater depth of knowledge of the therapy concerned and a reasonable level of confidence in the therapist.

While arguments continue about safety, efficacy and funding for complementary medicine, the patient perspective is often the one to which least attention is paid.

HOLISTIC NURSING IN PALLIATIVE CARE – THE WAY FORWARD?

In the UK, nurses have recently seen their role change. There have been changes in education and management plus extensive changes in NHS structure that are examined elsewhere in this book. Nursing is being critically appraised and assumptions are being challenged. Technology fragments nursing and dominates it at the expense of caring and of collective and individual values, all of which are necessary if healing is to occur. Nursing must embrace the qualitative side of healthcare and the therapeutic role. Holistic nursing is not new, but traditional hierarchical nurse

roles do not promote or encourage such an approach. Self-awareness lies at the heart of holistic nursing. Without the opportunity to explore this and develop skills as part of nursing education programmes, it is unreasonable to expect inexperienced nurses to learn from their seniors who have not been exposed to such skills themselves. New models of nursing attempt to address this by introducing holistic concepts, and try to provide a framework for integration into practice.

The overall dimension of valuing has global and personal implications, and holds within it five other interwoven dimensions. These are connecting, doing for, finding meaning, empowering, and preserving own integrity. The latter provides the emphasis missing from traditional models which still dominate practice. Exploring our emotions and subjective inner experiences as nurses helps us to develop appropriate coping strategies. Self-care is implicit, as is personal development, not only in terms of knowledge and skills but also of the psyche and the soul. Perhaps in the process of providing complementary therapies to patients, nurses are providing something precious for themselves: they are reclaiming an aspect of nursing that they perceive is no longer valued either by training and assessment procedures, or by purchasers of healthcare and managers. These are values that are concerned with healing, love, caring and compassion (Wright 1995). The training in, and practice of, complementary medicine may enhance intuitive and creative skills and thereby balance the high technological skills also required of nurses.

Some of the shared concepts and values of complementary medicine, holistic nursing and palliative care can be summarised as follows:

- A philosophy that is concerned with holism and holistic practice. Body, mind and spirit are all connected and have everything to do with health and well-being.

- The therapies emphasise a person's uniqueness and attempt to tailor treatment to meet varied and changing needs. This includes understanding and treating people in the context of their culture, their family and their community.

- The therapies include the use of therapeutic approaches that mobilise an individual's unique and innate capacity for self-healing at many levels, and support living and dying well.

- Holistic practice is based upon equal participation and partnership. There is a greater emphasis on helping people to understand and help themselves, education and self-care rather than dependence. This involves entering into a non-dependent relationship with the patient, and places demands upon its practitioners for maintaining boundaries and changing behaviour so that each remains well. Holistic practice transforms the practitioner as well as the patient.

- Illness can be viewed as a possible opportunity for discovery as well as misfortune if a person so chooses. The dying process is an essential journey for the soul, which embraces each person's spiritual belief.

- Holistic practice includes an understanding of the social and economic conditions that generate and maintain ill-health. There is a commitment to improve the therapeutic value of the environment in which healthcare takes place.

As the evidence of efficacy and benefit of complementary medicine and the therapeutic relationship increases, so nursing develops in therapeutic value.

PROFESSIONAL ISSUES
Safety and efficacy

Alternative and complementary medicine is emerging at a time when orthodox healthcare and practice are being scrutinised for evidence of both safety and efficacy. In 2000 a report from the House of Lords recommended that the government should establish several Centres of Excellence for complementary medicine and provide pump priming funds to fund centres for research. It is unlikely that this will take place in the near future or that good-quality evidence will become available in the short term to accelerate the integration of complementary medicine within the NHS.

In the meantime, nurses using complementary medicine should be practising within agreed protocols with written standards to ensure safety. Furthermore, with good evaluation tools and audit, results could be shared through organisations such as the Royal College of Nursing Forum on Complementary Medicine. These measures would promote the early stages of evidence-based practice in nursing.

When presenting a proposal to integrate a therapy into clinical practice, it must have clear aims that acknowledge the limitations as well as the benefits of any proposed therapy. Gaining team support is essential. The author believes that experiential learning remains the most powerful method of helping team members appreciate the benefits of the complementary approach. By offering and encouraging the uptake of a staff service, healthcare professionals can experience complementary approaches for themselves. At the same time, this provides managers with the opportunity to demonstrate the value that they place on their staff. It may even help to alleviate the stresses that carers experience in the provision of a palliative care service.

Training and competency

Most complementary therapy training in the UK does not meet an agreed standard and is variable. Many complementary medicine organisations are attempting to rationalise training standards and offer continuing education as well as codes of practice and disciplinary procedures. The Osteopaths Act 1993 and Chiropractors Act 1994 now regulate these professions. It is likely that acupuncture, homoeopathy and herbal medicine will seek similar protected status over the next decade. Self-regulation is most likely for the remaining smaller professional bodies that represent many complementary therapies. In the meantime most training courses in complementary medicine have not been designed with the nurse in mind. This may change slowly as training in complementary medicine is offered by universities, which specifically target healthcare professionals and link that education to an appropriate regulatory organisation.

Because nurses work in such a variety of complex environments and are governed by professional codes of conduct, they have additional responsibilities when using complementary medicine as an adjunct to their nursing skills. Each nurse has a professional responsibility to ensure that the level of training is adequate for practice in palliative care and that the practice is safe and in the patient's best interest. Training must be of a sufficient depth and duration to allow for both supervised practice and reflection.

Summary

- Funding, resources and research personnel for complementary medicine are lacking.
- Most trials in conventional medicine looking at safety and efficacy of a product or procedure are funded by the pharmaceutical industry or orthodox and well funded charities; none of these show a great interest in supporting complementary medical research.
- Large-scale research into complementary medicine requires government funding.

- Nurses who use complementary medicine must work within agreed protocols and standards of practice. This should include well designed evaluation tools and audit in order to promote evidence-based practice. Pilot studies could form an essential part of this evidence.
- No single intervention is intrinsically safe, and safety issues must take priority prior to planning.
- Each nurse has a legal obligation to demonstrate competence for the use of complementary medicine in a specific situation.
- Reflection on practice, good communication and clear documentation promote the use of complementary medicine.
- Gaining team support for complementary medicine is essential. Aim for resolution and understanding, not conflict.´
- Experiential learning introduces the benefits of complementary medicine to the team, encourages self-care and promotes the holistic delivery of care to patients.
- Costs must be assessed and funding obtained before the introduction of any meaningful complementary medicine service. Additional skills should be reflected in pay awards for nurses and equitable promotion opportunities maintained, as for any other nursing skill and responsibility.

CONCLUSION

Cancer provokes anxiety. The subjective experience of the person with cancer is not readily addressed by providers of healthcare, although cancer itself may be well treated. Nurses, especially cancer and palliative care nurses, have been at the forefront of attempts to soften the rigours of treatment, enhance the results of it, and offer supportive therapies by providing complementary medicine. The philosophies of complementary medicine, palliative care and holistic nursing share similar values and beliefs, making them natural team-mates. Holistic nursing does not compromise any of the basic principles of complementary medicine. It cannot, however, be adopted without radical reassessment of usual practices. Such change occurs slowly and takes time to implement. The role of complementary medicine is being explored in efforts to provide an integrated health service. Such a service must embrace the continuing biochemical, diagnostic and surgical advances with a wide range of therapeutic options from complementary medicine. Integration implies equal respect and partnership. Such attitudes will ensure that holistic principles are not subsumed by economic or political expediency and provide maximum benefit to patients. Healthcare professionals share the responsibility for ensuring that best practice is based on evidence that is qualitative and quantitative.

The next two decades will see many changes in both the treatment of cancer and its delivery. Hopefully, it will also provide a more powerful and nurturing service as well as a supportive environment for both patients and providers. Complementary medicine is a positive step forward, giving benefit to many, not least in the provision of comfort and hope.

References

Alimi D, Rubino C, Pichard-Leandri E et al 2003 Analgesic effect of auricular acupuncture for cancer pain: a randomised, blinded, controlled trial. Journal of Clinical Oncology 21:4120–4126

Barnett M 2001 Overview of complementary therapies in cancer care. In: Barraclough J (ed.) Integrated cancer care: holistic, complementary and creative approaches. Oxford University Press, New York, p 3–17

Bauer-Wu S, Healey M, Rosenbaum E et al 2004 Facing the challenges of stem cell/bone marrow transplantation with mindfulness meditation: a pilot study. Psycho-oncology 13:S10–S11

Blom M, Dawidson I, Fernberg J O, Johnson G, Angmar-Mansson B 1996 Acupuncture treatment of patients with radiation-induced xerostomia. Oral Oncology, European Journal of Cancer 32B(3):182–190

Booth L 2000 Vertical reflexology. Judy Piatkus, London

Botting D 1997 Review of the literature on the effectiveness of reflexology. Complementary Therapies in Nursing and Midwifery 5:123–130

British Medical Association 2005 Medicine in the 21st century – standards for the delivery of undergraduate medical education. BMA, London

Burke C, Sikora K 1992 Cancer: the dual approach. Nursing Times 88(38):62–66

Byers D C 1983 Better health with foot reflexology. Ingham Publishing, St Petersburg, Florida

Carlson L, Speca M, Patel K, Goodey E 2003 Mindfulness based stress reduction in relation to quality of life, mood, symptoms of stress and immune parameters in breast and prostate cancer outpatients. Psychosomatic Medicine 65:571–581

Clark D 2002 Between hope and acceptance: the medicalisation of dying. British Medical Journal 324:905–907

Cohen A J, Menter A, Hale L 2005 Acupuncture: role in comprehensive cancer care – a primer for the oncologist and review of the literature. Integrative Cancer Therapies 4(2):131–143

Coss R A, McGrath P, Caggiano V 1998 Alternative care: patient choices for adjunct therapies within a cancer center. Cancer Practice 3:176–181

Dobbs B Z 1985 Oncology nursing: alternative health approaches – reflexology part 6. Nursing Mirror 160(9):41–42

Eriksen L 1995 Using reflexology to relieve chronic constipation. A collection of articles. Danish Reflexologists Association, Kolding, Denmark

Ernst E, Resch K L, Mills S et al 1995 Complementary medicine – a definition. British Journal of General Practice 45:506

Ernst E, Filshie J, Hardy J 2003 Evidence-based complementary medicine for palliative cancer care: does it make sense? Palliative Medicine 17(8):704–707

Federation of Holistic Therapists 2005 FHT website. Online. Available: http://www.fht.org.uk/whats/a_reflexology_palliative_care.asp 21 June 2005

Filshie J, Redman D 1985 Acupuncture and malignant pain problems. European Journal of Surgical Oncology 11:389–394

Furnham A 2001 Can alternative medicine be integrated into mainstream care? Pharmaceutical Journal 266:367–369

Gambles M, Crooke M, Wilkinson S 2002 Evaluation of a hospice based reflexology service; a qualitative audit of patient perceptions. European Journal of Oncology Nursing 6(1):37–44

Grealish L, Lomasney A, Whiteman B 2000 Foot massage. A nursing intervention to modify the distressing symptoms of pain and nausea in patients hospitalized with cancer. Cancer Nursing 23(3):237–243

Grossman P, Niemann L, Schmidt S, Walach H 2004 Mindfulness based stress reduction and health benefits: a meta analysis. Journal of Psychosomatic Research 57:35–43

Gould A, MacPherson H 2001 Patient perspectives on outcomes after treatment with acupuncture. Journal of Alternative and Complementary Medicine 7(3):261–268

Hann D, Baker F, Denniston M, Entrekin N 2005 Long-term breast cancer survivors' use of complementary therapies: perceived impact on recovery and prevention of recurrence. Integrative Cancer Therapies 4(1):14–20

Helms J 1995 Acupuncture energetics: a clinical approach for physicians. Medical Acupuncture Publishers, Berkeley, California

Hodgson H 2000 Does reflexology impact on cancer patients quality of life? Nursing Standard 14(31):33–38

Hodkinson E 2001a The benefits of reflexology in palliative care. Reflexions 63:27

Hodkinson E 2001b Enhancing quality of life for people in palliative care settings. In: Mackereth P, Tiran D (eds) 2002 Clinical reflexology: a guide for health professionals. Churchill Livingstone, Edinburgh, Ch 14, p 181–189

House of Lords Select Committee on Science and Technology 2000 Complementary and alternative medicine – sixth report. The Stationery Office, London

Illich I 2003 Medical nemesis. 1974. Journal of Epidemiology and Community Health, 57(12):919–922

Kohn M 2003 Complementary therapies in cancer care. Abridged report of a study produced for Macmillan Cancer Relief. Macmillan Cancer Relief, London

Leng G 1999 A year of acupuncture in palliative care. Palliative Medicine 13:163–164

Lewith G T, Broomfield J, Prescot P 2002 Complementary cancer care in Southampton: a survey of staff and patients. Complementary Therapies in Medicine 10:100–106

Ma K W 1992 The roots and development of Chinese acupuncture: from prehistory to early 20th century. Acupuncture in Medicine 10(suppl):92–99

MacDonald G 1999 Medicine hands – massage therapy for people with cancer. Findhorn Press, Forres

Mackay N, Hansen S, McFarlane O 2004 Autonomic nervous system changes during Reiki treatment: a preliminary report. Journal of Alternative and Complementary Medicine 10(6):1077–1081

Mackereth P, Tiran D (eds) 2002 Clinical reflexology: a guide for health professionals. Churchill Livingstone, Edinburgh

McNamara P 1994 Massage for people with cancer. Cancer Support Centre, London

McNamara P 1999 Massage for people with cancer, 2nd edn. Cancer Resource Centre, London

Manocha R 2000 Why meditation? Australian Family Physician 29(12):1135–1138

Milligan M, Fanning M, Hunter S, Tadjali M, Stevens E 2002 Reflexology audit: patient satisfaction, impact on quality of life and availability in Scottish hospices. International Journal of Palliative Nursing 8(10):489–496

Molassiotis A, Yung H P, Yam B M, Chan F Y, Mok T S 2002 The effectiveness of progressive muscular relaxation training in managing chemo therapy induced nausea and vomiting in Chinese breast cancer patients: a randomized controlled trial. Support Care Cancer 10(3):237–410

Molassiotis A, Fernadez-Ortega P, Pud D et al 2005 Use of complementary and alternative medicine in cancer patients: a European survey. Annals of Oncology 16(4):655–663

Moore T 1992 Care of the soul; how to add depth and meaning to everyday life. Piatkus, London

Morris K T, Johnson N, Homer L, Walts D 2000 A comparison of complementary therapy use between breast cancer patients and patients with other primary tumour sites. American Journal of Surgery 179:407–411

National Institutes of Health 1997 Acupuncture. NIH Consensus Statement 15(5):1–34. Online. Available: http://consensus.nih.gov/1997/1997Acupuncture107html.htm 30 Jan 2007

NHS Confederation 1997 Complementary medicine in the NHS; managing the issues (research paper No 4). NHS Confederation, London

Ott M J, Norris R L, Bauer–Wu S M 2006 Mindfulness meditation for oncology patients: a discussion and critical review. Integrative Cancer Therapies 5(2):98–108

Petti F, Bangrazi A, Liquori A, Reale G, Ippolitti F 1998 Effects of acupuncture on immune response related to opioid-like peptides. Journal of Traditional Chinese Medicine 18(1):55–63

Pinder M, Pedro L, Thoedoray G, Tracy K 2005 Complementary healthcare: a guide for patients. Prince of Wales Foundation for Integrated Health, London

Price S, Price L 1995 Aromatherapy for health care professionals. Churchill Livingstone, New York

Rankin-Box D 1997 Therapies in practice; survey assessing use of complementary therapies. Complementary Therapies in Nursing and Midwifery 3:92–99

Rees R W, Feigel I, Vickers A, Zollman C, McGurk R, Smith C 2000 Prevalence of complementary therapy use by women with breast cancer: a population based survey. European Journal of Cancer 36:1359–1364

Sloman R 1995 Relaxation and the relief of cancer pain. Nursing Clinics of North America 30(4):697–709

Stephenson N L, Weinrich S P, Tavakoli A S 2000 The effects of foot reflexology on anxiety and pain in patients with breast and lung cancer. Oncology Nursing Forum 27(1):67–72

Tavares M 2003 National guidelines for the use of complementary therapies in supportive and palliative care. Prince of Wales Foundation for Integrated Health and National Council for Hospice and Specialist Palliative Care Services, London

Towlerton G, Filshie J, O'Brien M, Duncan A 1999 Acupuncture for the control of vasomotor symptoms caused by tamoxifen. Palliative Medicine 13(5):445

Vickers A J, Strauss D J, Fearon B, Cassileth B R 2004 Acupuncture for post-chemotherapy fatigue: a phase II study. Journal of Clinical Oncology 22:1731–1735

Walker L G, Walker M B, Ogston K et al 1999 Psychological, clinical and pathological effects of relaxation training and guided imagery during primary chemotherapy. British Journal of Cancer 80(1–2):262–268

Walker L G, Lind M J, Russell I T et al 2006 A randomised controlled study of the relative psychoneuroimmunological effects of relaxation therapy and guided imagery, alone and in combination, in patients with colorectal cancer (ongoing research project). Cancer Research UK, London

Watson S, Watson S 1997 The effects of massage – a holistic approach to care. Nursing Standard 11(47):45–47

Wright S G 1995 Bringing the heart back into nursing. Complementary Therapies in Nursing and Midwifery 1(1):15–20

Yang J H 2005 The effect of foot reflexology on nausea, vomiting and fatigue of breast cancer patients undergoing chemotherapy. Taehan Kanho Hakkoe Chi 35(1):177–185

Chapter 15

The changing face of nursing in palliative care

Audrey Rowe

INTRODUCTION

Palliative care is guided by the underpinning philosophy that focuses on achieving the best quality of life for patients and families within a holistic framework (National Institute for Clinical Excellence [NICE] 2004a). There is a growing impetus within healthcare strategy that recognises the need for all healthcare professionals to be able to apply these principles when caring for patients with supportive and palliative care needs (NICE 2004a). Nurses have a key function within this framework and the multiple facets of the nursing role in palliative care have been explored in several studies. Rittman et al (1997) explored the experience of nursing dying patients using a phenomenological approach. This identified that great importance is placed on knowing and journeying alongside the patient and family, maintaining hope, managing the disease process and ensuring quality of care. Thompson et al (2006) also examined nurse

Original chapter written by Sharon McNish has been added to and updated by Audrey Rowe.

perceptions of end-of-life care on an acute medical ward and demonstrated some commonality of findings, with key themes identified of being there with the patient and family, creating a safe haven, and managing care effectively. These findings are echoed in the work of Barnard et al (2006) in a qualitative study that examined the journey of palliative care nursing; nurses described their experiences as being about creating meaning, doing everything possible, working as a team and developing closeness with patients.

Hamilton & McDowell (2004) also highlighted that the palliative care nurse was central to the team approach, in coordinating care and ensuring effective communication between the team, patients and families. Nursing, therefore, has a unique and important role in achieving and striving for effective high-quality care for patients with advanced illness.

The need for care to be centred around the needs of the patient has been recognised in the Calman–Hine report (Department of Health [DoH] 1995) and the National Health Service (NHS) Cancer Plan (DoH 2000a). This has led to the development of more specialist clinical nursing roles within cancer and palliative care, such as tumour-specific clinical nurse specialists (CNSs) and nurse consultants. The importance of the role of the CNS in advancing patient care has also been identified within recent healthcare strategy (DoH 1995, 2000c, 2001).

These developments must also be viewed in partnership with more general healthcare strategy such as the NHS Plan (DoH 2000b) and 'Making a difference' (DoH 1999), which have placed nursing at the forefront of care and reiterated the need for the erosion of traditional role boundaries to meet the demands of the new NHS. This has been manifest in the creation of advanced nursing roles such as the nurse consultant and the nurse practitioner. The role of the healthcare assistant also merits consideration, in supporting health strategy and the registered nurse in such developments (Spilsbury & Meyer 2004).

EMERGING AND DEVELOPING NURSING ROLES WITHIN PALLIATIVE CARE

- Nurse consultant
- Clinical nurse specialist
- Role of the healthcare assistant

Evidence to support nursing roles within palliative care

Within palliative care there is limited evidence to support emerging nursing roles such as the nurse

consultant, with the predominance of the literature available concentrating on the role of the CNS in palliative care, which first emerged within the 1970s (Webber 2000). The palliative care CNS has had a significant impact on nursing roles within the specialty and across nursing in its broadest sense, with the role being regarded by many as a template for clinical nurse specialism (Johnston 2005).

The main focus of the chapter will therefore be on a literature-based analysis of the evidence to support the use of the CNS model in palliative care. Consideration will be given to the evidence for the use of the model and the role from post-holder, patient and stakeholder perspectives. The remainder of the chapter will discuss the emerging clinical roles within the specialty, such as the nurse consultant and the role of the healthcare assistant. Consideration will also be given to possible future developments in palliative care nursing.

OVERVIEW OF THE CLINICAL NURSE SPECIALIST IN PALLIATIVE CARE

CNS roles in palliative care are in the main funded for the first 3 years by the charity Macmillan Cancer Relief; thereafter, the NHS Trust where the post is located usually takes over funding. These nurses are often referred to as Macmillan nurses (Skilbeck & Payne 2003). Most palliative care CNSs work in either hospital or community settings, although a small minority are integrated in a dual remit across both settings. The development of posts has tended to be *ad hoc,* in response to local need and resources available (Clark et al 2002).

Initially the role was established to work predominantly with terminally ill cancer patients. Developments in cancer and palliative care and NHS reforms, as previously discussed, have precipitated changes to the role over the past 20 years (Seymour et al 2002). Influence from Macmillan Cancer Relief has widened the objectives of the role, involving patients at diagnosis and throughout the disease trajectory (Webber 2000). Government policy documents have further impacted on the role, with the reorganisation of cancer services, an endorsement of the importance of the specialist nurse role and multidisciplinary working (DoH 1995, 2000a, 2000c, NICE 2004a). The growing movement towards inclusive specialist palliative care for all patients with advanced illness irrespective of diagnosis must also be considered (National Council for Hospice and Specialist Palliative Care Services [NCHSPCS] 2003, NCPC 2005). This impetus for equity in care provision, where previously specialist palliative care has concentrated predominantly on patients with a cancer diagnosis, may also directly influence role development of the palliative care CNS.

Despite such directives, it would appear that these shifts in practice are gradual, with recent research suggesting that palliative care CNSs were still seeing only a small percentage of non-cancer patients (Skilbeck et al 2002). The initial funding of the majority of these posts by a major cancer charity has undoubtedly had a bearing on referral criteria; however, with the shift towards multiprofessional teams within the specialty and recognition that there is a pressing need to ensure parity of care for all dying patients, it is to be expected that these traditional boundaries will continue to be eroded (Skilbeck & Payne 2005). A recent survey of specialist palliative care services within England identified that 85% did accept patients with heart failure, with 59% also describing collaborative working practices between different service providers (Gibbs et al 2006), thus suggesting a gradual shift towards inclusive provision.

The role of the Macmillan nurse

The role of the Macmillan nurse appears to have evolved gradually into the model of the CNS (Corner et al 2003, Skilbeck et al 2002). This appears to be contributable to the political influences outlined above and resource pressures on the Macmillan nurse from the implication that palliative care should be available to all (Seymour et al 2002). Innovation in cancer treatments has led to improved symptom control and increased prognosis. There is a growing focus, therefore, on quality of life, equity of access to specialist palliative care, and recognition that the Macmillan nurse cannot be involved with every palliative patient (Webber 2000).

Macmillan Cancer Relief endorsed the adoption of the CNS model; although the evidence base used is unclear (Webber 1994), this framework for clinical nurse specialism appears to be widely accepted by Macmillan nurses (Skilbeck & Seymour 2002).

The clinical nurse specialist

The CNS model encompasses expert clinical practice, consultancy, education, leadership and research, and appears to have originated from the work of Hamric (1989). It is theorised that the CNS influences patient care by two methods: indirect care and direct care (Chuk 1997). By intervening in complex patient care, the CNS has a direct impact on patient outcomes. Indirect care occurs when the CNS influences prac-

tice and care delivery by consultancy, education, research and strategic involvement. The evidence base for these assumptions is limited, however (Castledine 1998, Sechrist & Berlin 1998, Wilson-Barnett & Beech 1994), and would appear to have evolved from policy influence and professional consensus (Manley 1997).

OVERVIEW OF THE EVIDENCE PERTAINING TO CLINICAL NURSE SPECIALISTS IN PALLIATIVE CARE

In analysing the evidence and literature pertaining to clinical nurse specialism and the palliative care CNS, distinct themes are evident. These include: perceptions of the specialist nursing role from post-holders, stakeholders and patient perspectives, organisation and analysis of CNS working, and evaluation of outcomes following intervention. The following subsection will discuss the literature relating to how CNSs in palliative care and generic CNSs perceive their nursing role. Examination of the literature surrounding the generic CNS and the palliative care CNS will allow deeper understanding of the multifaceted nature of the CNS role. The majority of the studies examining the palliative care CNS role sampled Macmillan nurses and their role. Palliative care CNSs will therefore be referred to as Macmillan nurses throughout the text.

HOW DO MACMILLAN NURSES PERCEIVE THEIR ROLE?

Subthemes identified within the literature pertaining to role perception are:

- workload pressure
- role conflict.

Workload pressure

Newton & Waters (2001) examined Macmillan nurse perceptions of stress in the role. Their findings were that Macmillan nurses experience a variety of stress relating to: pressure of workload, role ambiguity, and misunderstanding of the role by patients and professionals. Poor interprofessional relationships and deficient support systems were also discussed. The methodology for the study utilised open-ended questionnaire and semi-structured interview. The findings of this study have congruence with those of Jones (1999), who reported that pressure of workload and client group have a major impact on the functioning of the Macmillan nurse. This study utilised a small sample of five Macmillan nurses and used individual clinical supervision as a retrospective data collection method. The differing foci of the methodology and sample size of these studies must be taken into consideration when interpreting the findings for generalisability. These findings, however, are similar to results reported from several studies examining CNS perceptions of their role. Bousefield (1997) identified eight themes that impacted on CNS functioning, including role conflict, isolation, burnout and poor time management. This study used a small purposive sample of seven CNSs and employed a phenomenological approach. McCreadie (2001), in a study utilising a larger sample of 20 CNSs, also reported lack of support, increasing workload and isolation. These factors impinged on the ability of the participants to function in all aspects of the CNS model, with participants concentrating on direct patient care.

Booth et al (2003) used a questionnaire and focus groups to ascertain Macmillan nurses' practice development needs. Again, pressure of workload and a lack of understanding about the role were cited by respondents as factors that hinder practice development. Pressure of work is an important finding. The levels of intervention (Box 15.1) have been discussed by Newton & Waters (2001); these were intended to assist the specialist nurse in managing an increasing workload by transferring the predominance of direct patient care to primary carers (NCHSPCS 1996, Webber 2000), with the CNS acting in an advisory role and intervening only in complex cases. These studies, however, demonstrate that Macmillan nurses and CNSs struggle to disengage from direct patient care, for a variety of reasons, with the implication being that the levels of intervention utilised within palliative care may be perceived to be ineffective.

Role conflict

Seymour et al (2002) reported on the findings from semi-structured interviews with 44 Macmillan nurses, as part of an evaluative study of Macmillan nursing (Clark et al 2000). Main findings related to the changing nature of the patient care role, working in multiprofessional teams, and the role of education, research and audit. Post-holders identified strongly with the direct patient care role, feeling that it gave credibility and job satisfaction. Some participants who had been in post since the early days of Macmillan nursing, or who were very new into post, felt threatened by the 'rhetoric of clinical nurse specialism' and did not wish to disengage from direct patient care. The authors did not quantify the

> **Box 15.1** Levels of intervention (from NCHSPCS 1996, after P Caddow, Wellhouse NHS Trust Symptom Control Support Team, with permission from the National Council for Palliative Care)
>
> **LEVEL 1**
> Advice and information may be accessed by professional colleagues directly with the team. No contact with the patient will be made by the team.
>
> **LEVEL 2**
> The team may make a consultative visit, preferably jointly with the referrer. Such visits will be single, unless requested otherwise by the referrer, and further contact will be made with the professional carer only.
>
> **LEVEL 3**
> The team may make short-term interventions with the patient or family when specific problems need several visits. The intention is then to withdraw. Further referral may be made as necessary.
>
> **LEVEL 4**
> Ongoing, multiple-problem situations requiring continuing, regular assessment.

numbers of participants who held these views, however. Many reported a sense of overload, which concurs with the findings already discussed. This study, however, offers new insights into workload pressure, in that some Macmillan nurses may perpetuate the problem by concentrating solely on direct patient care to the detriment of any other aspects of the CNS model.

Bousefield (1997) described role conflict in the CNS role in terms of stakeholders having different expectations of the role and interprofessional rivalry. Aspects of workload pressure impinging on CNS functioning were not prominent in the discussion, rather that CNSs had to become adept at effective time management. McCreadie (2001) also discussed work prioritisation as being imperative for CNSs, in relation to managing an increasing workload. Perhaps the differing client focus of the generic CNS, as opposed to the Macmillan nurse's client group of advanced cancer patients, may explain the subtle differences in generic CNS and Macmillan nurse working.

The majority of the Macmillan nurses in the study by Seymour et al (2002) were striving to develop the consultative and educational aspects of the role. Education was recognised as being vital to empower generalist staff. Delivering such education, in some cases, was constrained by patient care demands, particularly in small teams with little secretarial support. This was recognised as a paradoxical situation by the participants in the study, as they realised that until the education was delivered on an ongoing basis direct patient care demands would continue to dominate. Post-holders reported feeling under-prepared for the delivery of formal education, and some actively avoided teaching. The study by Booth et al (2003) also supports this finding.

Generic CNSs were able to carry out education, although this was impinged upon by the direct care role (Gibson & Bamford 2001, McCreadie 2001).

Some Macmillan nurses reported that work demands and under-resourcing of ward staff meant that the Macmillan nurse may act as a substitute and that opportunities to engage in informal education through joint visits were limited (Seymour et al 2002). This phenomenon of the specialist nurse 'filling in gaps' was also reported by Bamford & Gibson (2000) in their study of generic CNSs. Clearly, this practice, although apparently commonplace, is an inappropriate use of resources and has implications for effective specialist nurse functioning and the quality of care delivery.

HOW DO MACMILLAN NURSES AND GENERIC CNSs ORGANISE WORKLOAD?

Subthemes identified in the literature examining the organisation and analysis of Macmillan nurse and generic CNS working are:

- referral and discharge patterns
- interventions and caseload.

Referral

Until recently, information about patterns of Macmillan nurse referral has been limited. Addington-Hall & Altmann (2000) examined the nature of patients referred to community specialist palliative care nurses and found that a large number of referrals were for 'emotional support'. A more recent study of referral patterns (Skilbeck et al 2002), as part of a wider study (Clark et al 2000), also reported that two-thirds of referrals were for 'emotional support'. Studies pertaining to detailed analysis of referral pat-

terns to generic CNSs were not evident within the literature retrieved.

Clark et al (2000) gathered prospective data on all new patients referred to 12 Macmillan services over an 8-week period. During the study, 814 new patients were referred, with a mean of 68 patients per service. The researchers commented on this high workload for a specialist service, which correlates with concerns amongst participants that their workload is predominantly direct patient care. The numbers of referrals generated by each service were quite different, with some anomalies being accountable because of differing team size. However, the researchers also discuss the heterogeneous nature of each service, with lack of a uniform approach to service delivery across the teams observed. This is attributed by the authors to the *ad hoc* nature of service development over the past 20 years. Analysis of the literature also reveals that generic CNS working is diverse and heterogeneous. This is partly due to the fluid nature of the role, but may also be attributable to the *ad hoc* development of CNS roles, often alongside medical consultants, with little structure or guidance (Castledine 2002).

Discharge

Discharge of patients is discussed by Clark et al (2002) and supported by qualitative data. Information about discharge patterns from generic CNSs was, again, not evident within the retrieved literature. Discharge occurs when the patient has completed an episode of care with the Macmillan nurse to resolve identified problems. Discharge is usually through mutual agreement with the patient and is instigated with the proviso that patients or primary carers may re-refer if necessary (Newbury & Hatherall 2004).

A reluctance to discharge patients was identified by Clark et al (2002); it was felt by the Macmillan nurses that these patients required ongoing support because of the progressive nature of their illness. The role of the primary carer in providing ongoing care was not discussed. Other teams in the study tended to discharge patients at the earliest opportunity, with the option to re-refer if necessary. Thus, the researchers again identified a diversity of working practices across the teams.

Newbury & Hatherall (2004) audited discharge patterns amongst a team of Macmillan nurses over a 6-month period. Findings were that Macmillan nurses within the team had different working practices for discharging patients, which is congruent with Clark et al (2002). However, this was a small-scale audit of one Macmillan nurse team. The authors identified that the audit lacked rigour because of the methods of data collection used; therefore, the results should be interpreted with caution. The results of these studies do, however, pose questions about the efficacy of methods of service delivery.

Interventions and caseload

As part of a wider study (Clark et al 2000), Skilbeck & Seymour (2002) reported on their findings of Macmillan nurse working. The specific nature of Macmillan nurse interventions and enactment of the direct care role were studied by utilising multiple sources of data in the form of a comparative case study approach. Prospective data from case notes and Macmillan nurse diaries, alongside the qualitative data obtained from the participant interviews and referral data, were analysed. Findings were that, on average, Macmillan nurses spend the majority of their time in direct patient care (56.6%). Very little time is spent on any other aspects of the CNS role, although the Macmillan nurses found it difficult to separate the educative and consultative aspects from the direct role to record within their diaries. This is acknowledged as a weakness in the methodology by the researchers and they advise caution in attaching weight to these results.

These findings are also reflected in the literature examining CNS working. A recent questionnaire survey of specialist and advanced nurses working in the UK identified that CNSs spend 60% of time in clinical work, with education, management and research being described as the other components fulfilled by post-holders (Ball 2005). This utilised a large sample with a 69% ($n = 507$) response rate, and the questionnaire used was piloted prior to use to determine validity. This study provides new information about the different advanced nursing roles that are evolving within the NHS. It suggests that these nurses make a difference to patient outcomes; however, this finding was based on the post-holders' perceptions rather than actual measurement of care outcomes, and might be viewed as a limitation of the study.

McCreadie (2001) found that CNSs identified the 'communicator–carer' role as being central to their practice. Other roles described that have congruence with the CNS model described by Hamric (1989) are clinician, educator/resource and research. The CNSs obtained greatest job satisfaction from the patient care role. Little time was spent in the research subrole, with only limited time given to education. The author

does not discuss the consultancy subrole, posing questions about generic CNS practice. The researcher acknowledges that using a semi-structured interview may have shaped the emerging theory prematurely, and that supplementing the study with participant observation may have added strength to the findings. Gibson & Bamford (2001) also identified that CNSs spend the majority of time in direct clinical care, with some time spent in education. Consultancy was not discussed, with little time being spent on research, although participants recognised its importance.

Clark et al (2000) also found that Macmillan nurses spent a large amount of time in liaison work with other health professionals to broker services for patients. Eighty-nine per cent of new referrals received a direct visit from the Macmillan nurse, with two-thirds of these receiving two or more subsequent visits. There was a wide variation in the number of visits patients received. The most common intervention recorded was emotional care. Such detailed analysis of generic CNS working was not apparent within the literature.

Skilbeck et al (2002) again reported the diverse nature of teams' working patterns and suggest that this warranted further investigation. This insight into Macmillan nurse working is in conflict with the theoretical suppositions of the CNS model, for several reasons suggested by the researchers, as follows. Team organisation and resource availability were highlighted, with teams that had a team leader and access to secretarial support functioning more effectively at CNS level. Inadequate preparation for the role and a lack of ongoing support was also discussed. The researchers felt that there was a 'potential tension in the adoption of the CNS model' by the Macmillan nurse. Clark et al (2002) suggested that the future role of the Macmillan nurse may require a complete reconfiguration of services. Clearly the current situation, whereby teams are providing an inequitable or suboptimal service in respect of fulfilling all the subroles of the CNS model, requires further clarification and guidance from key stakeholders (Clark et al 2002).

Analysis of the literature identifies that CNS and Macmillan nurses may not be fulfilling all aspects of the specialist nurse role. Hamric (1989) believes that, in order to practise effectively as a CNS, all subroles must be practised. This has also been proposed in several policy documents in the UK (DoH 2001, Royal College of Nursing [RCN] 2003). This has implications for effective patient care, as clearly an inability to function effectively as a CNS may not promote or influence best practice for a patient group.

DO MACMILLAN NURSES AND GENERIC CNSs MAKE A DIFFERENCE TO PATIENT OUTCOMES?

Corner at al (2003) discuss findings from the analysis of patient outcomes after intervention from the Macmillan nurse, as part of the wider study by Clark et al (2000). Findings were mixed, with positive outcomes recorded for a small majority of patients. The researchers justify the inability to carry out a randomised controlled trial (RCT) in this client group because the Macmillan service was well established and it would be deemed unethical to withhold such a service from advanced cancer patients. However, Hanks et al (2002) carried out a RCT to evaluate a hospital specialist palliative care team. Patients were randomised to either full access to the specialist palliative care team or indirect consultancy, whereby healthcare professionals had access only to telephone advice. Findings did not demonstrate statistically significant difference between the two groups, perhaps suggesting that indirect intervention is as efficacious as direct care. There were some reported problems with recruitment and control group contamination, however.

Clark et al (2000) utilised qualitative data generated from patient and carer interviews and nursing records. Quantitative approaches were also used to assess quality of life by using the Palliative Care Outcome Scale and the European Organisation for Research and Treatment of Cancer Quality of Life Questionnaire C30 (EORTC QLQ-C30) scale. Difficulties in conducting the research, as discussed by the authors, were that the majority of patients in the study were in the advanced stages of disease. The researchers felt that patients might not identify positive outcomes from Macmillan nurse intervention as much of the work could be hidden in brokerage of services for patients. The lack of a systematic approach to the completion of the Macmillan nurse case records also hindered data collection. The quantitative data were incomplete because of patient attrition, but suggested a significant improvement in patients' emotional well-being and anxiety levels in the week following referral. The authors recognise that these results may be biased, as the fitter patients were able to complete the assessments fully.

The researchers developed the approach to the analysis of the qualitative data. Case studies from each patient were compiled from the sources of data. A single narrative was developed of each patient's experiences over the 28-day period. Instances of care were identified, where there was evidence of the outcome of care, and analysed as to whether they were positive, equivocal or negative. Attempts were made by the researchers to strengthen validity by using several members of the research team to analyse the data. Some 55% of patient case studies were judged to have an overall balance of positive outcomes from Macmillan nurse intervention. The researchers called for further investigation in this field – and clearly further research is required.

Douglas et al (2003) also reported on the economic analysis of this study. Findings were that patients may have more positive nursing outcomes when they have intensive contact from Macmillan nurses, with less favourable outcomes identified for those with limited input. The authors suggest that if the findings were replicated that Macmillan nurses should have more direct care interventions with patients. The lack of evidence to support the utilisation of the CNS model is also discussed. This debate is expanded in a recent paper that suggests there is scope for extension of the palliative CNS role to one of leading patient care, because of the 'brokerage role' identified in previous research, although the difficulties of pursuing nurse-led care are discussed (Skilbeck & Payne 2005).

Skilbeck & Payne concede that there is need for further research to ascertain the most effective care model for palliative care patients, particularly in considering the needs of patients with other advanced illnesses as they may require different types of intervention across the disease trajectory. They propose that specialist palliative care need should be determined by complexity of symptoms rather than diagnosis. The levels of intervention (see Box 15.1) do prioritise intervention by specialist services to patients with complex needs; however, the specialist remains a consultant to the primary carer rather than leading care. Shifting to the model proposed by Skilbeck & Payne (2005) would have considerable resourcing implications as the CNS could potentially have a much larger caseload. An alternative model of care has recently been proposed (Daley et al 2006), whereby heart failure specialist nurses work collaboratively with specialist palliative care services, thus sharing the workload more effectively.

Other studies have examined generic CNS interventions. Tijhuis et al (2003) used a RCT to compare CNS intervention for patients with rheumatoid arthritis with day care and inpatient care. Findings were that there were no statistically significant differences between patients in any group. A study of CNS intervention in Parkinson's disease also found no significant difference between CNS follow-up and consultant-led follow-up for unproblematic patients (Reynolds et al 2000). In contrast, Forster & Young

(1996), in a RCT of stroke patients, found no significant benefits for patients or carers who were assigned to extra CNS support and intervention over a 12-month period. The researchers attributed the findings to the often intractable difficulties encountered by stroke patients.

These studies about CNS and Macmillan nurse working have shown some small benefits associated with direct intervention from specialist nurses. Deficits in the literature are identified in relation to evidence to support the use of the CNS model. None of the literature retrieved demonstrated the benefits that theoretically may occur from the indirect intervention from specialist nurses, for example through education, research and consultation. Whilst it may be difficult to capture this unique contribution to patient care, further studies that utilise an effective methodology are required to advance the evidence base available to support the existence of the Macmillan nurse and generic CNS.

This section has discussed the evidence base pertaining to the evaluation of patient outcomes after specialist nurse intervention and has highlighted the limitations of the current research. The large study carried out by Clark et al (2000) has made an important contribution to this evidence and has illustrated the difficulties that Macmillan nurses face within the current context.

HOW DO PATIENTS FEEL ABOUT MACMILLAN NURSES?

McLoughlin (2002) examined patients' and carers' experiences of the community palliative care CNS. All participants valued the input of the Macmillan nurse in several ways: being supportive, influencing care provision, and having specialist knowledge. Early referral and ongoing involvement was also highly regarded. However, participants displayed a lack of understanding of the palliative care CNS role and had preconceived ideas about the Macmillan nurse. Richardson (2002), in a phenomenological study of 12 palliative care patients, also reported that patients held the specialist palliative care nurse in high regard and valued the support provided.

Beaver et al (1999, 2000), in a study of perceptions of community services received during terminal illness, also reported a lack of understanding of the role of the Macmillan nurse amongst patients and carers. Patients valued the support and expertise of the Macmillan nurse, but infrequent visiting and being left to contact the Macmillan nurse if there was a problem were considered to be unhelpful. That patients and carers have high expectations and may

want a specialist service, even if they do not need it, was also acknowledged by the authors.

Communication between community services was identified as poor, with each professional suggesting something different and a lack of coordination evident. The findings of Jarret et al (1999) support these findings, with a lack of organisation of care and frequent crisis intervention reported by patients and carers. Poor communication between care sectors and health professionals was also evident. The Macmillan nurse was noted as having a positive influence on care and an ability to 'get things done', echoing the findings of Clark et al (2000) in the brokering of services and liaising with other professionals. Confusion about different nursing roles is also apparent in these patient and carer accounts. Inequity in service provision was noted by the researchers, with some, but not all, patients having a district nurse and even fewer having access to a Macmillan nurse.

Grande et al (1996), in contrast, in their study of 43 palliative care patients, found that perceptions of services received during terminal illness were predominantly positive, with no negative statements made about Macmillan nurses and very little about general practitioners and district nurses. The lack of negativity is acknowledged and considered by the researchers. Patients valued intervention from district nurses, and their knowledge and skills. Macmillan nurses were perceived to be invaluable in providing emotional support and information for the patient and family; this aspect was not mentioned in relation to any other member of the primary healthcare team. The authors argue that district nurses are well placed to offer this support to patients and that further education is required for patients and families about the different roles of healthcare professionals. These findings are strengthened by Raynes et al (2000), who used focus groups to ascertain terminally ill patients' views about the care they received. They reported that patients generally valued primary care services. Macmillan nurses were highly regarded, with the majority of participants wanting more, ongoing support from such nurses.

Analysis of patients' views and experiences of Macmillan nurses has revealed that patients generally value such nurses. A lack of understanding of the specialist nurse role is apparent, with patients feeling let down by infrequent or no intervention from a Macmillan nurse. A picture of inadequate service provision and organisation within primary care is evident. Clearly, more work is needed to ensure equity of access and effective organisation of care. The evidence in the literature for the effectiveness of the CNS model from the patient's perspective is limited. Patients may have little understanding of the role, and the impact of the indirect components of the CNS model is difficult to assess from the research. Patients do not seem to welcome discharge from the Macmillan nurse caseload, instead valuing ongoing support and specialist nursing care. The valuable role of the district nurse in providing ongoing supportive care also does not appear to be widely recognised by patients and carers.

HOW DO OTHER HEALTH PROFESSIONALS PERCEIVE THE ROLE?

Little evidence is available in the literature about stakeholder evaluation, with only three studies retrieved that examined the palliative care CNS in isolation; others investigated stakeholder views about palliative care services.

Jack et al (2002, 2003) reported findings from a study that evaluated the impact of the CNS in palliative care within the acute setting. Data were collected using standardized open-ended interviews. Findings were predominantly positive. Respondents felt that the supportive, advisory and educational roles of the CNS were beneficial, and this provides some evidence that stakeholders have an understanding of the CNS role and that some benefits were derived from the indirect care roles of the palliative care CNS. The longitudinal study of Clark et al (2000) used questionnaire survey and interviews of key stakeholders. Findings were in the main positive, with managers valuing the Macmillan role. Some conflict between managerial expectations and Macmillan nurse perceptions of the role were evident, in that managers may expect Macmillan nurses to move away from the direct care role to concentrate on influencing care across a wider spectrum through indirect care, thereby fulfilling the different facets of the CNS model.

SUMMARY OF DISCUSSION

The evidence underpinning the palliative care CNS is dominated by qualitative approaches, for which a hierarchy of evidence to evaluate the strength of such studies is not available (NICE 2004b). Several studies used a mixed methodology; this triangulation approach may strengthen the validity and credibility of the conclusions (Shih 1998). Other studies retrieved used questionnaire, survey or descriptive outcome measurements, which are considered to be weak evidence in the hierarchy of evidence (NHS Centre for

Reviews and Dissemination 2001). That palliative care may not lend itself to robust empirical studies is the topic of ongoing debate within the literature (Bailey et al 2002, Corner 1996, Keeley 1999, Wilkes 1998). This point is borne out by the low levels of research available about the role that can be classed as strong evidence. Caution is therefore required in attaching significant weight to the findings.

Diversity of Macmillan and CNS working

The evidence suggests that Macmillan nurses and CNSs work heterogeneously. Some teams are part of a wider multidisciplinary specialist palliative care team; others may consist of small numbers of Macmillan nurses with sessional medical support. It is to be expected that teams are gradually evolving into multidisciplinary specialist palliative care teams in line with national service frameworks (DoH 2000a).

Macmillan nurses and CNSs appear to have difficulties in fulfilling all aspects of the CNS model. Workload pressure from direct patient care appears to be the main determinant of working patterns, preventing fulfilment of the theory of specialist practice, as without education, consultancy and research the specialist is unable truly to empower the generalist. This will, therefore, impinge directly on effective service provision. The patient group served by the Macmillan nurse must also be regarded as an important factor in influencing CNS practice. Consideration must be given to the philosophy of palliative care, which aims to achieve holistic, high-quality care with the emphasis on quality of life (NICE 2004a). The current model of CNS practice may also not address the needs of palliative care patients across all disease trajectories, a factor that will increasingly require attention (Skilbeck & Payne 2005).

Macmillan nurses may also achieve greatest satisfaction from direct care and may feel under-prepared for other aspects of the CNS role, with resulting patchy CNS performance. Clearly, there is a need for further clarification of the direction of the Macmillan nurse role in specialist palliative care from the key stakeholders involved.

Does the evidence support the utilisation of the CNS model in specialist palliative care?

Evidence for the effectiveness of the CNS model in specialist palliative care appears to be weak. Evolution of the CNS model appears to be historical and in response to political and medical pressures

(Castledine 1998). A clear evidence base for the model is difficult to ascertain from the literature, thereby limiting conclusions.

Corner et al (2003) reported modest improvements in patient-perceived outcomes after Macmillan nurse intervention. Douglas et al (2003) also suggested that patients may benefit from increased face-to-face contact with the Macmillan nurse, perhaps suggesting that the CNS model may not be appropriate in this area. However, this provides relatively low-level (grade III) evidence for only the direct and consultative aspects of the CNS model. Using a qualitative approach, Jack et al (2002, 2003) reported satisfaction amongst stakeholders with the educative and consultative aspects of the role.

There is high-level evidence (grade I) for the utilisation of the CNS model in other specialties (Reynolds et al 2000, Tijhuis et al 2003). However, these trials also addressed only the direct care component of the CNS model. The challenge remains to find an appropriate methodology to capture the impact of functioning fully in all aspects of the CNS model, particularly in palliative care (Douglas et al 2003).

Research priorities for the CNS role in palliative care

Clearly, directions for future research must examine the most effective model of service delivery for specialist palliative care nurses. There is a lack of clarity in the literature about whether specialist nurses are meeting the needs of patients with advanced illness by adopting the CNS model. Some authors have suggested that the role should be extended to lead patient care (Skilbeck & Payne 2005), with patient need being identified by complexity of symptoms rather than diagnosis. Whilst this may offer improved satisfaction and care for patients, there is a need for further research to provide robust evidence to underpin specialist palliative care nursing service provision to allow evaluation of the most appropriate model of care for patients with advanced illness, particularly within the current economic climate within the NHS, where such specialist nursing roles are being scrutinised (Kelly & Trevatt 2006).

A randomisation methodology that compares indirect components of care (e.g. telephone consultancy) versus direct Macmillan intervention may allow more effective evaluation of the CNS role, and has been shown to be achievable by Hanks et al (2002). Conclusions may then be drawn about the efficacy of the CNS model in specialist palliative care.

Having examined and analysed the role of the CNS in palliative care as the main focus, the remainder of the chapter discusses the emerging roles within palliative nursing and suggests possible areas for future development for nursing within the specialty.

OTHER EMERGING ROLES WITHIN PALLIATIVE CARE NURSING

Nurse consultant

The nurse consultant role arose from 'Making a difference' (DoH 1999). This government policy proposed a new career framework for nurses. Recognition of the need to develop and extend nursing roles to meet the challenges of the new NHS is inherent within this policy. 'Making a difference' proposed four levels of nursing within the framework, from healthcare assistant, registered practitioner, through to senior registered practitioner and consultant nurse.

Consultant nurses were developed to allow experienced senior nurses to remain in clinical practice and have a focus to ensure improved outcomes for patients by service development and attention to quality of care. The posts have responsibility in four main areas: expert practice, professional leadership and consultancy; education and development; and practice and service development linked to research and evaluation. All posts have a commitment to ensuring that at least 50% of time is spent in clinical practice with patients and clients (DoH 1999).

Manley (1997) presents a conceptual framework for the role after conducting an action research study examining the advanced practitioner/nurse consultant role and suggests that:

> The skills and knowledge base of consultancy, underpinned by a strong nursing foundation, augmented by strong leadership and combined with the educator and researcher functions, are presented as the attributes of the advanced practitioner/consultant nurse.
>
> (Manley 1997, p 180)

This framework utilised the clinical nurse specialist model proposed by Hamric (1989) as a starting point in the absence of any other available framework to inform the job description for the nurse consultant role. Manley (1997) suggests that the role has marked similarities with the CNS model but also argues that it has a transformational leadership component, with strong links to development, management and research.

There is a dearth of strong evidence within the literature to date to support the use of the nurse consultant role, although this is to be expected with a new, emerging role. A national evaluative study of consultant nurses reported mixed findings, with the effects of role ambiguity, role conflict and problems with role boundary management voiced amongst the concerns. Some nurses did report high levels of job satisfaction and improved career and professional development opportunities (Guest et al 2001). This was a descriptive study, which utilised questionnaire, interviews and network analysis to examine the new role. Clearly there are parallels with the inherent problems previously discussed about the CNS role, and further research to define the role and evaluate the effectiveness of nurse consultants in improving patient outcomes is required. The study by Ball (2005), which surveyed nurses in advanced practice nursing roles, indicated that nurse consultants are involved in diagnostic and care coordination as well as the other subroles of research, education and management. This survey also reported high levels of job satisfaction amongst postholders. The model suggested by Skilbeck & Payne (2005) for an extended role for the palliative care CNS, to enable the CNS to lead care, clearly has some similarity with the nurse consultant role.

A literature search of Medline and Cinahl revealed very little literature that pertained to the palliative care consultant nurse. Blackford & Street (2001) examined the role of the Australian nurse consultant in palliative care in a qualitative study. Findings identified that there were also problems with role clarity and boundaries. Hekkink et al (2005), however, examined the role of the HIV nurse consultant using a validated questionnaire to ascertain patients' preferences and experiences of quality of care in relation to nurse consultants. Parallels may perhaps be drawn between the management of chronic illnesses such as cancer and HIV but the differing patient populations must be acknowledged. This study, however, gives a snapshot of patients' viewpoints in relation to the role. The findings were in the main positive, with patients valuing the nurse consultant.

The impact of implementing policy in the absence of evidence to support these new nursing roles must be acknowledged, for which the government has been subject to criticism. There appears to be an assumption that untested reforms will lead to improvement in patient care and outcomes (Bradshaw 2003). Particularly within palliative care, where the patient population is vulnerable, there is a need for ongoing research to underpin these roles in a robust manner.

Role of the healthcare assistant

The role of the healthcare assistant (HCA) has become more prominent in recent years because of the nursing and midwifery recruitment crisis, role expansion and the ongoing demands of the new NHS (Keeney et al 2005). The role was proposed as part of Project 2000 to assist qualified nurses following the instigation of supernumerary status for student nurses (Meek 1998). There are few data regarding the number of HCAs currently employed in the NHS and independent sector, with limited understanding of the skills and competencies of the workforce (Spilsbury & Meyer 2004, Thornley 2000). Often the role varies according to the clinical area, leading to ambiguity and conflict (McKenna & Hasson 2004). That HCAs are not professionally registered or regulated, requiring supervision from registered nurses, must also be considered a potential tension (Keeney et al 2005).

Studies have demonstrated that other healthcare professionals and patients value the role of the HCA (Keeney et al 2005, Meek 1998). These studies utilised small sample sizes, in differing clinical contexts; care is therefore required in generalising the findings. The main negative findings from these studies were the lack of role clarity and lack of preparation for the role.

In response to these perceived problems with the HCA role, some clinical areas have developed their own training programmes, which incorporate National Vocational Qualifications (NVQs) and are tailored to their clinical area (Arblaster et al 2004). NVQ programmes are vocational frameworks developed by the government that are competency based, allowing attainment of skills in the workplace (Meek 1998). The advent of Agenda for Change (DoH 2004), which identifies clear levels of skills and competencies for healthcare staff, must also be acknowledged as an important step in regulating nursing roles. There are two levels of HCA identified within the job profiles, described as 'clinical support worker' and 'senior clinical support worker' (RCN 2006). These different levels have competencies identified at NVQ level 2 and 3 respectively, recognising that there are different skill sets within non-registered nursing staff.

Within palliative care nursing the role of the HCA is well established anecdotally, although little evidence exists within the literature. A search of Medline and Cinahl revealed an absence of research that concentrated solely on the role of the HCA in palliative care. There is a clear requirement for further evaluation of the role within the specialty.

Marie Curie Cancer Care, which currently employs more than 900 HCAs in hospice inpatient units and as part of the community Marie Curie Nursing Service, has also taken steps to address some of these issues. Community HCAs newly in post undertake a 2-day introductory course on palliative care nursing. The charity has also recently published a code of conduct for HCAs; this does not take responsibility for accountability from the trained nurse but identifies standards of conduct expected of HCAs within the charity (Fraser 2005). HCAs have also taken part in a pilot study to obtain NVQ level 2 and 3, again helping to standardise knowledge and skills (Poppleton 2003). The development and implementation of an accredited competency framework for HCAs within the charity, linked to the new NVQ in health and social care (Skills for Health 2005a) and also containing competencies specific to palliative care, is ongoing. These developments highlight the emerging prominence of the HCA role in supporting palliative care nursing.

However, these developments, although commendable, do not address role ambiguity and the requirement for standard training and preparation for the HCA role on a national basis, an area that, whilst causing much debate within the nursing press (McKenna & Hasson 2004), requires robust action within government policy and adequate resourcing. The development of the 'Career framework for health' (Skills for Health 2005b), which proposes to standardise national occupational standards and competencies for use within the health sector, must be regarded as a significant development in role regulation. The publication of national minimum standards for care (DoH 2003) and the development of new inspection frameworks for care homes by the Commission for Social Care Inspection (CSCI 2006) identify definitive levels of qualifications required for care staff, with 50% of the workforce required to have NVQ level 2–3 by 2008. This standard will be necessary for continued care home/agency registration.

Clearly the HCA role is here to stay and will continue to impact on the care given to patients as trained nurses continue to extend their roles and the issues of recruitment and retention remain problematic. HCAs may perform the majority of direct patient care as traditional nursing roles are eroded; the importance of the role in palliative nursing, where caring and physically being with the patient are perceived to be valuable palliative nursing actions (Barnard et al 2006), must be considered carefully. Ongoing clarification of the role, regulation and preparation required for the HCA role is needed to safeguard both patient care and the HCA (McKenna & Hasson 2004, Spilsbury & Meyer 2004).

FUTURE DEVELOPMENTS WITHIN PALLIATIVE NURSING

The role of the nurse practitioner (NP) emerging within palliative care merits consideration (McHale 1998, Williams & Sidani 2001). Much discussion is evident within the American nursing literature about the NP role and the blurring of boundaries between other advanced practice nursing roles such as the CNS (Locsin 2002, Wright 1997). These authors argue that there is an impetus for combining the two roles to enhance patient care and reduce role overlap and ambiguity. Manley (1997), however, acknowledges the differences between the NP role and that of the CNS, with the CNS being a multidimensional role providing direct and indirect services and the NP being more unidimensional, focusing on direct care. This view is also supported by Williams & Sidani (2001), who state that NPs spend the majority of time in the clinical component of the role.

NP roles are well established in other care settings; NPs are professionally autonomous and may receive patients with undifferentiated and undiagnosed problems. The role encompasses diagnosis, treatment and planning of ongoing care for patients (Marsden et al 2003). The NP is perceived as an expert in the chosen area of clinical practice, and the role is multifaceted with subroles in education, research and consultation (Locsin 2002). This has obvious similarities and parallels with the CNS model described by Hamric (1989), but again illustrates the ambiguity surrounding different nursing roles and their relative functions.

Williams & Sidani (2001) examined the nature of the NP role in an American oncology palliative clinic by means of a case study design. Qualitative and quantitative data were collected from one NP and analysed to provide detail about the nature of the role. Findings were that this NP engaged less frequently in diagnostic and therapeutic procedures than other acute care NPs, with the role focusing on advanced nursing practice aimed at symptom management, maintaining quality of life and dignity. This again has parallels with the functions of the palliative care CNS. The limitations of this study must be acknowledged in that it examined only one NP role, but it does offer some insight into different advanced nursing roles within the specialty. In the UK, the NP role does not appear to have embraced palliative care, but it may offer mechanisms to improve patient care and innovative solutions to medical recruitment problems within specialist palliative care. The potential for the nurse consultant role to develop further also merits consideration, particularly in the light of the study recently reported by Ball (2005), which identified that nurse consultants were already engaging in diagnostic practice, care coordination and management.

McHale (1998) suggested that Macmillan nurses were moving towards an advanced practice role and proposed that the model should be replicated in American hospice care, with such nurses having direct management responsibility for patient care. This has not, however, happened with the Macmillan role in the UK, with such nurses continuing to use the levels of intervention (see Box 15.1). Skilbeck & Payne (2005) have suggested that there is a need for a shift in focus in the palliative CNS role, towards leading patient care. That this may offer improved care for patients with advanced illness merits consideration, but further evaluation of this proposal is required to ensure that the problems faced by palliative care CNSs in managing their current role are not magnified. Perhaps future developments will identify one advanced nursing role within palliative care that is inclusive of all of the current specialist roles, including the CNS, NP and nurse consultant, truly to champion high-quality patient care. This idea is supported by the Nursing and Midwifery Council (NMC 2005) in its guidance regarding the standard for post-registration nursing. This framework identifies one level of advanced practice, that of advanced nurse practitioner, with ten key role competencies that encompass facets of the CNS, nurse consultant and NP roles.

There is anecdotal evidence locally that innovative ways of role and service development are being used within palliative nursing (Box 15.2). Similarly, heart failure nurse specialists in Bradford have championed the development of a collaborative service for specialist palliative care (Box 15.3). This clearly illustrates how nursing can develop and lead palliative care to meet patients' needs in an innovative manner across both the malignant and non-malignant spectrum of advanced illness. Such innovation is also echoed in the work of Ball (2005), who found that nurses were evolving and developing their roles to improve the patient's experience and care.

CONCLUSION

This chapter has offered an overview and analysis of the literature surrounding some of the nursing roles within palliative care, in particular the CNS model of care. Analysis of the differing roles emerging within nursing and impacting on the specialty has identified the deficits within the evidence base to support these roles. Nevertheless there is some evidence to suggest that these roles can make a difference to patient care (Ball 2005, Beaver et al 1999, Clark et al 2000). Common themes running through the literature pertaining to

Box 15.2 Example of nursing innovation within palliative care

Nurses within the Marie Curie Hospice in Newcastle have undertaken a successful pilot project in which half of the hospice beds were identified as being nurse-led in response to medical recruitment problems and the nurses' desire to develop new and innovative ways of working. The team members have developed their nursing roles with the support of the education department, medical team and hospice management. This has enabled the hospice to continue to offer specialist palliative care, planned respite and rehabilitation. This project has now developed from nurse-led beds to nurse-led care, following the medical model with a named nurse rather than a named consultant leading care for specific patients. Linked to this are plans for the development of two advanced nurse practitioners in palliative care, who will lead nurse-led care within the hospice inpatient unit.

these roles are: lack of role clarity, role ambiguity, overlap, and a lack of patient and professional understanding about the roles. The differing titles and perceived roles may only add to the confusion, particularly in relation to advanced nursing practice, where clinical nurse specialists, nurse consultants and nurse practitioners may care for patients. Clearly there is a need to clarify and rationalise these titles and nursing roles, and ensure that further research is conducted to validate their use. It is clear from the literature that nursing roles will continue to evolve in response to changing demands and patient needs (Ball 2005).

Within palliative care, where quality of life and care is so important, we must not lose sight of the true essence of palliative nursing, that precious gift of just 'being' and caring alongside the patient and family (Thompson et al 2006). Aranda (2005) admonishes us against becoming engrossed in establishing the specialist nature of our nursing roles to the detriment of our efforts in striving to ensure that all share this knowledge about caring for dying patients effectively. Fullbrook (2005) also warns us that, in the rush to embrace these new nursing roles, the concept of 'caring' is being devalued and reduced to the lowest common denominator in healthcare. Within palliative care, whilst adapting to the changing face of nursing and all that it encompasses, there is a need to continue to strive for best quality of patient care and management by ensuring that such new roles have proven benefit to patient outcomes.

Box 15.3   Description of the Bradford Heart Failure Palliative Care Service

In 2002, each of the Bradford Primary Care Trusts appointed a heart failure nurse specialist (HFNS). The nurses formed a team whose aim was to support people at home after a hospital admission for heart failure.

None of the nurses appointed had specialist palliative care experience but felt that providing (or facilitating) good supportive and palliative care was an important part of their role. They made links with the local specialist palliative care services and attended their multidisciplinary meetings. They also collaborated educationally, delivering joint sessions for primary care teams and organising events at which palliative care and heart failure staff could learn from one another.

One of the palliative care consultants has been involved with the HFNS team from its outset, being a member of the district-wide steering group and championing the collaboration of these services at a local and national level.

Thanks to modest additional non-cancer funding, a support group for people with heart failure and their carers has been set up in the hospice day centre. Run by the HFNSs, patients attend every other week. The group provides social interaction and informal emotional support, group relaxation and breathing training, one-to-one professional support as necessary, and a rolling programme of structured sessions covering drugs, nutrition, exercise, psychological well-being and benefits advice. It has proved popular and has high scores on evaluation.

So far, direct involvement of the specialist palliative care services has been required for less than 20% of the HFNSs' patients. The HFNSs have become capable of coordinating care until death for many of their patients. Additional support sometimes takes the form of just telephone advice or a joint visit from a palliative care consultant or Macmillan nurse, and experience has demonstrated that high-quality palliative care can be facilitated or provided by HFNSs with support from the existing specialist palliative care services.

Acknowledgements and thanks for writing this service case study to Dr Andrew Daley, Consultant in Palliative Medicine, Bradford Teaching Hospitals NHS Foundation Trust, and Mary Crawshaw-Ralli, Heart Failure Nurse Specialist, Bradford City Primary Care Trust.

References

Addington-Hall J, Altmann D 2000 Which terminally ill cancer patients receive care from community specialist palliative care nurses? Journal of Advanced Nursing 32(4):799–806

Aranda S 2005 Specialist palliative care nursing – an oxymoron? International Journal of Palliative Nursing 11(3):107–108

Arblaster G, Streather C, Hugill L et al 2004 A training programme for healthcare support workers. Nursing Standard 18(43):33–37

Bailey C, Froggatt K, Field D et al 2002 The nursing contribution to qualitative research in palliative care 1990–1999: a critical evaluation. Journal of Advanced Nursing 40(1):48–60

Ball J 2005 Maxi nurses. Advanced and specialist nursing roles. Results from a survey of RCN members in advanced and specialist nursing roles. Online. Available: http://www.rcn.org.uk/publications/pdf/maxi_nurses_advanced.pdf 30 June 2005

Bamford O, Gibson F 2000 The clinical nurse specialist: perceptions of practising CNSs of their role and development needs. Journal of Clinical Nursing 9(2):282–292

Barnard A, Hollingum C, Hartfiel B 2006 Going on a journey: understanding palliative care nursing. International Journal of Palliative Nursing 12(1):6–12

Beaver K, Luker K A, Woods S 1999 The views of terminally ill people and lay carers on primary care services. International Journal of Palliative Nursing 5(6):266–274

Beaver K, Luker K A, Woods S 2000 Primary care services received during terminal illness. International Journal of Palliative Nursing 6(5):220–227

Blackford J, Street A 2001 The role of the palliative care nurse consultant in promoting continuity of end-of-life care. International Journal of Palliative Nursing 7(6):273–278

Booth K, Luker K A, Costello J et al 2003 Macmillan cancer and palliative care specialists: their practice development support needs. International Journal of Palliative Nursing 9(2):73–79

Bousfield C 1997 A phenomenological investigation into the role of the clinical nurse specialist. Journal of Advanced Nursing 25:245–256

Bradshaw P L 2003 Modernising the British National Health Service (NHS) – some ideological and policy considerations. Journal of Nursing Management 11:85–90

Castledine G 1998 Clinical specialists in nursing in the UK: the early years. In: Castledine G, McGee P (eds) Advanced and specialist nursing practice. Blackwell Science, Oxford p 1–22

Castledine G 2002 The development of the role of the clinical nurse specialist in the UK. British Journal of Nursing 11(7):506–508

Chuk P K 1997 Clinical nurse specialists and quality patient care. Journal of Advanced Nursing 26(3):501–506

Clark D, Corner J, Normand C et al 2000 Macmillan nursing in hospital and community settings: an evaluation of service delivery, costs and outcomes. Sheffield Palliative Care Studies Group, Sheffield

Clark D, Seymour J, Douglas H R et al 2002 Clinical nurse specialists in palliative care. Part 2. Explaining diversity in organisation and costs of Macmillan nursing services. Palliative Medicine 16:375–385

Commission for Social Care Inspection 2006 About CSCI. Online. Available: http://www.csci.org.uk/about_csci.aspx 9 Nov 2006

Corner J 1996 Is there a research paradigm for palliative care? Palliative Medicine 10:201–208

Corner J, Halliday D, Haviland J et al 2003 Exploring nursing outcomes for patients with advanced cancer following intervention by Macmillan specialist palliative care nurses. Journal of Advanced Nursing 41(6):561–574

Daley A, Matthews C, Williams A 2006 Heart failure and palliative care services working in partnership: a report of a new model of care. Palliative Medicine 20:593–601

Department of Health 1995 A policy framework for commissioning cancer services. HMSO, London

Department of Health 1999 Making a difference: strengthening the nursing, midwifery and health visiting contribution to health and healthcare. HMSO, London

Department of Health 2000a The NHS Cancer Plan: a plan for investment, a plan for reform. DoH, London

Department of Health 2000b The NHS Plan. DoH, London

Department of Health 2000c The nursing contribution to cancer care. DoH, London

Department of Health 2001 Nurse specialists, nurse consultants, nurse leads: the development and implementation of new roles to improve cancer and palliative care. DoH, London

Department of Health 2003 Domiciliary care: national minimum standards. Online. Available: http://www.dh.gov.uk/PublicationsAndStatistics/Publications/PublicationsPolicyAndGuidance/PublicationsPolicyAndGuidanceArticle/fs/en?CONTENT_ID=4083661&chk=H57QMv 31 Jan 2007

Department of Health 2004 Agenda for change. Online. Available: http://www.dh.gov.uk/PolicyAndGuidance/HumanResourcesAndTraining/ModernisingPay/AgendaForChange/fs/en 6 May 2006

Douglas H R, Halliday D, Normand C et al 2003 Economic evaluation of specialist cancer and palliative nursing: Macmillan evaluation study findings. International Journal of Palliative Nursing 9(10):429–438

Forster A, Young J 1996 Specialist nurse support for patients with stroke in the community: a randomised controlled trial. British Medical Journal 312:1642–1646

Fraser N 2005 Marie Curie cancer care code of conduct for healthcare assistants. Marie Curie Cancer Care Nursing News Issue 8 (April):8–9

Fullbrook S 2005 Role of the 'ordinary 'nurse: concept of qualified caring. British Journal of Nursing 13(12):733

Gibbs L M E, Khatri A K, Gibbs J S R 2006 Survey of specialist palliative care and heart failure: September 2004. Palliative Medicine 20:603–609

Gibson F, Bamford O 2001 Focus group interviews to examine the role of the clinical nurse specialist. Journal of Nursing Management 9:331–342

Grande G E, Todd C J, Barclay S I G et al 1996 What terminally ill patients value in the support provided by GPs, district nurses and Macmillan nurses. International Journal of Palliative Nursing 2(3):138–143

Guest D, Redfern S, Wilson-Barnett J et al 2001 A preliminary evaluation of the establishment of nurse, midwife and health visitor consultants. Online. Available: http://www.kcl.ac.uk/content/1/c6/01/13/70/paper7.pdf 7 Feb 2007

Hamilton F, McDowell J 2004 Identifying the palliative care role of the nurse working in community hospitals: an exploratory study. International Journal of Palliative Nursing 10(9):426–434

Hamric A 1989 History and overview of the CNS role. In: Hamric A B, Spross J (eds) The clinical nurse specialist in theory and practice, 2nd edn. Grune & Stratton, New York, p 3–18

Hanks G W, Robbins M, Sharp D et al 2002 The impact study: a randomised controlled trial to evaluate a hospital palliative care team. British Journal of Cancer 87:733–739

Hekkink C F, Wigersma L, Yzermans et al 2005 HIV nursing consultants: patients' preferences and experiences about the quality of care. Journal of Clinical Nursing 14:327–333

Jack B, Oldham J, Williams A 2002 Impact of the palliative care clinical nurse specialist on patients and relatives: a stakeholder evaluation. European Journal of Oncology Nursing 6(4):236–242

Jack B, Oldham J, Williams A 2003 A stakeholder evaluation of the impact of the palliative care clinical nurse specialist upon doctors and nurses, within an acute hospital setting. Palliative Medicine 17:283–288

Jarret N J, Payne S A, Wiles R A 1999 Terminally ill patients' and lay-carers' perceptions of community-based services. Journal of Advanced Nursing 29(2):476–483

Johnston B 2005 Overview of nursing developments in palliative care. In: Lugton J, Kindlen M (eds) Palliative care: the nursing role, 2nd edn. Churchill Livingstone, Edinburgh, p 1–32

Jones A 1999 'A heavy and blessed experience': a psychoanalytic study of community Macmillan nurses and their roles in serious illness and palliative care. Journal of Advanced Nursing 30(6):1297–1303

Keeley D 1999 Rigorous assessment of palliative care revisited: wisdom and compassion are needed when evidence is lacking. British Medical Journal 319:1447–1448

Keeney S, Hasson F, McKenna H et al 2005 Nurses', midwives and patients' perception of trained health care assistants. Journal of Advanced Nursing 50(4):345–355

Kelly D, Trevatt P 2006 NHS finances. Cancer Nursing Practice 5(8):14–17

Locsin R C 2002 Quo vadis? Advanced practice nursing or advanced nursing practice? Holistic Nursing Practice 16(2):1–4

Manley K 1997 A conceptual framework for advanced practice: an action research project operationalising an advanced practitioner/consultant nurse role. Journal of Advanced Nursing 6(3):179–190

Marsden J, Dolan B, Holt L 2003 Nurse practitioner practice and deployment: electronic mail Delphi study. Journal of Advanced Nursing 43(6):595–605

McCreadie M 2001 The role of the clinical nurse specialist. Nursing Standard 16(10):33–38

McHale H K 1998 The role of the advanced practice nurse in hospice care. Kansas Nurse 73(3):1–2

McKenna H, Hasson F 2004 Patient safety and quality of care: the role of the health care assistant. Journal of Nursing Management 12:452–459

McLoughlin P A 2002 Community specialist palliative care: experiences of patients and carers. International Journal of Palliative Nursing 8(7):344–353

Meek I 1998 Evaluation of the role of the health care assistant within a community mental health intensive care team. Journal of Nursing Management 6(1):11–19

National Council for Hospice and Specialist Palliative Care Services 1996 Palliative care in the hospital setting. Occasional Paper 10. NCHSPCS, London

National Council for Hospice and Specialist Palliative Care Services 2003 Palliative care for adults with non-malignant diseases: developing a national policy. Briefing no. 12. NCHSPCS, London

National Council for Palliative Care 2005 20:20 Vision: the shape of the future for palliative care. NCPC, London

National Institute for Clinical Excellence 2004a Guidance on cancer services: improving supportive and palliative care for adults with cancer: the manual. NICE, London

National Institute for Clinical Excellence 2004b Guidance on cancer services: improving supportive and palliative care for adults with cancer: the research evidence. NICE, London

Newbury J, Hatherall C A 2004 Audit on discharging patients from community specialist palliative care nursing services. International Journal of Palliative Nursing 10(1):24–31

Newton J, Waters V 2001 Community palliative care clinical nurse specialists' descriptions of stress in their work. International Journal of Palliative Nursing 7(11):531–540

NHS Centre for Reviews and Dissemination 2001 Undertaking systematic reviews of research on effectiveness: CRD's guidance for those carrying out or commissioning reviews. Online. Available: http://www.york.ac.uk/inst/crd/report4.htm 1 May 2006

Nursing and Midwifery Council 2005 Implementation of a framework for the standard for post registration nursing. NMC, London

Poppleton A 2003 How do I turn my vocation into a NVQ? Marie Curie Cancer Care Nursing News Issue 2 (Sept):10

Raynes N V, Leach J M, Rawlings B et al 2000 Using focus groups to seek the views of patients dying from cancer about the care they receive. Health Expectations 3:169–175

Reynolds H, Wilson-Barnett J, Richardson G 2000 Evaluation of the role of the Parkinson's disease nurse specialist. International Journal of Nursing Studies 37:337–349

Richardson J S 2002 Health promotion in palliative care: the patients' perception of therapeutic interaction with the palliative nurse in the primary care setting. Journal of Advanced Nursing 40(4):432–440

Rittman M D, Paige P, Rivera J et al 1997 Phenomenological study of nurses caring for dying patients. Cancer Nursing 20(2):115–119

Royal College of Nursing 2003 A framework for adult cancer nursing. RCN, London

Royal College of Nursing 2006 Agenda for change. Job profiles. Online. Available: http://www.rcn.org.uk/agendaforchange/payconditions/jobprofile/ 5 May 2006

Sechrist K, Berlin L 1998 Special article: Role of the clinical nurse specialist: an integrative review of the literature. American Association of Critical-Care Nurses Clinical Issues: Advanced Practice in Acute & Critical Care 9(2):306–324

Seymour J, Clark D, Hughes P et al 2002 Clinical nurse specialists in palliative care. Part 3. Issues for the Macmillan nurse role. Palliative Medicine 16:386–394

Shih F J 1998 Triangulation in nursing research: issues of conceptual clarity and purpose. Journal of Advanced Nursing 28(3):631–641

Skilbeck J, Payne S 2003 Emotional support and the role of clinical nurse specialists in palliative care. Journal of Advanced Nursing 43(5):521–530

Skilbeck J, Payne S 2005 End of life care: a discursive analysis of specialist palliative care nursing. Journal of Advanced Nursing 51(4):325–334

Skilbeck J, Seymour J 2002 Meeting complex needs: an analysis of Macmillan nurses' work with patients. International Journal of Palliative Nursing 8(12):574–582

Skilbeck J, Corner J, Bath P et al 2002 Clinical nurse specialists in palliative care. Part 1. A description of the Macmillan nurse caseload. Palliative Medicine 16:285–296

Skills for Health 2005a S/NVQs awards and qualifications. Online. Available: http://www.skillsforhealth.org.uk/qualifications-3.php 5 May 2006

Skills for Health 2005b A career framework for health. Online. Available: http://www.skillsforhealth.org.uk/careerframework/ 5 May 2006

Spilsbury K, Meyer J 2004 Use, misuse and non-use of health care assistants: understanding the work of health care assistants in a hospital setting. Journal of Nursing Management 12(6):411–418

Thompson G, McClement S, Daeninck P 2006 Nurses' perceptions of quality end-of-life care on an acute medical ward. Journal of Advanced Nursing 53(2):169–177

Thornley C 2000 A question of competence? Re-evaluating the roles of the nursing auxiliary and health care assistant in the NHS. Journal of Clinical Nursing 9(3):451–458

Tijhuis G J, Zwinderman A H, Hazes J M W et al 2003 Two year follow-up of a randomized controlled trial of a clinical nurse specialist intervention, inpatient and day patient team care in rheumatoid arthritis. Journal of Advanced Nursing 41(1):34–43

Webber J 1994 A model response . . . Macmillan nursing services. Nursing Times 90(25):66–68

Webber J 2000 The evolving role of the Macmillan nurse. Macmillan Post holders' Handbook. Macmillan Cancer Relief, London

Wilkes L 1998 Palliative care nursing research: trends from 1987–1996. International Journal of Palliative Nursing 4(3):128–133

Williams D, Sidani S 2001 An analysis of the nurse practitioner role in palliative care. Canadian Journal of Nursing Leadership 14(4):13–19

Wilson-Barnett J, Beech S 1994 Evaluating the clinical nurse specialist: a review. International Journal of Nursing Studies 31(6):561–571

Wright K 1997 Advanced practice nursing: merging the role of the clinical nurse specialist and nurse practitioner roles. Gastroenterology Nursing 20(2):57–60

Further reading

Brykczynska G 2002 The critical essence of advanced practice. In: Clarke D, Flanagan J, Kendrick K (eds) Advancing nursing practice in cancer and palliative care. Palgrave, Hampshire, p 20–42

Johnston B M 2005 Introduction to palliative care: overview of nursing developments. In: Lugton J, McIntyre R (eds) Palliative care: the nursing role, 2nd edn. Elsevier, Edinburgh, p 1–29

Seymour J 2004 What's in a name? A concept analysis of key terms in palliative care nursing. In: Payne S, Seymour J, Ingleton C (eds) Palliative care nursing: principles and evidence for practice. Open University Press, Maidenhead p 55–74

Chapter 16

Looking after yourself

Fiona Setch

INTRODUCTION

> I say, I say, I say
>   How do you stop a conversation at a party?
>   By admitting that you work with people who are dying . . .
>   (Fiona Setch, on numerous occasions from 1989 to today)

Does that strike a popular chord for you?

Death, dying, bereavement and loss remain taboo subjects for most of Western society, and within healthcare the traditional medical model can still view death as a failure to cure. Vachon (1997) highlights that stress and burnout exists in palliative care, but is generally less than in other specialties. This may be due to the recognition of the inherent stress of working within palliative care that resulted in support programmes being built into the work from the beginning. But things have changed and have constantly evolved since 'the beginning', as specialist palliative care units are responding and developing to meet the needs not only of those patients with cancer, AIDS and motor neurone disease (MND), but also with other illnesses such as end-stage cardiac, respiratory, renal and neurological diseases. Increasing numbers of younger patients with complex family dynamics are being referred to palliative care services.

The aim of this chapter is to provide you with the opportunity to:

- identify the specific stressors within palliative care and the potential impact on your work
- explore your existing support strategies and how these can be developed further to enhance your work

- focus on professional support mechanisms such as clinical supervision, training and reflective practice to complement your personal support strategies
- review your current practice and perform your own personal action plan to improve looking after yourself.

There are several exercises to complete to explore the issues involved in looking after yourself. To do this you will find the following useful:

- paper and pens (differently coloured highlighter pens)
- time and space
- to be open and honest with yourself
- to have access to a friend or colleague to discuss issues that may come up for you
- a sense of humour!

Paper and coloured pens are used as life is seldom black and white; you may want to highlight different parts of your experience.

A useful model to think about when reading this chapter and performing the exercises is Kolb's adult learning cycle (Fig. 16.1). In this model, you have an *experience* such as a critical incident at work and you take time to *reflect* on what happened and why. You then focus on *concluding and understanding* about the incident and how you can transfer the learning to the next time you have the same or a similar experience. The final and most important part of the learning cycle is to *plan active experimentation.*

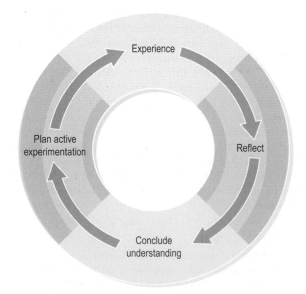

Figure 16.1 Kolb's adult learning cycle (adapted from Kolb 1984).

In the film 'Dead Poets' Society' Robin Williams portrays a teacher who challenges conventional teaching methods. During one scene he asks his students to stand on their desks rather than sit at them to view the classroom from another angle. During this chapter, I would like to invite you to look at your ideas of support from a different perspective. Whatever your role is within palliative care nursing, the aim in this chapter is that you will have an increased awareness of your own individual support needs and a personal action plan on how you are going to have those needs met. Stotter (1997) suggests that the quality of care given to patients is dependent on the extent to which carers feel cared for. Staff support should be an integral part of specialist palliative care.

WHAT IS STRESS?

There are many words, thoughts and images associated with stress including:

- unique to individuals
- can be pleasant and exciting
- a state we experience
- keeps us on our toes for survival – fight or flight
- physical manifestations of stress – can affect all parts of the body
- a 21st century problem
- affects everybody in some shape or form
- battle fatigue
- an unpleasant experience provides stressors that lead to burnout
- just part and parcel of the world of work nowadays
- overload
- burnout
- in extreme cases depression, career change.

The word stress is derived from the Latin word *stringere,* meaning to draw tight. One of the pioneers of the medical understanding of stress, Hans Selye (1956), wrote:

> The word stress, like success, failure or happiness, means different things to different people.

The Health and Safety Executive (2000) defined stress as:

> The adverse reaction people have to excessive pressures or other types of demands placed on them.

Outside pressures are known as stressors. They contribute to the physiological stress reaction that involves complex metabolic, endocrine, cardiovascular and neurological adaptations of the body to stress-inducing events that can lead to illness or exhaustion.

Problems arise when stress is maintained over a lengthy period of time, as this can result in burnout. 'Battle fatigue' and 'burnout' are terms used specifically to describe staff stress when caring for patients who are dying.

During 1997, the government commissioned a report about the well-being of healthcare workers, entitled 'Improving the health of the NHS workforce' (Williams et al 1998). This report revealed new information about the ill-health of both the environment and those providing care in the NHS, and amongst its recommendations was that staff should be encouraged to look after their own health. Caregivers need to recognise that it takes a whole person to respond day after day to the holistic needs of other people. Within healthcare, workloads, lack of resources and staff shortages have become major stressors on general healthcare. There are also specific stressors for palliative care workers.

STRESS SPECIFIC TO PALLIATIVE CARE

Language is extremely powerful. How often do we read media headlines such as 'Linda McCartney loses valiant fight against cancer'? There is an implicit assumption of failure in this headline, which can act as a stressor in caring for dying people. For patients, words like cancer and death conjure up images of horror (Fig. 16.2). Few people in society actually know what happens when someone dies, other than what they have read about or seen on television.

Part of the 'battle fatigue' described by Vachon (1997) is the constant normalising and processing of the patient's and their loved ones' anxieties – as well as the healthcare worker's own feelings as a human being who happens to work as a nurse.

Murray Parkes (1998) advocates that, in order to help those who are dying, we must be prepared to get close to them, to share their fears and to stay with them in their fear. This involves a deep level of communication, which offers the double-edged sword of being both an absolute privilege and a sometimes painful experience.

Twycross (1995) suggests that there are several challenges that are inevitable in palliative care:

- facing your own mortality
- facing your own limitations, personally and professionally

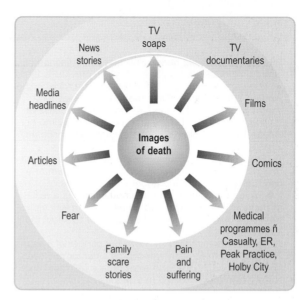

Figure 16.2   Images of death.

- sharing control
- learning to be with patients rather than doing things for them
- dealing honestly with your emotions.

Some of these issues are illustrated in Case Studies 16.1 and 16.2.

Personal reflections on the case studies

In the two case studies, I was carer, friend and a large part of Sue's support system while at work, being charge nurse, clinical supervisor and part of several staff members' support systems. In relation to the patient Colin, I was nurse, carer and confidante, and support-giver to his family and partner.

I am sharing these personal experiences as they taught me an invaluable lesson about the absolute importance of personal support, support systems and the essential role of clinical supervision, although, in retrospect, it was not until some time had passed that I became aware of what my own needs were. I am well aware that I came very close to burnout and was in danger of:

- becoming physically and emotionally exhausted
- feeling worn out
- losing my enthusiasm
- doubting my abilities to provide leadership
- doubting my abilities to care for patients
- becoming cynical, disillusioned and angry
- dreading going to work.

Case Study 16.1 Caring for Sue

Sue is a 33-year-old nurse. She had been diagnosed with non-Hodgkin's lymphoma 3 years previously while working and travelling in New Zealand, after which she worked in Somalia for Save the Children Fund for 2 years. Sue returned to the UK, was in the process of buying her home in Bristol and was 2 months into her Health Visiting Diploma when the lymphoma became aggressive.

Following chemotherapy and a period of remission of 3 months, the lymphoma recurred in the form of a cerebral lymphoma. Sue underwent 3 months of intensive radiotherapy and chemotherapy. As a result of these treatments she had numerous admissions to the same oncology ward, where she got to know the staff very well.

Sue's immediate carers were her partner of 5 years, Richard, who had been working as a doctor overseas, and two close friends who were nurses. All three carers were particularly involved in Sue's care.

Sue was in denial about her health, having fertility treatment and planning a beach holiday in Greece in 3 months' time with Richard. She deteriorated suddenly, lapsed into unconsciousness and died 24 hours later in the arms of her partner – her two friends camped out in the day room. All three carers were very stoical and appeared to be 'holding it together'.

Sue's friends requested that they care for her after death. They washed and dressed her in her favourite clothes and put on her make-up and jewellery. All unnecessary clinical equipment was cleared away from Sue's room and replaced by aromatherapy oils and music. When Sue's room was ready, they invited the nursing staff to say goodbye. After they had completed this, the carers spent their own private time with Sue and left the hospital ward.

REFLECTION POINT
1. If you were one of the nurses on this oncology unit, involved in caring for Sue, what would some of the issues of care be for you?
2. What feelings do you think you would be experiencing during Sue's care?

Issues
Sue: an inspirational young woman
Age identification
Peer – a fellow nurse
Personal identification
Sue starting a new life – career, new home
Partner – a doctor – knowledgeable
Close friends are nurses
Carers very stoical
Sue's denial of illness, death
Fertility treatment
Length of hospital visits
5 months of intensive nursing
Sue very friendly with staff
Sudden deterioration
Carers took control at time of death

Carers performed last offices

Carers invited nurses to say goodbye. What a beautiful death! Sadness

Feelings
Sadness
This could be me/one of my friends
Personal identification
Help!
This is so unjust!
Sue and carers knowledgeable – challenged
How to help carers?
How would I cope?
Does she need to know her reality?
Can only be there for Sue to talk
Privilege to know Sue – but hard
Going to be really hard when Sue dies
Sharing of intensive time with Sue
Quick death, better quality of life, relief
Sadness for self, Richard and friends – slightly disempowered
On reflection, best thing for them; privileged to be able to facilitate this

---

The turning point for me was a clinical supervision session, during which I became empowered to identify what I needed to do to avoid becoming stressed further. Clinical supervision was then, and is today in my current role, one of my main support mechanisms and I will discuss clinical supervision in more detail later in the chapter.

STAFF SUPPORT

In January 2005, the leading Mental Health UK Charity, Mind, commissioned research on the extent of the problem of work-based stress in England and Wales, and what could and should be done about it. This report 'Stress and mental health in the workplace' (Mind 2005) had amongst its key recommendations:

- There should be on-the-job support and mentoring schemes.
- Employees should be provided with genuine control over their work and an appropriate degree of self-management of workload.

Within healthcare there are several sources of staff support including:

Case Study 16.2   Care for the carer

Fiona, a 28-year-old staff nurse, receives a letter from one of her best friends, Sue, who is currently nursing in New Zealand. The letter contained the news that she has been diagnosed with non-Hodgkin's lymphoma but not to worry, as it is not aggressive and she is asymptomatic.

Over the next 3 years they correspond regularly and meet up whenever Sue is home. Fiona is now working as a nurse in a London residential unit, caring for people with HIV/AIDS.

Sue talks to Fiona about living with cancer, sharing her disease progress, and her hopes and fears. Their close friendship deepens.

Two years later, Fiona is promoted to charge nurse on the unit. She enjoys her work tremendously, finding it extremely challenging, managing a 24-bed unit, being part of a dynamic charge nurse team and clinical supervisor for a team of 10 trained nurses, as well as undertaking some patient care. Sue has recently returned to the UK and is starting her health visiting training in Bristol.

Sue's cancer suddenly becomes aggressive. Several months later, her condition deteriorates suddenly. She is very depressed and Fiona spends as much time with Sue as she can. As a result, Fiona is physically tired and emotionally drained. Fiona recently spent a week's holiday visiting Sue and accompanying her for radiotherapy treatments, as well as 'girlie' things like watching Wimbledon tennis together, shopping, eating out, and many hours of talking and just spending time together.

On her first shift back at work after visiting Sue, Colin, a patient whom Fiona had known and nursed for 4 years, was admitted for terminal care. Fiona had been his 'key nurse' in her previous job.

After hand-over, Fiona receives a telephone call from her mother with the unexpected news that an old family friend has died suddenly. Fiona has a clinical supervision appointment with her line manager at 3pm.

REFLECTION POINT
1. What are the issues facing Fiona?
2. How do you think that clinical supervision could be supportive to Fiona?

Issues facing Fiona
- Sadness at the illness of Sue
- Sue's illness has brought their existing friendship even closer
- Personal identification
- Emotionally tired due to job stress and supporting Sue
- Over-extending personal resources, spending a week's holiday with ill friend
- Overwhelming situation – on return to work
- Sadness at Colin's deterioration in health
- Feeling unable to cope with the sudden death of an old family friend
- Feeling guilty that she wasn't coping
- Wanting to be there for Colin and his family – but knowing she would burst into tears . . .
- Feeling guilty
- Feelings of inadequacy

How clinical supervision could support Fiona
- By providing a confidential space, uninterrupted, away from the unit, to focus on what was occurring
- Giving a space to focus on the impact of how personal life was affecting professional practice
- Enabling reflection on the critical incident of Colin's deterioration and how, despite being involved in Colin's care for so long, another team member could be his key nurse
- Giving direction to 'practise what she preached' to the staff she supervised and to take some time out to attend family friend's funeral and be able to be there when Sue died
- Providing the opportunity to explore and review her support systems and an action plan on how she might cope with the challenging time ahead
- Validating Fiona as a human being and her skills as a professional nurse
- Acknowledgement that this was a very difficult, painful time – that was the way it was, but it would pass

---

- line management
- induction and mentoring
- annual appraisal
- clinical supervision
- peer support
- reflective practice groups and critical incident reviews
- team meetings
- occupational health services
- counselling services
- education and training opportunities.

The organisation that you work for may well provide some or all of the above; however, if you are not aware of what your own individual support needs are, you may not feel supported or able to access the support services that are available. For example, a Trust may have allocated clinical supervisors for all district nurses and sent memos out, but if the district nurses have never experienced clinical supervision and know little about it they are unlikely to take up this opportunity for support.

If you expect your organisation to know what you want and need, you may be setting the organisation up to fail, as the most important starting point for you to determine your support needs is you!

Each of us has our own individual experience of life, our nursing, our own values and expectations, so that our experiences and expectations of staff support will be different.

During times of stress, our network of support can help us to cope with the demands placed on us. Our contacts can act as a buffer, by relieving us of some of the pressure – or as a safety valve, by providing an outlet for feelings.

Support network mind map

> No man is an island, entire of itself,
>   Every man is a piece of the continent, a part of the main.
>
> (John Donne 1571–1631)

For this exercise you will need a large piece of paper and pens.

Step 1

Write your name in the middle of the page and draw a circle around it.

Step 2

Think of your existing support structures.

Draw in the main branches – these are the main categories that make up your network. Label them. For an example, see Figure 16.3.

Step 3

Having identified the main categories, the next step involves drawing smaller branches from the large ones with specific people who give you support (Fig. 16.4). Your named people can be anyone who supports you. For example:

- *Work* – your manager, team members, other colleagues, peers, a support group, the organisation
- *Family and friends* – your partner, parents, children, siblings, pets, extended family, friends

- *Professional* – union, general practitioner, supervisor, counsellor, aromatherapist
- *Interest* – social, church, sports, education, charity work, club

Only include the names of people that you would actively seek support from.

Step 4

With differently coloured pens, write a 'W' next to the names of people who help you to resolve your work-related problems.

Step 5

Reflect on your support network. For someone to be able to support you, they need to know what your needs are. For example, sometimes you may need simply to tell the story of an event, without interruptions, questions or suggestions; whereas on another occasion you will need/want to be challenged.

On both occasions, the person listening is not telepathic. Therefore, you need to communicate your needs clearly, otherwise you could unknowingly be setting up both yourself and the person listening to fail, and end up feeling frustrated, angry and even less supported than you felt originally.

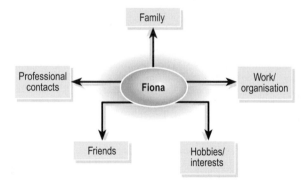

Figure 16.3   Support network mind map: example of step 2.

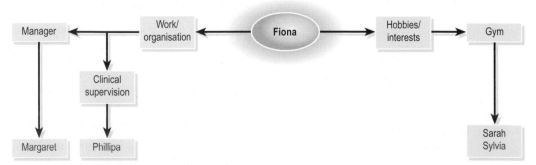

Figure 16.4   Support network mind map: example of step 3.

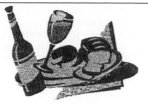

The Support Menu

Starter

Peer Support

Reflective Diary

Quiet Space … Time for Yourself

Exercise

Planning a Holiday

Main Course

Reflection in Action

Reflective Practice

Clinical Supervision

Annual Appraisal

Education & Training

Critical Incident Reflection

Coaching

Counselling

Sweet

Support Group

Teaching

Aromatherapy

Social Outing – a Drink, Meal or Coffee

'One of your Treats'

Being on Holiday

In order to assert your needs, you need to be clear about who is capable of providing what to you in specific examples. Complete Table 16.1 to identify who is involved in your support structure.

Having completed this exercise:

- What are your initial thoughts on your individual support system?
- Does your support system give you the right type of support, with a balance between work and emotional issues?
- Are there enough people in it?
- What gaps exist, if any?
- Are you in danger of making too many demands on too few people?
- Are there any surprises?
- What changes would you like to make?
- How will you go about it?

SUPPORT MENU

Earlier in the chapter, I mentioned the film 'Dead Poets' Society'. Like Robin Williams' teacher, I would like to invite you to stand on your desk and view your support from a different perspective.

You have just identified your existing support strategies. This is an excellent starting point to think about looking after yourself – if you are not well supported yourself, how can you support others effectively?

A method of thinking about your support strategies is to envisage options like an enticing restaurant menu. Imagine you are visiting your favourite restaurant. You open the menu and are faced with a sumptuous choice of starters, main courses and sweets. On some occasions you may want to choose a starter and main course, or on others just a main course or for the full works – starter, main course and sweet! I would like to present to you the Support Menu.

Examples from the starter menu might be writing in your reflective diary, or it may involve a quiet 5 minutes of relaxation. From the main course menu, education and training can be tremendously supportive. It is my observation that issues-based multi-disciplinary training provides an excellent forum for constructive, supportive teamwork, as the following comments made following a 1-day experiential 'Caring for the dying' course illustrate.

What have been the benefits of attending this session?

- Sharing experiences with others
- An increased awareness of my own feelings surrounding death and dying

Table 16.1   Support structure

Types of support	Person who provides support
Accepting Someone who listens to you, non-judgementally and without giving advice	
Personal support Unconditional support for you even though they may not be in agreement with what you are doing – your own personal backing group!	
Personal challenge Someone who asks you incisive questions, checking out your attitudes, feelings and behaviour	
Work-oriented support and challenge Someone who knows your job, can help you identify strengths and cope with difficulties	
Crisis work A skilled professional who can listen appropriately (e.g. counsellor, occupational health nurse)	

- Time to focus on the activities of daily working life that have become normal
- Time out to discuss the stresses of caring for the dying
- Time out together to think and explore
- A space for personal reflection
- Knowing that most of my feelings are shared by others
- Time out from the working environment and sharing a good laugh with colleagues.

Are there any changes you intend to make to your practice as a result of attending this training?

- To support each other more – demonstrate that we are there for each other
- Allow more time to think quietly and gather thoughts
- Attend reflective practice more often
- Try to accept and give a higher priority to my own needs
- Arranging agreed time to support colleagues and not just snatching a minute or so
- Not to rely on bumping into a supportive colleague in the corridor for support any more – making time for each other.

From my own Support Menu I would like to share a starter, main course and sweet. As a starter I suggest two pocket-sized self-help books, 'Take care of yourself' (Sach 1997) and 'The little book of calm' (Wilson 1996). I find these texts both inspirational and very practical, as they are filled with exercises and 'thoughts for the day'.

Rest your fingers

One of my favourite exercises, which I practise myself and with others, is called 'rest your fingers'. Ensure that you are sitting comfortably with both feet on the floor. Take a deep breath in and slowly exhale. Close your eyes. Gently rest your thumbs and fingers of one hand against the thumbs and fingertips of the other, with just the lightest touch. Breathe slowly, count to 60, and invite the calm to be with you! (Adapted from Wilson 1996.)

My main course choices are reflection in action and clinical supervision.

Reflection in action

This is a tool that can be used in preparation for clinical supervision, as part of reflective practice or as a stand-alone critical incident review. Think of a critical incident and complete the format outlined in Table 16.2; it will help you clarify your position and evaluate the learning that was in it for you.

Clinical supervision

I am passionate about clinical supervision as I have first-hand experience of how effective, dynamic and empathetic clinical supervision can be. From the case scenarios earlier in this chapter, I have already mentioned that it was clinical supervision that was the turning point for me, and prevented me from becoming another nurse suffering from burnout who appeared as a statistic in a report on stress at work.

Table 16.2   Reflection in action (J Sweetenham, unpublished work, 1997)

R	**Recognise significant thoughts/feelings** What are you thinking? How are you feeling?
E	**Explore the significant elements** What is significant in your thoughts/feelings? About the context of the situation?
F	**Focus on your response** How did you respond to the situation? How do you feel about your response?
L	**List the relevant underlying knowledge/experience/ assumptions** What prior knowledge/experience/assumptions led you to respond in this way?
E	**Evaluate the validity of that knowledge/experience/assumptions** Did that prior knowledge/experience/assumptions help you?
C	**Clarify what you have learned** What does this new learning do to your previous knowledge/experience/assumptions?
T	**Transfer this learning to new situations** What will the new learning help you do in the future?

There are numerous definitions of clinical supervision which include the following key themes. Supervision is:

- a process
- a regular, protected time
- a confidential space
- a facilitated reflection on clinical practice
- a process which enables the supervisee to achieve, sustain and develop high-quality practice
- a supervisee-led agenda
- a part of lifelong learning.

Bond & Holland (1998) conclude that clinical supervision should continue throughout a nurse's career, in whatever direction – clinical practice, research, education or management.

The definition that I use is breaking the word down into 'super' and 'vision', because that it is what clinical supervision is – a brilliant way of focusing on your work from another perspective.

Clinical supervision has many functions, which include:

- self-awareness and interpersonal relationships
- personal management
- problem-solving
- support
- education

- reflection
- analysis of situations
- planning
- development.

The benefits of receiving clinical supervision include:

- having a 'sounding out space', confidentiality
- experience of a supportive, confidential relationship
- improving patient care by reflecting on practice, looking at skills, achievements and challenging situations, focusing on self
- providing clarity of direction – set aims and objectives
- the opportunity to take 'time out', take a step back to reflect
- valuing personal achievements.

Although clinical supervision has been around within nursing for the past 20 years, there remain several blocks to clinical supervision, which include:

- lack of knowledge
- lack of trust and confidentiality
- time
- fear that 'it' will be challenging
- new concept
- more change
- lack of enthusiasm
- it may 'open up a can of worms'
- being judged
- who will do it?

There are specific issues and challenges of working in palliative care that clinical supervision can help with. These include:

- the curse of perfectionism – are you ever too hard on yourself?
- younger patients with complex social and psychological problems
- personal identification with patients
- multiple complex problems
- euthanasia
- many skilled staff may be involved in one patient – problems of power, feeling deskilled, communication problems
- intense time in patients' lives – that you work with day in and day out
- multiple bereavements
- working with death, dying, bereavement and loss – day in, day out
- impact on personal life.

Within palliative care, whatever our roles, we all strive for the very best for our patients. Perhaps it is because we are focusing on quality of life with a short timespan? Are we caretakers of a living museum? Trying to ensure that the whole scene – patient, family and carers – has the best of everything, and our patients are remembered exactly as they want to be?

From my personal experiences of being both clinical supervisee and clinical supervisor, I believe that clinical supervision is an essential component of nursing.

There are several models of clinical supervision. Table 16.3 summarises popular approaches to the delivery of clinical supervision. Different organisations have different approaches and ideas about the implementation of clinical supervision.

The following quotes are from nurses who have been receiving clinical supervision:

'I have been receiving telephone supervision for 3 years now, and it is the one phone call a month that I can't wait to take . . . since it is really for me – and about my professional learning needs. I know that I am communicating with my supervisor and she is committed to enabling me to understand and learn more about my potential and how I reflect on these developments. Supervision for me is active, dynamic and essential to my essence of care – it is what underpins my Working Life!'

(Kate, senior nurse)

'In my second clinical supervision session, I took a patient who I was having a crisis of confidence about. I had been asked to go into a nursing home to give advice to the nursing staff about pain relief. Sarah was a 50-year-old woman who had multiple sclerosis and what was described as 'intractable pain'. After assessing Sarah, I returned to my place of work troubled that I had not really done very much. When my supervisor asked me more about Sarah, we

Table 16.3 Approaches to the delivery of clinical supervision, and their relative advantages and disadvantages

Approach	Advantages	Disadvantages
One to one Face to face or telephone	Exclusive time making it easier to build trust Confidentiality and privacy increased No competition with peers for time, etc. Able to negotiate personal needs and work at own pace Can be monitored easily	Can be expensive There may be a lack of suitably qualified supervisors Can intensify problems within the supervisory relationship May be too intense for some supervisees Could encourage dependency Evaluation and feedback from one person's perspective only
Peer	More accessible Peers often have more clinical credibility Could build on existing good relationships Promotes ownership of supervision	Can be difficult to organise Could become an opportunity for a chat Can be collusive Boundaries difficult to keep to There can be competition to get needs met
Triad	Cost effective as a supervisor is shared for two supervisees Can promote learning from peer Mutual support Can be less intense than one to one	Sharing the time, therefore reducing the time available Reduced privacy and confidentiality Peers could collude against supervisor
Group	As above plus the opportunity to learn from the group process Increases the range of supervisory techniques available	As above plus the dynamics of the group may interfere or be destructive Supervisor requires group facilitator skills and an understanding of group dynamics Not all are suited to group work Difficulty of newcomers entering the group Group dynamics may temporarily block the task
Peer group	As above plus may enhance team relationships	As above but without a designated supervisor the group dynamics may easily become destructive as rivalry for leadership becomes unmanageable
Team	As with group plus may enhance team relationships	As for group but can address only limited clinical issues owing to multiprofessional backgrounds of the group

came up with a long list of the losses in her life which included her husband who was her main carer, best friend and the love of her life, her home and possessions, what little independence that she had left, her mobility, her dignity, her daughter Pat had recently gone away to university . . . all that, and Sarah had pain. When I looked at this long list of losses I realised that my expectations had been unrealistic; that I had thought that sorting Sarah's pain was probably her main problem, when in fact it was almost at the bottom of her list of problems and issues. I continued seeing Sarah and several weeks later I was able to share with my supervisor and celebrate my achievement at helping the nursing home staff alleviate her pain, but my real joy and cause for celebration was that Sarah smiled and told me a joke and all I had done was take time to listen to her . . . In this situation clinical supervision helped me see my patient's situation from a different perspective, be more realistic in my expectations of myself and, most importantly, provided me with the opportunity to celebrate Sarah's smile and joke!'

(Gill, community nurse)

If you are not receiving clinical supervision, ask yourself the question 'Why not?' I suggest you find out what is available in your area of work.

All it takes is for two people to start talking about clinical supervision; obviously, you need to know about the concept and principles, and there are some excellent resources available. A good way to begin is to find someone who has experience of clinical supervision or is interested in the concept – if you wait for others to provide it, you may be waiting a long time; so *carpe diem* – seize the day!

From my Support Menu, the sweet menu I would like to share with you is *10 treats*. Close your eyes and think of 10 things that you like doing for yourself that do not involve a lot of either time or money. Write down your list, which may include:

- a relaxing bath
- gardening
- walking the dog
- stroking your cat
- listening to a relaxation tape
- fishing
- watching a favourite TV programme
- cooking
- listening to music.

When you have compiled your list, look at it and visualise yourself enjoying your individual daily treats. Imagine how very happy and relaxed you feel when you do them.

Try to do at least one every day – and enjoy treating yourself.

This exercise was the gift of Jim Kukendyall, a clinical psychologist who facilitated a ward-based support group of which I was a member.

SO WHAT NEXT?

In this chapter I have outlined specific stressors within palliative care nursing. I chose to share my own personal experiences, as I believe in leading by example. By sharing my experience of how specific issues and challenges of working in palliative care affected me, I hope that it may help you in your work.

You also have had the opportunity to explore your existing support strategies and I have provided some examples of alternative strategies that you may choose to think about.

PERSONAL ACTION PLANNING

In the adult learning cycle (see Fig. 16.1), active experimentation and planning for the next time you experience an event is a crucial part of learning. In 'looking after yourself', it is the difference between learning from your mistakes or taking them with you into your next experience.

There will be some very practical steps that you can take immediately, such as:

- identifying your existing support strategies
- giving yourself permission to think about yourself before thinking of supporting others.

There will be other steps that may take some time, such as finding a clinical supervisor and starting clinical supervision. Take some time to write down the steps that you are going to take to look after yourself .

The approaches I have outlined in this chapter may not have been part of your working life up to now. My challenge to you is to take the time for yourself – I can guarantee it will improve your quality of work life, and have a knock-on effect on your whole life.

I would like to share a poem that has given me much inspiration since I heard it at a nursing conference in 1991.

Risks

To laugh is to risk appearing the fool
To weep is to risk appearing sentimental
To reach out to another is to risk involvement

To expose feelings is to risk exposing your true self
To place your ideas, your dreams before a crowd is to risk their loss
To love is to risk not being loved in return
To live is to risk death
To hope is to risk despair
To try is to risk failure
But risks must be taken
Because the greatest hazard is to risk nothing
The person who risks nothing, does nothing, has nothing and is nothing

They may avoid suffering and sorrow but they cannot learn, feel, change, grow, love or live, chained by their certitudes
They are slaves; they have forfeited their freedom
Only a person who risks is truly free!

(Richard Rector 1991, unpublished)

When you invest time in yourself, you will be looking after yourself. As a result, you will be more equipped to support your patients and colleagues, and to 'bring comfort and hope'.

References

Bond M, Holland S 1998 Skills of clinical supervision for nurses. Open University Press, Buckingham

Donne J 1963 In: Cohen J M, Cohen M J (ed.) The Penguin dictionary of quotations. Penguin, Harmondsworth

Health and Safety Executive 2000 The scale of occupational stress: the Bristol Stress at Work Study. Contract research report. HSE Publications, London

Kolb D 1984 Experiential learning: experience as the source of learning and development. Prentice Hall, Engleswood Cliffs, New Jersey

Mind 2005 Stress and mental health in the workplace. Mind Publications, London

Murray Parkes C 1998 Coping with loss, the dying adult. BMJ Publications, London

Sach P 1997 Take care of yourself. Penguin, Harmondsworth

Selye H 1956 The stress of life. McGraw-Hill, New York. Accessed online http://en.wikipedia.org/wiki/Hans_Selye 6 May 2007

Stotter D 1997 Staff support in healthcare. Blackwell Science, Oxford

Twycross R 1995 Introducing palliative care. Radcliffe Medical Press, Oxford

Vachon M 1997 Recent research into staff stress in palliative care. European Journal of Palliative Care 4(3):99–103

Williams S, Michie S, Pattani S 1998 Improving the health of the NHS workforce: report of the partnership on the health of the NHS workforce. Nuffield Trust, London

Wilson P 1996 The little book of calm. Penguin, Harmondsworth

Index

Page numbers in **bold** refer to illustrations and tables